Adaptation in
SPORTS TRAINING

Atko Viru

CRC Press
Boca Raton   Boston   London   New York   Washington, D.C.

Library of Congress Cataloging-in-Publication Data

Adaptation in sports training / author, Atko Viru
      p. cm.
    Includes bibliographical references and index.
    ISBN 0-8493-0171-8
    1. Sports--Physiological aspects. 2. Adaptation (Physiology)
I. Viru, A. A.
RC1235.A335 1995
612'.044—dc20   94-20219
                                                           CIP

ACKNOWLEDGMENTS

The author gratefully acknowledges the valuable technical aid by Ms. Amanda Kriit, Ms. Kadri Kivistik, and Ms. Aino Luik. The author would also like to thank Professor Bengt Saltin for valuable suggestions.

PREFACE

A great amount of results has accumulated on changes in the organism induced by systematically performed exercises. The changes take place on the levels of cellular structures, tissues, organs, and body building. The changes extended from the metabolic processes and their molecular mechanisms up to functional capacities of cellular structures as well as of organs and their systems. Pronounced alterations have been found in the mechanisms of control of bodily functions and metabolic processes, including levels of cellular autoregulation, hormonal regulation, and neural regulation.

There have never been any serious doubts that at least most of the training-induced changes express adaptation to conditions of enhanced muscular activity. Convincing results have been obtained establishing specific links between changes in the organism and performance level in various sports events. Consequently, the nature of training has to be considered in introducing adaptive changes in the organism which ensure an increase in performance capacity. It is also suggestible that training increases the capacities of adaptation mechanism, creating thereby a foundation for health promotion and a general increase in working capacity. Therefore, training experiments provide material not only for analysis of physical training but also for improved understanding of adaptation processes and increase of the body's adaptivity all-in-all.

In this volume a discussion of adaptive changes induced by systematically performed exercises is presented. the available results of physiological and biochemical studies are systematized according to the following leit-motif:

- Adaptation to various influences or demands on the organism consists of specific homeostatic regulation and (if the influence is strong enough) activation of the mechanism of general (unspecific) adaptation.
- The mechanism of general adaptation ensures mobilization of the organism's energy and protein resources and activation of the body's defense faculties.
- Both homeostatic regulation and general adaptation need the interference of hormonal regulation and neural regulation into cellular autoregulation.
- Through the mobilization of protein resources, extended opportunities for adaptive protein synthesis are provided by the activity of the mechanism of general adaptation.
- The adaptive protein synthesis ensures the development of most active cellular structures and the increased number of enzyme molecules concerned to the activity of these structures; hence the foundation for the transition from acute adaptation to continuous stable adaptation.
- Since the adaptive protein synthesis is specifically related to the activity of cellular structures during acute adaptation, the specific effect of each training exercise is founded on the production of metabolic inductors for specific protein synthesis.
- While the training exercises used determine the specific choice for adaptive protein synthesis and thereby for training-induced changes, the total load of training sessions determines the activation of endocrine systems and through the produced hormonal inductors the amplification of the adaptive protein synthesis.
- The mentioned considerations make it possible to develop the guidance of training practice.

Atko Viru

THE AUTHOR

Atko Viru, D.Sc., is Professor of Exercise Physiology at the Institute of Exercise Biology, The University of Tartu, Tartu, Estonia.

Dr. Viru graduated from the University of Tartu in 1955 and received the degree of Candidate of Biochemical Sciences (Ph.D.) in 1963. In 1970 he obtained the degree of Doctor of Biological Sciences from the Academy of Sciences of Estonia.

Dr. Viru began teaching at the University in 1959. He became Associate Professor in Exercise Physiology in 1966. He was made Head of the Department of Sports Medicine in 1967 and held that position until 1971. In 1971 he became Professor and Head of the Department of Sports Physiology. From 1973 to 1989 he was Dean of the Faculty of Physical Education.

Dr. Viru is Corresponding Editor of the journal *Biology of Sport* and member of the Editorial Board of the *International Journal of Sports Medicine* and *Sports Medicine, Training and Rehabilitation*. He has lectured at universities in Bologne, Heidelberg, Prague, Stockholm, Jyväskylä, Santiago, Buenos Aires, Rome, Moscow, St. Petersburg, Kiev, Tashkent, Volgograd, Stavropol, and Yakutsk. He is a member of the New York Academy of Sciences, the Estonian Physiological Society, the Estonian Biochemical Society, and the Estonian Society of Endocrinology. From 1989 to 1991 he served as Chairman of the Estonian Physiological Society. From 1989 to the present he is President of the Estonian Olympic Academy and Vice President of the Estonian Olympic Committee.

Dr. Viru has published more than 400 papers in the field of physiology and biochemistry of adaptation to muscular activity. He is the author and co-author of four books published in Estonian, and four in Russian. In 1985 CRC Press published his *Hormones in Muscular Activity* in two volumes.

TABLE OF CONTENTS

Chapter 5
Specific Nature of Training on Skeletal Muscles

Chapter 6
Specificity of Training Effects on Aerobic Working Capacity and the Cardiovascular System

Chapter 7
Specificity of Training Effects on Control Functions and the Connective Tissue

Chapter 8
Molecular Mechanisms of Training Effects

Chapter 9
Gender Differences in Training Effects

Chapter 10
Physiological Aspects of Selected Problems of Training Methodology (Training Tactics)

Chapter 11
Physiological Aspects of Selected Problems of Training Methodology (Training Strategy)

Chapter 1

GENERAL OUTLINES OF ADAPTATION PROCESSES AND THE BIOLOGICAL NATURE OF EXERCISE TRAINING

ADAPTATION AND TRAINING

Muscular activity belongs to the group of factors closely related to adaptation processes in the organism. Every exercise triggers acute adaptation processes necessary to adjust body functions to the corresponding level of elevated energy metabolism. Adjustments are also necessary to avoid harmful alterations in the internal milieu of the organism. In turn, all these adjustments enable exercise performance and to a great extent determine the performance level. Systematic repetitions of exercises induce long-term stable adaptation that is founded on structural and metabolic changes, making possible increased functional capacities.

HOMEOSTATIC REGULATION

Since the publications of C. Bernard[1] and W.B. Cannon,[2,3] it is well recognized that adaptation to life conditions and to any kind of bodily activity is always directed towards maintaining or restoring the constancy of the body's internal milieu. For this purpose certain specific reactions are introduced. The integrated sum of these reactions was defined by W.B. Cannon[2,3] as homeostatic regulation. However, only some of the parameters of the body's internal milieu are kept at a constant level, while others vary to a great extent. Accordingly, the rigid and plastic constants of the internal environment were discriminated.[4] The rigid constants have a very narrow range of fluctations between the resting and activity levels, deviations from which cannot be associated with maintenance of life. The plastic constants can change to a great extent. Often their changes are necessary to compensate for the influences on the rigid constants or to restore their activity (Figure 1-1). The changes of plastic constants may also reflect the mobilization of bodily resources for certain activities. However, there are also special mechanisms responsible for the limitation of alterations of plastic constants and for restoration of the resting levels.

The main rigid constants are temperature, pH, osmotic pressure, and contents of ions, water, and pO_2. It is simple to notice that there are conditions which determine the optimal activity of enzymes. This enables us to understand the importance of the constancy of rigid constants. Without the necessary conditions which ensure the optimal activity of enzymes, metabolic processes will be disturbed and possibilities of maintaining life will be reduced.

Homeostatic regulation is affected through controlling factors at the level of cellular autonomic, hormonal, and neural regulation. According to contemporary knowledge, the homeostatic function may be extended to many hormones and other bioactive substances in cooperation with processes triggered by direct nervous influences. In various cases, behavioral responses are included into homeostatic regulation as well.

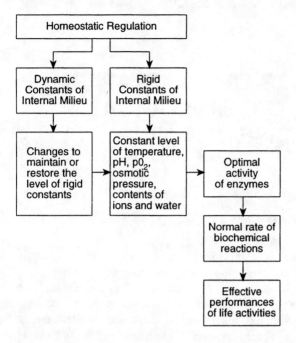

FIGURE 1-1. Homeostatic regulation (see text).

MECHANISM OF GENERAL ADAPTATION

Adaptive processes cannot be limited by specific homeostatic reactions. In many cases nonspecific alterations, independent of the specific nature of the activity, are observable. The nonspecific character of adaptation is expressed by the theory of W.B. Cannon[5] about the emergency function of the sympatho-adrenal system. L.A. Orbeli[6] discussed the adaptive-trophic function of sympathic innervation. Originally, nonspecific adaptation processes were conceptualized by H. Selye.[7] An extensive study of nonspecific adaptation responses enabled him to establish the stress reaction as a sum of nonspecific responses of the body to any strong demands made upon it.

The nonspecific adaptation responses constitute the mechanism of general adaptation[8,9] (Figure 1-2). The major components of the mechanism of general adpatation are: (1) mobilization of the body's energy reserve, (2) mobilization of the protein resources, and (3) activation of the body's defense faculties (immunoactivities etc.). As a result, increased possibilities will be provided on the one hand, for homeostatic regulation, and on the other hand, for actualization of any necessary bodily activities, including muscular exercises.

MOBILIZATION OF METABOLIC RESOURCES

The main principle of metabolic control is that the substrate/product ratio determines the activity of enzymes catalyzing respectively the conversing of a substrate (S) into a certain product (P) and the reaction in the opposite direction:

$$ S \xrightarrow{e_1 \rightarrow} P $$
$$ \xleftarrow{\quad \leftarrow e_2 \quad} $$

The increase of the substrate as well as the decrease of the product stimulate enzyme e_1 activity (catalyzes the conversion of the substrate S into the product P) and inhibit enzyme e_2 (catalyzes the opposite process) activity. The substrate can be converted into the product if the activity of enzyme e_1 surpasses the activity of enzyme e_2. The opposite situation will emerge in the decrease of the substrate and the increase of the product. Then an inhibition of enzyme

FIGURE 1-2. A scheme of adaptation to stressor. In response to stressor both specific homeostatic mechanisms and the mechanism of general adaptation are activated. The latter consists in mobilization of energy reserve, protein resources, and defense faculties. The mobilization of the body's energy reserve increases the possibilities for energy attaining of homeostatic responses. The mobilization of protein resources enables us to use an additional energy reserve as well as to induce rapid synthesis of enzyme proteins, which are necessary for actualizing the specific homeostatic mechanism, mobilization of energy reserve, and activation of immunologic responses and other defense faculties. Increased functional activity for actualizing the specific homeostatic reactions creates a specific induction of protein synthesis. After acute action of stressors it is expressed in adaptive synthesis of structure and enzyme proteins in conjunction with increased protein turnover. As a result the possibilities for concrete homeostatic response improve. This means the transition from short-term rapid adaptation to a stable continuous adaptation that is mainly pronounced in cases of repeated action of stressors.

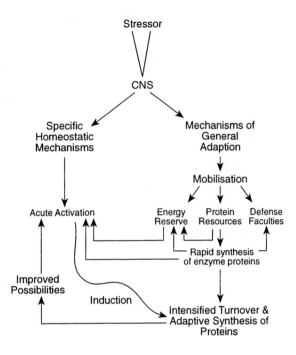

e_1 and a stimulation of enzyme e_2 occurs. Due to that the reaction stops and is replaced by the opposite reaction.

Actually cellular autoregulation is more complicated. In most cases the regulation is actualized in the course of the whole metabolic pathway or metabolic cycle. In a number of cases the reaction is inhibited not by the immediate product, but by the product of some subsequent reactions. Moreover, besides the accumulation of the products, the inhibitory role also belongs to some other results of reactions (changes of intracellular pH, ionic composition, availability of coenzymes, etc.).

The onset of the intensification of glycogen degradation is determined by the activity of glycogen phosphorylase. The opposite process depends on the activity of glycogen synthase. Both enzymes exist in active and inactive forms. The actual enzyme activity depends on the ratio between active and inactive forms. The stimulation of enzyme activity consists of converting inactive forms into active ones. The inhibition is actualized by the conversion of active forms into inactive enzymes. As the main aim of glycogenolysis is the energy supply of ATP resynthesis, it is natural that the main stimulators of glycogen phosphorylase activity are the low level of ATP and high levels of ADP and AMP. Calcium and sodium ions as well as acetylcholine also increase the activity of glycogen phosphorylase. The liberation of acethylcholine and the increased levels of cytoplasmic calcium and sodium ions are the initial events of excitement of the cell, including excitement of the muscular cell that initiates the concentration. Hence, cellular activity itself rapidly adjusts energy production to meet the increasing needs. Nevertheless, the role of the substrate/product ratio is obvious: the intensity of the reaction catalyzed by glycogen phosphorylase decreases with the reduction of the intracellular glycogen store (substrate) and with the accumulation of glucose-6-phosphate (product of the next reaction). At the same time glucose-6-phosphate activates glycogen synthesis.

In further glycogenolysis an important stage is the conversion of fructose-6-phosphate into fructose-1,6-diphosphate. The reaction is catalyzed by phosphocfructokinase (PFK). Its activity is stimulated by the high level of fructose-6-phosphate (substrate), ADP and AMP, as well as by the low level of fructose-1,6-diphosphate (product). The reaction is inhibited by an increase in the ATP content.

If the intensity of glycogenolysis surpasses the intensity of oxidation processes, a part of pyruvate is converted into lactate. The latter inhibits a number of enzymes of gluconeogenesis (PFK etc.) as a product of the metabolic pathway; the inhibition is also due to the concomitant accumulation of hydrogen ions.

Using glycogenolysis as an example, it is easy to understand that cellular autoregulation is directed towards the immediate satisfaction of cellular needs, on the one hand, and towards the exclusion of pronounced changes in the cellular compartment on the other hand. Thus cellular autoregulation is important for the resting state. However, it is not suitable for an overall mobilization of cellular and bodily resources. If we continue the analysis of glycogenolysis, it is worth pointing to the results showing that in isolated skeletal muscles the events concomitant with the initiation of contraction stimulate glycogenolysis only for a short time.[10,11] Agreeing results were also obtained in humans.[12] Obviously the inhibitory factors oppose the stimulatory action of acetylcholine, Na^+ having entered the cell, as well as of Ca^{++} released from the sarcoplasmic reticulum. The exclusion of lactate accumulation and the reduction of intracellular pH by the inhibition of glycogenolytic processes has a positive value for the resting state. However, it also eliminates the chances of athletes to compete in races of 400 and 800 m or in swimming of 100 and 200 m, as well as to participate in intensive activities during an ice-hockey match, etc.

The overall mobilization of cellular and bodily resources requires the interference of *hormonal regulation* with cellular autoregulation (Figure 1-3). The main aim of *hormonal regulation* is to adjust the metabolic processes to the level corresponding to the actual needs of life activities, despite the opposite effects of cellular autoregulation. This aim is achieved through the action of hormones on the activity of enzymes.

The hormone effects on enzyme activities are realized in two ways. First, in a number of cases the structure of the enzyme molecule changes under the influence of a hormone due to which the enzyme activity increases or decreases. In many cases the corresponding change consists in either phosphorylation or dephosphorylation of the enzymne molecule. A second possibility is the change in the number of enzyme molecules through hormone reaction. A number of hormones are capable of inducing or inhibiting the synthesis of enzyme proteins, resulting in an increase or decrease in the number of enzyme molecles. In some cases hormones are able to either intensify or suppress the degradation of enzyme proteins.

It has been demonstrated that in skeletal muscles during their activity a pronounced glycolysis occurs under the influence of adrenaline on the activity of glycogen phosphorylase.[11,13,14] Obviously, this is the mechanism that enables athletes to perform short-term competitive exercises. Through the action of hormones on enzyme activities, the mobilization of hepatic glycogen stores, lipids and protein resources are also actualized during prolonged exercises.

Hormonal regulation is also necessary for performing the tasks of homeostatic regulation during muscular activity. Through hormonal actions, constant levels of ions and water are maintained in intra- and extracellular compartments (see Chapter 4). A constant level of glucose in the blood is also maintained with the aid of hormonal regulation.

The production of hormones by endocrine glands is primarily regulated with the aid of feedback systems: a high level of hormone suppresses and a low level stimulates the activity of corresponding endocrine systems. However, rapid adjustments of metabolic processes according to changes in bodily activities and environmental conditions require a quicker interference of hormones with cellular autoregulation than it occurs due to the feedback regulation of hormone production. The necessary rapid changes in hormone levels are evoked by *nervous regulation* of endocrine functions (Figure 1-4). Some of the endocrine glands are directly supplied by functional nerves, the excitement of which causes changes in hormone secretion. For instance, excitement of the *n. splanchnicus* results in rapid adrenaline secretion by the adrenal medulla at the beginning of exercise (see Chapter 3). The activities of other

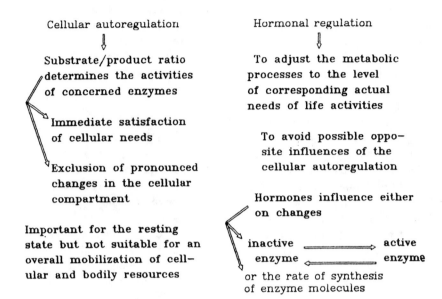

FIGURE 1-3.   Metabolic control by cellular autoregulation and hormonal regulation.

endocrine glands are altered by a two-step system: (1) hypothalamic neurosecretory cells produce neurohormones (liberins or statins) which stimulate or inhibit the release of pituitary trophic hormones, (2) pituitary trophic hormones stimulate the activity of peripheral endocrine glands.

There are also possibilities for direct nervous influence on metabolic processes without any hormonal interference. One such possibility is the flow of axonplasma by the nerves. It was thought that the axonplasma contains compounds stimulating or inhibiting the synthesis of certain regulatory and other proteins. A number of metabolic changes are caused by mediator compounds released from nerve endings to the extra- and intracellular compartments. It is also assumed that changes in the electrical activity of the cellular membrane due to nervous impulses may lead to the transcription of synthesis of some proteins.[15]

ACUTE AND LONG-TERM ADAPTATION

Exercises performed by athletes during training sessions or competitions evoke adjustments belonging to the group of acute adaptation processes. These processes include both homeostatic regulatory responses and changes coordinated by the mechanism of general adaptation. Every exercise results in an increased oxygen demand and a necessity to eliminate the CO_2 produced. Accordingly, the activity of cardiovascular and respiratory systems has to increase. The bigger the role of anaerobic glycogenolysis in ATP resynthesis, the higher is the need for homeostatic means in order to avoid an increase in the concentration of H^-. Augmented energy metabolism results in increased heat production. Adjustments at the level of thermoregulation have to follow. Increased perspiration alters water and electrolyte balances. Again, necessities arise for related homeostatic responses (see Chapter 3). It is also necessary to maintain euglycemia (see Chapter 3).

When exercise intensity or duration increases over certain threshold values, an overall mobilization of energy and protein resources (activation of the mechanism of general adaptation) takes place.

Structural and functional changes developing in the organism of an athlete during prolonged periods of training express long-term adaptation. In order to stimulate the long-term adaptive changes, it is necessary to synthesize a number of new molecules of proteins. The corresponding adaptive protein synthesis concerns the structural proteins of the most active cellular structures and the enzyme proteins of the main metabolic pathways during the acute adaptation (e.g. during performance of exercise). Thereby the nature of training exercises determines the locuses for long-term adaptational changes (see Chapter 6).

The adaptive protein synthesis needs: (1) creation of inductors acting on the cellular genetic apparatus and calling forth the specifically related synthesis of the concerned proteins, (2) supply of synthesis processes by 'building materials' (amino acids and precursors for synthesis of ribonuclear acids), (3) destruction of the old, physiologically exhausted cellular elements, and (4) supply of synthesis processes by energy. The first task will be fulfilled by the metabolic changes during exercise as well as by hormonal changes during and after exercise (see Chapter 8). An essential role here belongs to protein catabolism.[16] All other tasks are deeply related to activation of the mechanism of general adaptation. Therefore, the load of training sessions has to be sufficiently high to activate the mechanism of general adaptation including the pronounced alterations in endocrine functions.

During the recovery period after training sessions or competitions, the body's energy reserves and protein resources can be extensively used for the adaptive synthesis of enzyme and structural proteins in order to restore the functional capacity of cellular structures (see Chapter 4). The enlargement of active cellular structures and thus an improvement of the functional capacity is actualized in consequence of post-exercise synthetic processes.

THE NATURE OF EXERCISE TRAINING

Sports training consists of exercises performed systematically in order to improve physical abilities and acquire skills connected with the technique of the performance of the sports event (Figure 1-5). Experience, and to a certain extent, the results of related studies suggest to the coach which exercises are necessary. Testing of physical abilities, visual evaluation of the performance technique, and competition results will indicate how effective the training was. When exercise training is used for health promotion in people of various ages or for stimulation of harmonic physical development in children and adolescents, the usual approach is the same: more or less justified exercises are performed to achieve the corresponding goals.

This usual understanding leaves a gap between exercise and the effects of its systematical repetition. Moreover, in regard to the guidance of training, an essential problem arises due to the fact that a couple of months is necessary before the training effects are revealed in physical abilities and physical working capacity to a measurable extent. Therefore, only delayed feedback information on training effects may be obtained by tests of physical

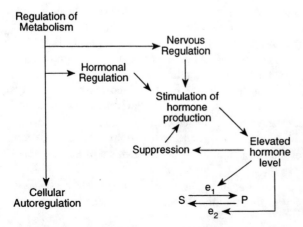

FIGURE 1-4. Three levels of regulation of metabolism.

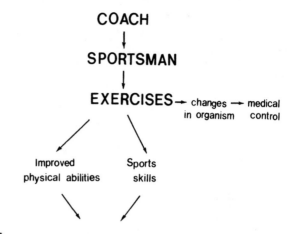

FIGURE 1-5. A usual approach to understanding training.

abilities and competition results. Moreover, the main shortcoming of this feedback information is that the concerned changes reflect an integral action of various exercises, training methods, and regimes.

The situation will significantly change if we consider that (a) all training effects are founded on exercise-induced changes in the organism (Figure 1-6),[17] and (b) there exists a specific dependence of each change on the exercise nature, intensity and duration.[18]

The background for this approach originates from the following results of physiological and biochemical studies:

1. A number of changes and peculiarities in the organism distinguish the top athlete, the 'homo olympicus', from the sedentary person, the 'homo sedentarius'. Changes and peculiarities are established on levels of cellular structures, metabolic processes and resources, functions and morphological characteristics of various organs, and coordination of the organism's activities. In a number of cases quantitative relationships between the concerned changes and performance estimates are established.[19-25]

2. Training experiments as well as cross-sectional studies indicate that certain changes necessary to improve the physical abilities are induced by systematical exercising.[19-25]

3. The character, intensity, and duration of training exercises as well as the peculiarities in the involvement of various muscles and motor units are determinants of adaptive changes in the organism when the exercise is systematically repeated (see Chapter 5).

4. The foundation for the specific dependence of changes in the organism on the exercises used is the exercise-induced adaptive protein synthesis.[19,26-30] It was hypothesized that the metabolite accumulation and hormonal changes during and after exercise are inductors for the specific synthesis of proteins. The latter warrants the increase in the most active cellular structures and the augmentation of enzyme molecules catalyzing the most responsible metabolic pathways[27] (see Chapter 8).

Thus, each training exercise results in specific changes in the organism, necessary to obtain the goal of the training. Collectively, the changes caused by various exercises warrant an increased level of sport performance, or a good physical development, or health promotion.

In the practical organizing of training, the main advantages of using the scheme presented in Figure 1-6 are: (1) each exercise will be performed in order to achieve a concrete goal in the form of a certain change in the organism, and (2) the resulting changes make it possible to check the effectiveness of each exercise (or at least group of exercises).

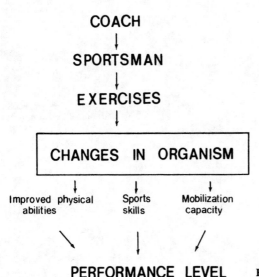

COACH
↓
SPORTSMAN
↓
EXERCISES
↓

CHANGES IN ORGANISM

Improved physical   Sports   Mobilization
abilities   skills   capacity

PERFORMANCE LEVEL   **FIGURE 1-6.**   An accomplished understanding training.

In this way, 'blind' exercising will be avoided and training will become a well-controlled process. The changes in the organism are not only goals. They will serve as the means for the operative feedback control of the training effectiveness (Figure 1-7). This will be a specific feedback allowing evaluation of the effect of the concrete exercises used.

The practical use of this approach requires of us to know what changes are necessary in order to achieve the aim of training. When the aim is top level performance in sports, the answer can be obtained by (1) an analysis of the factors limiting performance in the corresponding event, and (2) studies on top level athletes enabling to constitute a model of their organism (Figure 1-8).

During the period of 10 to 12 years required by a prepubertal boy or girl to become a champion, the top performance level and records will improve. Therefore, the level of top results today will not be sufficient for success after 10 years. Accordingly, the limiting structural, metabolic, and functional parameters have to allow more. In this regard most complications arise due to the possibility that improvement of the record is not always found on the quantitative changes in the limiting parameter. We cannot exclude the possibility that the qualitative changes in interrelation between various factors may contribute to further progress in records. For example, performance in endurance events is limited by the functional capacity of the system responsible for oxygen transport, oxidation capacity of skeletal muscles, efficiency of energy processes, functional stability of related processes, and anaerobic capacity (see Chapters 5 and 6). The stabilization of the highest values of cardiac performance and maximal oxygen uptake in top athletes during the last 20 years suggests that the opportunities for further improvement on the level of the oxygen transport system are exhausted. Therefore, it must have been other factors that have made possible the progress in sports results during this period.

The top level of sports results depends on training as well as on genetic peculiarities. Therefore, the tasks of training and of sports selection have to be discriminated. However, it must be emphasized that there are no genetically induced factors that directly determine the level of sports results in any event. The positive (or negative) significance of genetic factors becomes apparent in training. There exists a dual interrelation. Training makes possible the use of genetically induced manifestations in the improvement of sports performance. At the same time the effectiveness of training in various directions depends on the susceptibility of the organism to the training action of various exercises. It is assumed that susceptibility to training action is related to the genetic program.[31,32] It is rather likely that this susceptibility

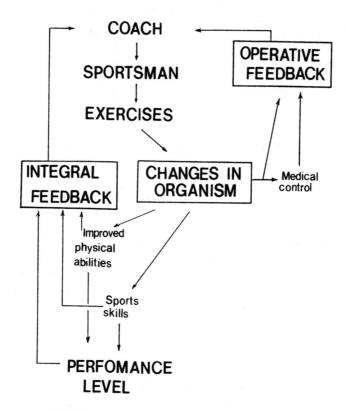

FIGURE 1-7. Integral and operative feedback in training.

is a manifestation of the sensitivity of the cellular genetic apparatus to the action of various inductors of the adaptive protein synthesis. Besides the important role of the genotype in the corresponding sensitivity, the conditions of individual life and particularly previous muscular activity (maybe already at preschool age) may phenotypically induce corrections.

Undoubtedly there also exist genetically induced factors that are not or are to a small extent influenced by training. It is meaningless to train for endurance events in the prevalence of fast-twitch glycolytic fibers or for power events in case of the opposite ratio between fast- and slow-twitch fibers. Likewise, it is hopeless to dream of becoming a basketball star and not have the precondition of being tall. Among genetically induced peculiarities in body building, an important role must belong to the variation in the attachment of muscle tendons on bones. The resulting differences in the ratio between the length of arms of double-armed levers have to favor, in some cases, the application of forces of muscle contraction. The opposite ratio has to be favorable for high velocity movements.

The tasks of training have to be distributed rationally during the whole period of 10 to 12 years. *Training strategy* has to determine how to distribute the tasks, taking into account the organism's development during adolescence. It means that the most favorable periods have to be found for inducing the necessary structural, metabolic, and functional changes. To training strategy also belongs the distribution of various tasks and within a year by training periods, and within training periods by mezo- and microcycles of training. Carrying out the induction of necessary changes is part of *training tactics*. Accordingly, the most rational ways for the organizing of training microcycles and training sessions have to be found. And finally the necessary training methods and exercises have to be chosen.

Despite the variability of the aims of training, in each case it is effective only if the exercises are performed systematically during a long period. Most exercises cause an arousal effect and stimulate the production of opioid peptides. By these actions exercise performance is connected with positive emotions. However, there are a number of cases when exercises result in negative feelings, when they have to be continued despite a developing fatigue. Therefore, a well-motivated attitude and strong will power is necessary to warrant the actual effectiveness of training. Consequently, carrying out the training process is related not only to biological changes in the organism but also depends on the educational means and psychological influences.

MODEL OF THE TOP ATHLETE

The data presented above give good opportunities to establish rather precisely what the limiting factors in most events are. A more complicated task is the quantitative aspect, to know the concrete level of the most responsible functions and processes needed to set a record or to reach a certain performance. The most serious complication arises from the situation that a lot of related research has been based on complicated methods, often including studies that involve animals, as well as experiments where certain organs have to be isolated. Even the findings from studies conducted with athletes are frequently unsuitable for a wider use of a performance model because sophisticated equipment and laboratory techniques are needed for practical application. Consequently, there are two different models in existence for high performance athletes:[33] (1) an ideal model, reflecting all the factors involved in a performance capacity and based on scientific research findings and (2) a realistic model, based on practically measurable indices.

For constitution of realistic models in various sports events, an analysis of the competition exercise has to be done. On one hand, the main characteristics of necessary muscle contractions and peculiarities of coordination of muscular activity have to be taken into consideration. On the other hand, it is important to establish the pathways of energy attaining muscle activity. The main pathway of ATP resynthesis can be presupposed by the fact that the relationship between exercise intensity and duration determines this pathway. In exercises with maximal duration up to 2 min a great role in ATP resynthesis belongs to anaerobic processes. In exercises with maximal duration from 2 to 8 min the role of aerobic processes gradually increases. In more prolonged exercises the ATP resynthesis is founded greatly on aerobic processes. Correlations between the results in various running distances and VO_2max or maximal oxygen debt confirmed that up to the 800 m race the maximal oxygen debt is more highly correlated with performance than VO_2max. In longer distances the significance of VO_2max as a factor of performance increases and correspondingly the significance of maximal O_2 debt decreases (Figure 1-9).[34] When we take into account that anaerobic processes consist in anaerobic glycogenolysis and phosphocreatine breakdown, the prevalence of the latter has to be accounted in exercises of maximal intensity. The duration of these exercises is possible up to 30 s. Figure 1-10 gives a generalized scheme of the dependence of the predominant mechanism of ATP resynthesis on the relative intensity of exercise.

Difficulties exist in determining the predominant mechanism of ATP resynthesis in sports games. It is necessary to bear in mind that the sportsman's activity during sports games consists of phases of high activity and relief. The relief phases are induced by (1) relatively passive participation in the team's activity, (2) 'time outs' or other stops during the game, or (3) change of players. Depending on the game, the duration of high activity phases is different. It was specially estimated that their mean duration is 8 s in volleyball,[36] 28 s in basketball,[37] and 36 s in ice hockey.[38] Correspondingly it is possible to suggest that during the phases of high activity the main pathway of ATP resynthesis is breakdown of phosphocreatine in volleyball, breakdown of phosphocreatine in combination with anaerobic glycogenolysis in basketball, and predominantly anaerobic glycogenolysis in ice hockey. This suggestion agrees with the calculations presented by E.L. Fox and D.K. Mathews.[21] They assumed that the relation between ATP resynthesis by phosphocreatine breakdown plus anaerobic glycogenolysis,

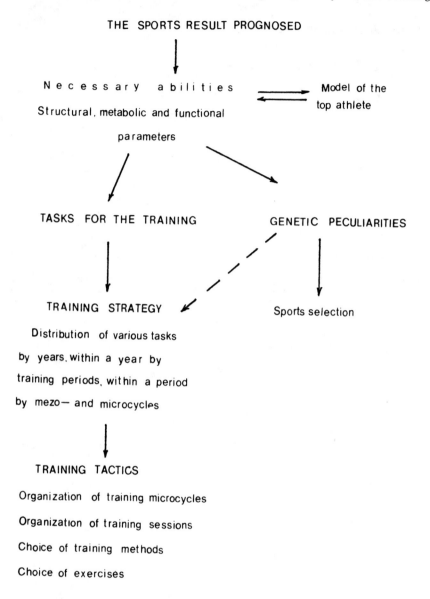

THE SPORTS RESULT PROGNOSED

Necessary abilities ⟶ Model of the top athlete

Structural, metabolic and functional

parameters

TASKS FOR THE TRAINING GENETIC PECULIARITIES

TRAINING STRATEGY Sports selection

Distribution of various tasks

by years, within a year by

training periods, within a period

by mezo— and microcycles

TRAINING TACTICS

Organization of training microcycles

Organization of training sessions

Choice of training methods

Choice of exercises

FIGURE 1-8. A generalized approach to the training organization.

anaerobic glycogenolysis plus oxidative phosphorylation and solely oxidative phosphorylation are in basketball 85 + 15 + 0, in football (soccer) 80 + 20 + 0, in ice hockey 95 + 5 + 0, in tennis 70 + 20 + 10, and in rugby 90 + 10 + 0. However, it is impossible to agree with a low significance in oxidative phosphorylation during the whole period of the game. The rate of efficiency of oxidative phosphorylation during passive phases determines the degree of restoration of the phosphocreatine store and elimination of lactate and thereby the readiness for the subsequent phase of high activity. Accordingly, a high correlation was found between playing activity and VO_2max in ice hockey players.[39] In qualified squash players possessing a high level of aerobic performance capacity, the blood lactate concentration increased during the so-called drill training session less than in a sportsman with a lower aerobic capacity.[40]

The mechanisms of ATP resynthesis can be evaluated by their highest rate, maximal capacity, and efficiency (Table 1-1). In this Table the anaerobic threshold has not been indicated. Without any doubt, exercise intensity at the anaerobic threshold is the most

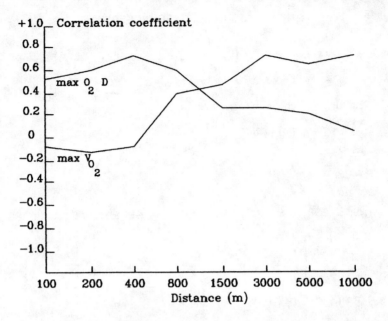

FIGURE 1-9. Correlations between competition velocity in various running distances and VO₂max (solid line), as well as between velocity and maximal oxygen debt. On the ordinate — r, on the abscissa — distance in m (a log scale). (From Volkov, N.I., *Human Bioenergetics in Strenuous Muscular Activity and Pathways for Improved Performance Capacity in Sportsmen,* Anokhin's Inst. Normal Physiol., Moscow, 1990. With permission.)

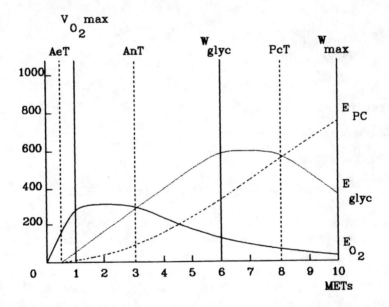

FIGURE 1-10. The rate of energy production by various mechanisms (cal·min⁻¹·kg b.wt.) in dependence of the relative intensity of exercise (METs). E_{pc} — phosphocreatine mechanism; E_{gluc} — anaerobic glucolysis; Eo_2 — oxidative phosphorylation; AT — aerobic threshold; VO₂max — level of maximal oxygen uptake; AnT — anaerobic threshold; W_{glyc} — maximal rate of anaerobic glycolysis; P_cT — threshold of phosphocreatine mechanism; and W_{max} — the highest rate of work output. (From Volkov, N. I., *Human Bioenergetics in Strenous Muscular Activity and Pathways for Improved Performance Capacity in Sportsmen,* Anokhin's Inst. Normal Physiol., Moscow, 1990. With permission.)

essential criterion (see Chapter 6). Accordingly, as a criterion for measuring the capacity of oxidative phosphorylation the maximal duration of exercise performed at the anaerobic threshold can be advised.

The main qualities of the human physical working capacity are aerobic endurance, anaerobic endurance, speed, power, and strength. Each sports event needs these qualities in various proportions. Therefore our next task is to clarify these proportions. According to the results of the corresponding analysis the model of the top sportsman in each event consists of criteria presented in Tables 1-2 to 6. These Tables are generalized schemes of determinants of the main qualities of the human physical working capacity. First, one can find integral indices. However, when the integral indices do not indicate improvement or reveal regression, a more detailed analysis should be made using the related indices. This is also advisable when the progress turns out to be smaller than expected. Detailed analysis has to suggest complementary exercises or changes in the usage of the training method.

Table 1-1. Bioenergetic Criteria for Working Capacity of Athletes

	Oxidative phosphorylation	Anaerobic glycogenolysis	Phosphocreatine mechanism
Intensity (power)	VO_2max, critical power output level	Maximal rate of lactate production and excess CO_2 formation, highest power output in 'pure' anaerobic exercise (30–60 s)	Maximal power output during 3–7 s, rate of phosphocreatine degradation
Capacity	Maximal amount of O_2 supply of exercising muscles, maximal exercising time on VO_2max level	Maximal amount of lactate accumulation, total O_2 debt, the highest pH shift	Alactic O_2 debt, accumulation of free creatine, time of all-out exercise at the highest levels of power output
Efficiency	Velocity constant of initial 'tuning' of VO_2, coefficient of mechanical efficiency	Mechanical equivalent of lactate formation	Velocity constant of alactic O_2 debt payment

From Volkov, N. I., *Tests and Criteria for Evaluation of Endurance in Sportsmen,* Central Inst. Phys. Cult., Moscow, 1989 (in Russian). With permission.

Table 1-2.   **A Generalized Scheme of Determinants of the Main Qualities of the Human Physical Working Capacity: Significance of Determinants of Aerobic Metabolism**

	Endurance		Speed	Power	Strength
	Aerobic	Anaerobic			
Oxygen supply of muscles	High	Relative	Negligible	Negligible	Negligible
Integral index					
Maximal oxygen uptake[41]					
Detailed indices					
Heart volume (x-ray photograph)					
Echocardiographic characteristics					
Maximal cardiac output					
Maximal stroke volume					
Maximal muscle blood flow					
Coronary blood capacity					
Degree of muscle capillarization					
Blood volume					
Total hemoglobin content					
Lung ventilation characteristics					
Oxygen diffusion in lungs					
Most simple indices					
Harvard step test[42]					
PWC170[43]					
Cooper's 12-min test[44]					
Oxygen utilization	High	Relative	Negligible	Negligible	Negligible
Integral index					
Exercise intensity at anaerobic threshold[45, 46]					
Detailed indices					
Total volume of mitochondria (biopsy)					
Activity of oxidation enzymes (biopsy)					
Maximal arteriovenous difference of oxygen					
Most simple index					
Conconi's test for anaerobic threshold[47]					

Table 1–3. A Generalized Scheme of Determinants of the Main Qualities of the Human Physical Working Capacity: Significance of Determinants of Anaerobic Metabolism

	Endurance		Speed	Power	Strength
	Aerobic	Anaerobic			
Anaerobic glycogenolysis	Relative	High	Relative	Negligible	Negligible
Integral indices					
Wingate test with lactate determination[48,49]					
Volkov's maximal lactate test[50]					
Detailed indices					
Highest lactate level and pH shift in muscles (biopsy) or blood after competition exercise					
Blood base excess determination					
Buffer capacity assessment					
Exercise-induced activation of glycolytic enzymes (biopsy)					
Content of pH-resistant isozymes					
Capacity for adrenaline output, maximal rate of adrenaline output					
Most simple indices					
Wingate test without lactate determination[48,51]					
Bosco test (decrease of power output from the first to the fourth 15-s period)[52]					
Phosphocreatine mechanism	Negligible	Relative	High	High	Relative
Integral indices					
Margaria staircase test[53]					
Maximal power output measurement					
Detailed indices					
Phosphocreatine kinase activity in muscles (biopsy)					
Dynamics of muscle phosphocreatine in exercise of high intensity[54]					
Most simple indices					
Margaria staircase test[53]					
Bosco test (power output during the first 15 s)					

Table 1-4. A Generalized Scheme of Determinants of the Main Qualities of the Human Physical Working Capacity: Significance of Energy Stores and Functional Stability

	Endurance		Speed	Power	Strength
	Aerobic	Anaerobic			
Energy stores					
Direct measurement					
Muscle glycogen content (biopsy)	High	High	Relative	Negligible	Negligible
Muscle phosphocreatine content (biopsy)	Negligible	High	High	Relative	Relative
Indirect assessment					
Blood glucose dynamics during prolonged exercise					
Mobilization of extramuscular energy stores	High	High	Negligible	Negligible	Negligible
Detailed indices					
Blood glucose dynamics during competitive exercise					
Blood free fatty acids and glycerol dynamics during competition exercise compared to lactate change					
Blood alanine dynamics during competition exercise					
Muscle tissue sensitivity to energy-mobilizing hormones (biopsy)					
Adipose tissue sensitivity to lipolytic hormones (biopsy)					
Interrelation of adrenaline, somatotropin, glucagon, cortisol and insulin changes during competition exercise					
Functional stability	High	High	Relative	Negligible	Negligible
Integral indices					
Indices of capacity of ATP resynthesis mechanisms (see Table 1-1)					
Dynamics of VO_2 during competition exercise[41]					
Detailed indices					
Dynamics of cardiorespiratory functions, hormone levels, EMG indices etc. during competition exercise					
Stability of Na,K-pump					
Most simple index					
Dynamics of working capacity (force or power output or speed) during competition exercise					

Table 1-5. **A Generalized Scheme of Determinants of the Main Qualities of the Human Physical Working Capacity: Significance of Determinants of Muscle Function**

	Endurance		Speed	Power	Strength
	Aerobic	**Anaerobic**			
Muscle composition					
Measurement of ratio of muscle fibers of various types (biopsy)					
% slow-twitch oxidative fibers	High	Negligible	Negligible	Negligible	Negligible
% fast-twitch oxidative-glycolytic fibers	Relative	High	Relative	Relative	Negligible
% fast glycolytic fibers	Negligible	Relative	High	High	High
Muscle strength					
Integral indices					
Voluntary strength of various muscle groups and strength after supramaximal electrical stimulation					
Assessment of strength deficit[55]					
Detailed indices					
Ultrasonic assessment of muscle hypertrophy					
Measurement of cross-section area of muscle fibers of various types (biopsy)					
Force output per cross-section of muscle					
Concentration of contractile proteins (biopsy)					
Myosin ATPase activity (biopsy)					
Maximal value of integral EMG during contraction					
Most simple indices					
Strength test according to competition activity					
Calculation of lean body mass on basis of measurement of specific gravity of the body[56]					
Ratio of a sum of various strength tests to the lean mass[57]					

Table 1-6. A Generalized Scheme of Determinants of the Main Qualities of the Human Physical Working Capacity: Significance of Determinants of Motor Unit Coordination and Homeostatic Regulation

	Endurance		Speed	Power	Strength
	Aerobic	Anaerobic			
Motor unit coordination	Relative	Relative	High	High	High
Integral index					
EMG characteistics of various movements[58,59]					
Detailed indices					
Interrelation of EMG of antagonist muscles in various movements					
Force-velocity curve in dynamic movements					
Force-time curve in static efforts					
Integral EMG ratio to force output and velocity of movement					
Assessment of spinal motor reflexes					
Most simple index					
Force-velocity and force-time relations in performing competition exercise[60]					
Homeostatic regulation of water-electrolyte balance	High	Relative	Negligible	Negligible	Negligible
Integral index					
Dynamics of water, sodium and potassium contents in muscles (biopsy) and blood during competition exercise					
Detailed indices					
Dynamics of water, sodium and potassium excretion by urine and sweat during competition exercise					
Maximal perspiration rate					
Dynamics of blood concentration of hormones, regulating water and sodium-potassium balance					
Most simple index					
Dynamics of body weight in various exercises					
Power of muscle contraction	Relative	Relative	High	High	Relative
Integral indices					
Maximal power output measurement					
Margaria staircase test					
Detailed indices					
Time needed to produce various levels of force output					
Force-velocity curves of various muscles					
Force-time curves in maximally rapid movements					
Maximal integral EMG at contraction with various velocities or forces					
Maximal rate of Ca^{2+} sequestering by SR					
Most simple indices					
Various power tests according to competition exercise					
Speed of movements	Negligible	Relative	High	High	Relative
Integral indices					
Speed of various movements					
Detailed indices					
Speed of movements at various levels of resistance					
Time of initiation of the contraction					
Time for initiation of relaxation					
Time needed to achieve the highest integral EMG					
Time of single movements					
Time of maximal relaxation					
Indices of nervemuscular lability and excitability					

Table 1-6 (continued). **A Generalized Scheme of Determinants of the Main Qualities of the Human Physical Working Capacity: Significance of Determinants of Motor Unit Coordination and Homeostatic Regulation**

| | Endurance | | | | |
	Aerobic	Anaerobic	Speed	Power	Strength
Maximal rate of calcium uptake by SR					
Maximal rate of Na,K-pump					
Most simple indices					
Assessment of the highest frequency of various movements					
Agility test according to competition exercise					

REFERENCES

1. **Bernard, C.**, *Lecons sur les Phénomènes de la Vie Communs aux Animaux et aux Végétaux*, Vol.1, Liberaire, J.-B., Ed., Baillièrs et Fils, Paris, 1878.
2. **Cannon, W.B.**, Organization of physiological homeostasis, *Physiol. Rev.*, 9, 399, 1929.
3. **Cannon, W.B.**, *The Wisdom of the Body*, Kogan, P., Ed., Trench, Trubner, London, 1932.
4. **Anokhin, P.K.**, General principles of the formation of the body's defense adaptations, *Vestnik Akad. USSR*, 17(2), 16, 1962 (in Russian).
5. **Cannon, W.P.**, *Bodily Changes in Pain, Hunger, Fear and Rage*, Appelton-Century, Crofts, New York, 1929.
6. **Orbeli, L.A.**, Review of the theory about the sympathetic innervation of skeletal muscles, organs of sense, and central nervous system, *Sechenov Physiol. J. USSR*, 15, 1, 1932 (in Russian).
7. **Selye, H.**, The physiology and pathology of exposure to stress, *Med. Publ., Montreal*, 1950.
8. **Viru, A.**, *Hormonal Mechanisms of Adaptation and Training*, Nauka, Leningrad, 1981.
9. **Viru, A.**, Mechanism of general adaptation, *Med. Hypothesis*, 38, 296, 1992.
10. **Conlee, R.K., McLane, J.A., Rennie, M.J., Winder, W.W., and Holloszy, J.O.**, Reversal of phosphorylase activation in muscle despite continued contractile activity, *Am. J. Physiol.*, 237, R291, 1979.
11. **Richter, E.A., Ruderman, N.B., Gavras, H., Belur, E.R., and Galbo, H.**, Muscle glycogenolysis during exercise: dual control by epinephrine and contractions, *Am. J. Physiol.*, 242, E25, 1982.
12. **Chasiotis, D., Sahlin, K., and Hultman, E.**, Regulation of glycogenolysis in human muscle at rest and during exercise, *J. Appl. Physiol.*, 53, 708, 1982.
13. **Arnall, D.A., Marker, J.C., Conlee, R.K., and Winder, W.W.**, Effect of infusing epinephrine on liver and muscle glycogenolysis during exercise in rats, *Am. J. Physiol.*, 250, E641, 1986.
14. **Spriet, L.L., Ren, J.M., and Hultman, E.**, Epinephrine infusion enhances muscle glycogenolysis during prolonged electrical stimulation, *J. Appl. Physiol.*, 64, 1439, 1988.
15. **Iljin, V.S., and Protasova, T.N.**, Biochemical foundations of homeostatic mechanisms, in *Homeostasis*, Gorizontov, P.D., Ed., Medicina, Moscow, 1976, 93 (in Russian).
16. **Mader, A.**, A transcription-translation activation feedback circuit as a function of protein degradation, with the quality of protein mass adaptation related to the average functional load, *J. Theor. Biol.*, 134, 135, 1988.
17. **Viru, A.**, How to understand the training, *Modern Athlete and Coach*, 32(2) 1994.
18. **Viru, A., and Viru, M.**, The specific nature of training on muscle: a review, *Sport Med. Training Rehab.*, 4, 79, 1993.
19. **Hollmann, W., and Hettinger, T.**, *Sportmedizin — Arbeits and Trainingsgrundlagen*, Schattauer, Stuttgart, 1976.
20. **Jakowlew, N.N.**, *Sportbiochemie*, Barth, Leipzig, 1977.
21. **Fox, E.L., and Mathews, D.K.**, *Physiological Basis of Physical Education and Athletics*, 3rd ed., W.B. Saunders, Philadelphia, 1981.
22. **Saltin, B., and Gollnick, P.D.**, Skeletal muscle adaptability: significance for metabolism and performance, in *Handbook of Physiology, Skeletal Muscle*, Peachy, L.D., Adrian, R.H., and Geiger, S.R., Eds., American Physiological Society, Bethesda, 1983, 555.
23. **Shephard, J.R., and Åstrand, P.-O.**, Eds., *Endurance in Sport*, Blackwell Scientific Publications, Oxford, 1992.
24. **Costill, D.L., Maglischo, E.W., and Richardson, A.B.**, *Swimming*, Blackwell Scientific Publications, Oxford, 1992.
25. **Komi, P.V.**, *Strength and Power in Sport*, Blackwell Scientific Publications, Oxford, 1992.

26. **Poortmans, J.R.**, Effects of long lasting physical exercises and training on protein metabolism, in *Metabolic Adaptations to Prolonged Physical Exercise*, Howald, H., and Poortmans, J.R., Eds., Birkhäuser, Basel, 1975, 212.

27. **Viru, A.**, The mechanism of training effects: an hypothesis, *Int. J. Sports Med.*, 5, 219, 1984.

28. **Poortmans, J.R.**, Protein metabolism, in *Principles of Exercise Biochemistry*, Poortmans, J.R., Ed., Karger, Basel, 1988, 164.

29. **Booth, F.W.**, Perspectives on molecular and cellular exercise physiology, *J. Appl. Physiol.*, 65, 1461, 1988.

30. **Booth, F.W., and Thomason, D.B.**, Molecular and cellular adaptation of muscle in response to exercise: perspectives of various models, *Physiol. Rev.*, 71, 541, 1991.

31. **Bouchard, C., and Malina, R.M.**, Genetics and olympic athletes, *Med. Sci. Sports Exercise*, 18, 28, 1984.

32. **Bouchard, C., Boulay, M.R., Simoneau, J.A., Lortie, G., and Pérusse, L.**, Heredity and trainability of aerobic and anaerobic performance. An update, *Sports Med.*, 5, 69, 1988.

33. **Viru, A.**, A high performance model, *Modern Athlete and Coach*, 25(3), 27, 1987.

34. **Volkov, N.I.**, *Human Bioenergetics in Strenuous Muscular Activity and Pathways for Improved Performance Capacity in Sportsmen*, Anokhin's Inst. Normal Physiol., Moscow, 1990.

35. **Volkov, N.I.**, *Tests and Criteria for Evaluation of Endurance in Sportsmen*, Central Inst. Phys. Cult., Moscow, 1989 (in Russian).

36. **Belyayev, A.V.**, *A study of training and competition loads in volleyball*, Thesis of acad. diss., Central Institute of Physical Culture, Moscow, 1974 (in Russian).

37. **Koryagin, V.M.**, *A study of competition and training loads in basketball-players of high qualification*, Thesis of acad. diss., Central Institute of Physical Culture, Moscow, 1973 (in Russian).

38. **Godik, M.A.**, *Control of Training and Competition Loads*, FiS, Moscow, 1980 (in Russian).

39. **Guminsky, A.A., Tarasov, A.V., Elizarova, O.S., and Samsonov, O.A.**, A study of aerobic and anaerobic indices in ice-hockey players, *Teor. Prakt. Fiz. Kult.*, 11, 39, 1971 (in Russian).

40. **Urhausen, A., Coen, B., Weile, B., and Kindermann, W.**, Sportmedizinische Leistungsdiagnostik and Trainings-steuerung in Rückschlagspielen, *Leistungssport*, 20, 29, 1990.

41. **Åstrand, P.-O., and Rodahl, K.**, *Textbook of Work Physiology*, McGraw-Hill, New York, 1977.

42. **Brouha, L.**, The step test. A simple method of measuring physical fitness for muscular work in young men, *Res. Quart.*, 14, 31, 1943.

43. **Wahlund, H.**, Determination of the physical working capacity, *Acta Med. Scand.*, 132 (Suppl. 215), 1948.

44. **Cooper, K.H.**, A means of assessing maximal oxygen uptake, *JAMA*, 203, 135, 1968.

45. **Mader, A., and Heck, H.**, A theory of the metabolic origin of "anaerobic threshold", *Int. J. Sports Med.*, 7 (Suppl. 1), 45, 1986.

46. **Mader, A.**, Evaluation of the endurance performance of marathon runners and theoretical analysis of test results, *J. Sports Med. Phys. Fitness*, 31, 1, 1991.

47. **Conconi, F., Ferrari, M., Ziglio, P.G., Droghetti, P., and Codeca, L.**, Determination of the anaerobic threshold by a noninvasive field test in runners, *J. Appl. Physiol.*, 52, 869, 1982.

48. **Bar-Or, O., Dotan, R., Jubar, O., Rotstem, A., Karlsson, J., and Tesch, P.**, Anaerobic capacity and muscle fiber type distribution, *Int. J. Sports Med.*, 1, 89, 1980.

49. **Jacobs, I.**, Blood lactate implications for training and sports performance, *Sports Med.*, 3, 10, 1986.

50. **Volkov, N.I., Shirkovets, E.A., and Barilkevich, V.E.**, Assessment of aerobic and anaerobic capacity of athletes in treadmill running tests, *Eur. J. Appl. Physiol.*, 34, 121, 1975.

51. **Vandewalle, H., Pérès, G., Heller, J., and Monod, H.**, All out anaerobic capacity tests on cycle ergometer, *Eur. J. Appl. Physiol.*, 54, 222, 1985.

52. **Bosco, C., Luhtanen, P., and Komi, P.V.**, Simple method for measurement of mechanical power in jumping, *Eur. J. Appl. Physiol.*, 50, 273, 1983.

53. **Margaria, R., Aghemo, P., and Rovelli, B.**, Measurement of muscular power (anaerobic) in man, *J. Appl. Physiol.*, 21, 1662, 1964.

54. **Hirvonen, J., Rehunen, S., Rusko, H. and Härkönen, M.**, Breakdown of high-energy phosphate compounds and lactate accumulation during short supramaximal exercise, *Eur. J. Appl. Physiol.*, 56, 253, 1987.

55. **Kots, J.M.**, Methods of investigation of muscular apparatus, *Teor. Prakt. Fiz. Kult.*, 9, 31, 1972 (in Russian).

56. **Siri, W.E.**, The gross composition of the body, *Adv. Biol. Med. Phys.*, 4, 239, 1956.

57. **Halling, U., and Viru, A.**, Human special strength and its ontogenetic dynamics, *Teor. Prakt. Fiz. Kult.*, 9, 32, 1981 (in Russian).

58. **Bigland-Ritchie, B.**, EMG/force relation and fatigue of human voluntary contraction, *Exercise Sport Sci. Rev.*, 9, 75, 1981.

59. **Sale, D.**, Neural adaptation in strength and power training, in *Human Muscle Power*, Jones, N., McCartney, N., and McComas, A., Eds., Human Kinetics Publ., Champaign, 1986, 281.

60. **Komi, P.V.**, Training of muscle strength and power: interaction of neuromotoric, hypertrophic and mechanical factors, *Int. J. Sports Med.*, 7 (Suppl.) 10, 1986.

Chapter 2

HORMONES IN ADAPTATION TO PHYSICAL EXERCISES (HORMONAL RESPONSES TO EXERCISE)

BLOOD HORMONAL ENSEMBLE DURING EXERCISE

The task of hormonal regulation is to interfere with cellular autoregulation in order to achieve a pronounced mobilization of bodily resources and functions and to warrant an effective homeostatic regulation (see Chapter 1, p. 4). Thus, hormonal responses are essential both for specific homeostatic regulation and for activation of the mechanism of general adaptation (Figure 2-1). During performance of exercises, hormones have an important function in mobilization of energy and protein resources and homeostatic control (see Chapter 3). They are also essential in regulation of recovery processes after exercise (see Chapter 4). Training effects depend on hormonal influences both on transcription and translation, in the adaptive protein synthesis (see Chapter 8).

A great amount of data is concerned with hormonal changes in the blood during exercise.[1-8] Figure 2-2 sums up the main effects of various exercises on the endocrine system. If in the case of some hormone responses there is a good accordance between the results of various authors, in regard to other responses there exists a pronounced discrepancy. These discrepancies were not excluded by the general use of radioimmunological methods possessing a high level of both accuracy and specific nature. Consequently, in order to evaluate the actual hormonal changes one must take into account the possibility that there exists a number of factors that determine the response as well as a number of conditions that modulate the response. They both can be connected with the individuality of persons, the parameters of performed exercise, and the conditions in which exercise is performed.

STABILITY AND VARIABILITY IN HORMONAL RESPONSES TO EXERCISE

In order to determine the stability and variability of hormonal responses to exercise, a number of hormones were repeatedly determined in 82 male persons during a 2-h exercise on the bicycle ergometer at the level of 60% VO_2max.[9] Results show that some hormone responses are common and stable (Figure 2-3) while others are connected with great interindividual differences. According to individual analysis of the obtained data, a rise was common in the concentration of aldosterone and somatotropin both in trained and untrained persons and of corticotropin in trained persons. Common and stable responses were also decreases in insulin and C-peptide. In most of the previous studies a pronounced increase in aldosterone[10-15] and somatotropin,[16-20] and decrease in insulin[21-26] and C-peptide levels [22,27] were commonly detected. Only during short-term anaerobic exercise a drop in insulin may be absent,[10,26,28,29] as well as after exercises of extreme duration a rise in the somatotropin level has not always been observed.[29-31] In these cases the stable and common responses of insulin and somatotropin are altered to variable ones. A common corticotropin rise has been suggested.[32,33] However, a number of persons were found who did not reveal corticotropin response during prolonged exercise.[20] An exercise-induced response is the increased secretion of corticoliberin by hypothalamic neurosecretory cells.[34]

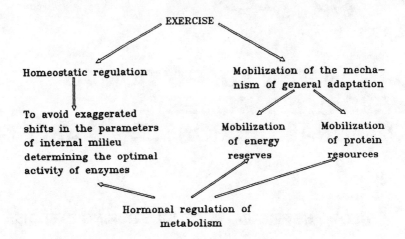

FIGURE 2-1.   Tasks of hormonal regulation in exercise.

There is no doubt that catecholamine responses[21,35-43] and probably also glucagon,[24,35,41,44,45] vasopressin,[12,14,46,47] renin,[10,12-15,46-48] angiotensin II,[10,13] and atrial natriuretic peptide[49-51] responses belong to the group of common endocrine changes during exercise. A pronounced increase was found in the melatonin level during prolonged exercise.[52,53] The magnitude of this response varies in dependence of lighting as well as of body mass and age.[53]

The changes in hormone levels that are common to all persons exhibit an inter-individual variability, but only in the magnitude of changes and in some minor characteristics of the dynamics, e.g. in the dynamics of somatotropin level either a rise throughout a 2-h exercise was observed, or a rise up to a constant niveau that was maintained until the exercise was stopped; or there was an initial rise, then a constant niveau, and during the final stage of exercise a moderate diminution.[9]

A great intraindividual variability[9] as well as various changes in the group's mean values have been observed in cortisol [20,29,30,52,54-59] and testosterone[52,55,57,60-63] levels. Five variants have been found in the dynamics of cortisol concentration (Figure 2-4)[9]: (1) an initial increase that was changed after 20 to 30 min of exercise by a decrease down to the basal level or below it, (2) biphasic increases (peak values during the first 30 min and at the end of exercise, with a decrease after the first peak), (3) a monophasic increase during the whole period of exercise, (4) a lack of alterations or a moderate decrease during the first 20 to 60 min of exercise and a pronounced increase during the second hour of exercise, and (5) a decrease during the whole period of exercise. As alterations in the corticotropin level were characterized mainly by a biphasic increase, the dynamics of corticotropin and cortisol coincided only in the second variant. In the first variant the adrenal cortex did not respond to the second corticotropin peak, in the fourth variant to the first peak and in the fifth variant to either peaks.

Nevertheless, there are two cases when the cortisol response to exercise is stable and common. First, a pronounced rise in the cortisol level is commonly observed during and/or after short-term exercise, the intensity of which is above the anaerobic threshold.[38,57,58,64-67] The other case is exercise lasting more than 2 to 3 h.[15,29,31,32,68-71] These facts together suggest that the typical cortisol dynamics is a biphasic increase during exercise whereas the first increase depends on exercise intensity and the second one on its duration. If the first peak is of short duration, the second rise in the cortisol concentration seems to be characterized by maintaining the high level for a long time.

An increase in the β-endorphin level is common during short-term high-intensity exercise.[72-75] However, during prolonged exercise the situation is analogous to changes in the cortisol concentration. A pronounced variability is evident[76-78] due to which some authors

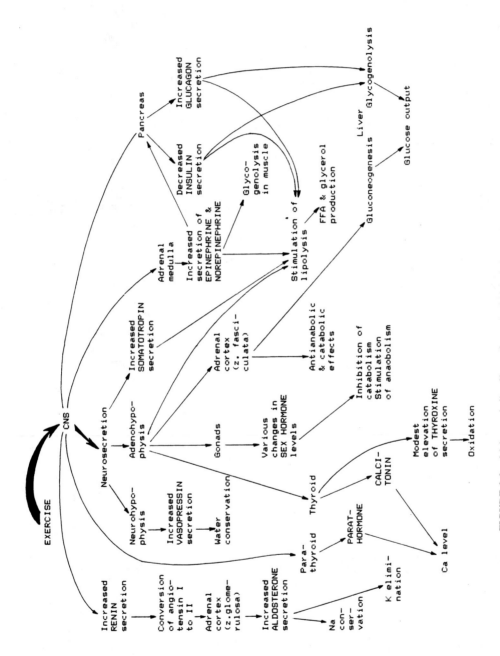

FIGURE 2-2. Main metabolic effects of exercise-induced changes in endocrine functions.

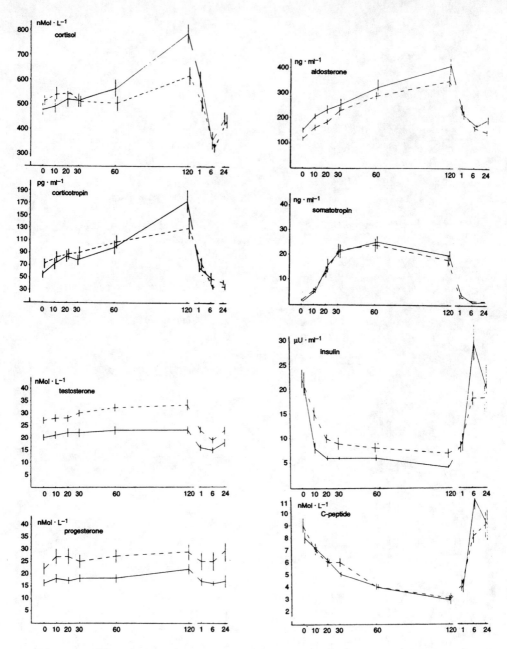

FIGURE 2-3. Stable hormonal responses to 2-h cycling exercise. Solid lines — endurance athletes, interrupted lines — untrained persons. (From Viru, A., Karelson, K., and Smirnova, T., *Int. J. Sports Med.,* 13, 230, 1992. With permission.)

obtained an elevated β-endorphin level[76,77,79] but the others did not find a significant change[72,75,78] at the end of prolonged exercise. During a 2-h exercise at 60% VO₂max approximately the same variants of β-endorphin level dynamics were observed in regard to the cortisol pattern: (1) an increase during the first 30 min followed by a decrease below the initial values, (2) a biphasic increase (peak values at the 30th and 120th min), (3) an increase only during the 2nd hour of exercise, and (4) a decrease during the whole period of exercise (Figure 2-5).[80]

The results obtained during the 2-h exercise did not allow us to establish any common variants in either testoterone nor progesterone dynamics.[9] However, there are also data

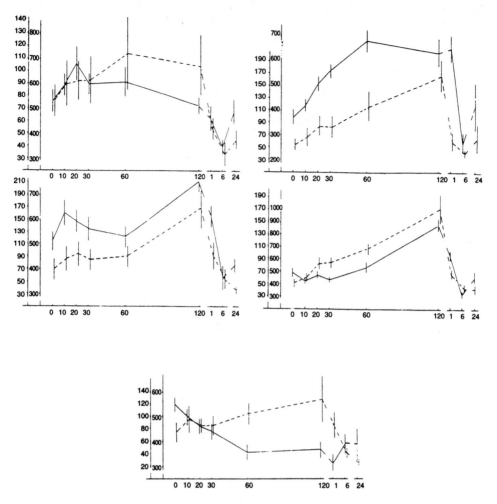

FIGURE 2-4. Five variants of cortisol dynamics during 2-h cycling exercise. Solid lines — cortisol dynamics, interrupted lines — corticotropin dynamics. (From Viru, A., Karelson, K., and Smirnova, T., *Int. J. Sports Med.,* 13, 230, 1992. With permission.)

suggesting that during short-term exercise the testosterone level increases while during prolonged exercise it decreases.[60,81] Cumming et al.[65] observed a significant elevation of the testosterone level in man with a short-term progressive cycling exercise up to the maximal intensity. The same group of investigators found a decreased testosterone concentration in cases of maximal intensity swimming in male and female swimmers.[82] A constant rise in the progesterone level has also been reported.[83]

A common increase in the estradiol concentration has been noted in women in some papers or in some groups[84-87] but in others no exercise-induced elevation has been found.[52,84] In women, exercise seems to raise progesterone[84,86,87] and prolactin [87] levels too. The marathon race resulted in a common rise in the testosterone level, but various changes in the progesterone and estradiol levels.[88] In men, the prolactin response to exercise seems to be quite variable[20,89] despite some reports indicating a common and stable increase.[65,83,90] Exercise-induced responses in the blood level of lutropin and follitropin are variable both in men[10,20,60,62,84,91] and women.[52,84-87] There exist data about an increase in some persons and a decrease in others.[60,62,87,88] In a recent study the decline in the lutropin level was preceded by an increase in the corticoliberine concentration in the blood. It was suggested that the lutropin decrease was caused by the gonadotropin-depressant property of corticoliberine.[34]

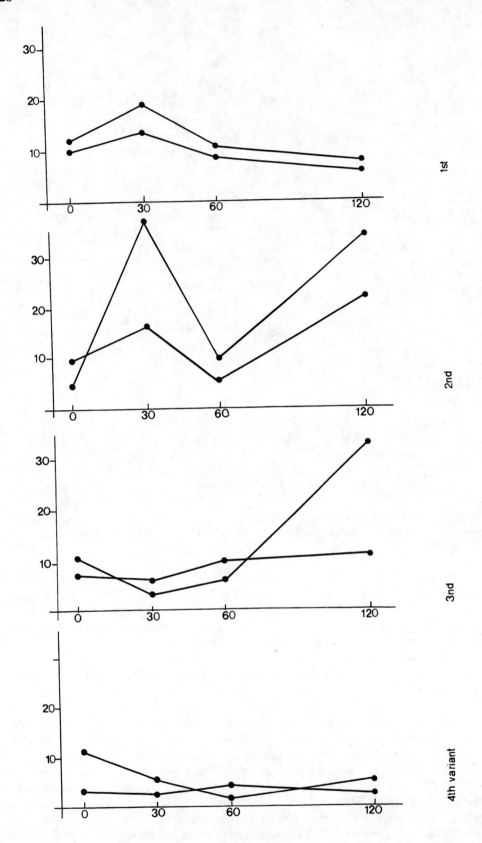

The exercise-induced responses of thyroid hormones[60,92-96] as well as those of thyrotropin[60,94-96] are rather variable.

Do the various variants of hormone responses to exercise indicate a different quality of adaptation? Theoretical analysis of various experimental data allowed us to suggest that the functional systems in whose activity the endocrine functions participate, contain not only alterations in the production of related hormones for 'private regulation', but also a complicated cooperation of actions by the 'attending regulation'. The latter is actualized by (1) modulating regulation influencing the number and state of cellular receptors, (2) metabolic regulation influencing through other receptors cellular metabolism and thus changing the realization of private regulation, and (3) regulation of the synthesis of proteins participating in the actualization of private regulation. The existence of the regulation of hormonal signal on two levels — on the level of cells producing the signal molecules, and on the level of receptors receiving the signal — makes variability of tactics of adaptive responses possible.[97] Therefore, the variability of responses seems to be completely natural. Nevertheless, this seems to happen if there are no strong demands on hormonal regulation. In cases where a decisive role belongs to hormonal regulation, the hormone response is common and stable.

THE RATE OF HORMONAL RESPONSES

In exercise-induced hormonal changes fast responses, responses of a modest rate, and responses with a lag-period can be discriminated (Figure 2-6). Fast response is characterized by a rapid increase in the concentration of hormones in the blood plasma within the first few minutes of exercise. Typical examples of these responses are rapid rises in catecholamine,[98,99] corticotropin,[64,66,74] and cortisol[38,100,101] concentration. A 6-s exercise at the highest possible power output level was sufficient to result in increases in adrenaline and noradrenaline concentrations.[102] Significant increases in plasma adrenaline were observed immediately after exercises causing exhaustion within 3.31 or 0.78 min and 15 min after exercises causing exhaustion within 0.1 min. In all cases significant increases in plasma noradrenaline were observed immediately after exercise.[103] Immediately after a 1-min anaerobic test adrenaline and noradrenaline concentrations were increased by 7.1 and 7.4 times the starting value.[104] Corticotropin and β-endorphin response was detected 5 min after the 1-min test.[104] While catecholamine response is elicited by direct action of sympathetic nerves to the adrenal medulla and by liberation of noradrenaline from the sympathetic nerve endings for increased release of pituitary trophic hormones, an increased secretion of corresponding liberins is necessary. A 13-min incremental exercise induced a rise in the serum corticoliberine level, associated with an increase in the corticotropin concentration.[34]

Responses of modest rate are characterized by a gradual increase in the hormone concentration which may continue up to the end of exercise or even for a longer time. In other cases the gradual increase during the first period of exercise is followed by a leveling-off to a constant niveau. Examples are increases in aldosterone,[9,10,15] renin,[10,15] and angiotensin II.[10,15] An initial lag period preceding the onset of changes has been described in regard to somatotropin,[16,19] insulin,[23-25] glucagon,[24,43] and calcitonine[125] response. Determination of hormone concentration by 10-min intervals during the first 30 min of exercise (at 60% VO_2max) confirmed the lag period in regard to somatotropin and insulin responses. However, it was only revealed as a possibility but not as a common characteristic of the response. Most frequently the lag period was found in the somatotropin response. In the insulin response the lag period was observed only in 25% of untrained persons and in 15% of athletes.[9]

FIGURE 2-5. Four variants of β-endorphin dynamics during 2-h cycling exercise. Each variant is characterized by two representative cases. (From Viru, A., Tendzegolskis, Z., and Smirnova, T., *Endocrin. Exp.*, 24, 63, 1990. With permission.)

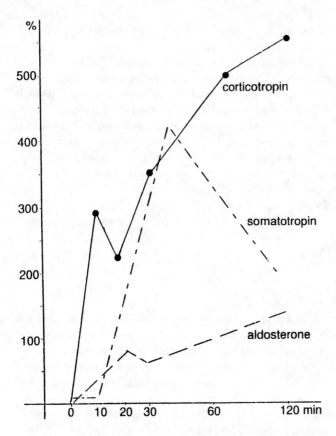

FIGURE 2-6. Individual dynamics of corticotropin (solid line), aldosterone (interrupted line) and somatotropin (interrupted line with dots) in an untrained person. The alterations of corticotropin level belong to the group of fast responses, of aldosterone — to the group of responses of a modest rate, and of somatotropin — to the group of responses with a lag period. (From Viru, A., *Int. J. Sports Med.*, 13, 201, 1992. With permission.)

Results were also obtained indicating that the response of the same hormone may have various kinetics depending on exercise intensity. For instance, short-term anaerobic exercises of high intensity cause a somatotropin response of a rather fast rate.[10] Even the glucagon response may be quite rapid in these exercises.[58]

It has been suggested that there are two types of mechanisms for activating the endocrine function at the beginning of exercise. One of them is responsible for a rapid activation, the other for a delayed activation.[5] The mechanism of rapid activation has to be connected with the functions of nervous centers and a high rate transfer of nervous influences to endocrine glands. The result of starting the mechanism of rapid activation is fast hormone responses. The mechanism of delayed activation is dependent on some effects of exercises which are cumulative. This mechanism determines the final hormone levels in the blood. If the rate of hormone changes in the first minutes of exercise depends on the degree of activity of the mechanism of rapid activation, the magnitude of hormone change depends on the mechanism of delayed activation. The response which occurs after the lag period is probably due to the lack of activity of the mechanism of rapid activation.

According to Galbo's[3] interpretation, at the onset of exercise, impulses from working muscles and motor centers modulate the activity in higher centers of the central nervous system in accordance with the relative work load. In turn, these centers elicit increased secretion of some pituitary hormones and increased sympatho-adrenal activity, controlling the changes in the secretion of subordinate endocrine cells (Figure 2-7). During continued exercise, hormone responses are modulated by impulses from receptors sensing temperature, intravascular volume, oxygen tension, and glucose availability. In this way the mechanisms of rapid activation (fast nervous component) and of delayed activation (slow internal milieu component) can be discriminated and their nature understood.

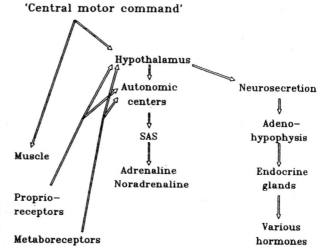

FIGURE 2-7. Control of endocrine functions during exercise by central motor command and impulses from proprioreceptors and metaboreceptors.

The importance of the function of cerebral motor centers has been evidenced by the results of experiments using tubocurarine, which weakens the skeletal muscle and increases the voluntary effort necessary to produce a certain work output. In partially curarized men a higher central command has been associated with exaggerated catecholamine, somatotropin, and corticotropin responses at a given submaximal work load and oxygen uptake.[6,7,99,105] The role of the slow internal milieu component has been stressed by the theory of glucostatic control of hormonal responses to exercise (see p. 36). It has been suggested that at least in intensive exercise a significant stimulus for activating the endocrine function may arise from metaboreceptors of skeletal muscles sensitive to the accumulation of anaerobic products.[6,7,106]

DETERMINANTS OF HORMONAL RESPONSES

SIGNIFICANCE OF EXERCISE INTENSITY

Most hormone responses are dependent on exercise intensity. First of all, this has been convincingly demonstrated in regard to catecholamine responses. A curve-linear relationship between exercise intensity and both adrenaline and noradrenaline levels (Figure 2-8) has been established in a number of studies.[36,38,40,58,104,107] Up to the relative intensity of 50 to 70% VO_2max, catecholamine changes are only modest or are not detectable. A pronounced increase in adrenaline and nordrenaline concentrations is followed by a further increase in exercise intensity.[36,37,40,58,104,107] Thus, there exists a certain level of exercise intensity that triggers the catecholamine response. This exercise level may be termed *threshold intensity for hormonal response*. Simultaneous determination of lactate levels suggests that threshold intensity for the catecholamine response is closely related to the aerobic threshold.[40,104]

Most data show that an increase in the blood cortisol concentration is displayed if the intensity of exercise exceeds 60 to 70% VO_2max.[15,37,54,58,108-110] Almost the same is revealed in regard to alterations of corticotropin[73,108,111] and β-endorphin.[73,111] Threshold intensity of the activation of the pituitary-adrenocortical system is also closely related to the anaerobic threshold. A close relationship has been found between lactate levels on the one hand and cortisol,[109,110] corticotropin, and β-endorphin[111] levels on the other hand. However, differently from the catecholamine response, in several cases the investigators have failed to obtain results showing any further dependence of adrenocortical activation on the intensity of exercise beyond the threshold load.[56,110,112] The data of Barwich et al.[113] suggest that a high level of hydrogenic ions may suppress cortisol secretion. However, during over-threshold exercises the activation of the pituitary-adrenocortical system is determined by the amount of

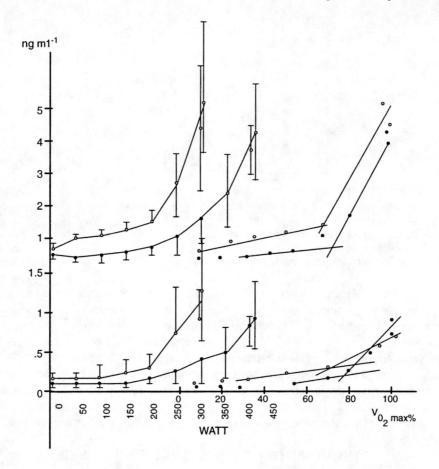

FIGURE 2-8. Blood catecholamine levels during exercise with gradually increased intensity (expressed as W on the left side and as % VO_2max on the right side) in trained (VO_2max 65.8 ± 4.7 ml·min⁻¹·kg⁻¹, closed circles) and untrained persons (VO_2max 49.2 ± 9.8 ml·min⁻¹·kg⁻¹, open circles). Constructed from results of M. Lehmann et al.[40]

utilized possibilities for anaerobic glycogenolysis rather than by the actual intensities of exercise: less intensive but more prolonged aerobic-anaerobic exercise caused a higher lactate accumulation than a brief intensive anaerobic exercise. A pronounced activation of this endocrine system was established only in the first exercise.[109]

During under-threshold exercises a decline in the blood cortisol level was noticed[15,54] that was, reasonably, related to the augmented rate of cortisol elimination from the blood.[114]

A linear relationship has been found between renin activity and exercise intensity[47] that was interpreted by the dependence of renin production on the function of the sympatho-adrenal system.[3] The renin response was found at exercise intensities of 60 and 80% VO_2max, but not at 25 and 40% VO_2max.[115]

There are data about the dependence of other hormone responses on exercise intensity, but a clear-cut dependence has not been demonstrated. When the intensity of exercise corresponded to 20% VO_2max, a drop in the plasma insulin level was noted only with a fat-rich diet, but not with a standard or high-carbohydrate diet. When the load was 50 or 70% VO_2max, a significant reduction in the insulin concentration was detected with all diets without any further dependence on the intensity of exercise.[25] Exercise intensities of 40% VO_2max[37] and 47% VO_2max[116] seemed to be enough to cause a decline in the insulin concentration.

The existence of a threshold intensity for somatotropin response and its dependence on exercise intensities has been evidenced in several studies.[19,58] This threshold intensity has been reported to be about 33% VO_2max[19] or between 40 and 70% VO_2max.[37] During intermittent exercise causing a rise in blood lactate over 4 mmol·l⁻¹, the somatotropin concentration increased more than during continuous exercise associated only with the initial elevation of the lactate level up to 2 mmol·l⁻¹. [117]

It has also been suggested that work intensity is a factor determining testosterone response:[118] work intensity was found to be positively correlated with increases in the plasma testosterone concentrations.[119] According to Jezová[120] plasma testosterone level was elevated at the exercise intensity of 4 W/1 kg of body weight but not at 1.5, 2.0, or 2.5 W/kg.

During prolonged exercise at 45% VO_2max the aldosterone concentration rose less than during exercise at 60% VO_2max;[15] 20-min cyclic exercises elicited an aldosterone response when the exercise intensity was at least 40% VO_2max.[115] During incremental exercise an increase in aldosterone concentration was found at lower exercise intensitites than the cortisol response.[121] However, there are a number of factors that influence aldosterone production. Comparison of the effects of various exercises for improved endurance showed that if there were thresholds by exercise intensity to elicit an aldosterone and somatotropin rise as well as an insulin drop in the blood, they had to be substantially lower than the anaerobic threshold.[122]

The vasopressin response was found at exercise intensities of 60 and 80% VO_2max but not at 25 and 40%. The plasma level of atrial natriuretic peptide increased at all four exercise intensities.[115]

An elevation in the estradiol level was found after 20 min of rather moderate exercise (30 to 35% VO_2max) but only in the post-ovulatory phase.[86]

SIGNIFICANCE OF EXERCISE DURATION

A considerable amount of results demonstrate the dependence of the magnitude of hormone responses on exercise duration.[5] Of course, if the dynamics of hormone responses is characterized by a continuous rise, the increase in the hormone concentration has to reach a higher level with the prolongation of exercise. The situation changes in the following cases: (1) if the dynamics of hormone response is characterized by leveling off to a stable level or by a change in the hormone rise with a decline and (2) if exercises of various intensities are compared. In more intensive exercises an enhanced hormone response is possible when it develops more quickly. At the same time the maximal possible duration of exercise decreases with a rise in exercise intensity. Therefore, when exercise duration is sufficient for a hormone response to reach the peak values, the magnitude of hormone responses is determined by exercise intensity. However, when the time until peak values of the hormone level exceeds exercise duration, the actual hormone level during brief highly intensive exercise is lower than during less intensive but more prolonged exercise, despite the less rapid development of hormone response. In several studies it has been found that in exercises of various intensity and duration the latter might mask the significance of intensity; the hormone responses were more pronounced in more prolonged but less intensive exercises.[29,123]

At the onset of exercise, impulses from working muscles and motor centers elicit an increased sympatho-adrenal activity and enhanced secretion of hypothalamic liberine, followed by the release of pituitary tropic hormones and increased activity of corresponding peripheral endocrine cells. These changes depend on the intensity of muscular activity. These changes in their turn determine the rate of the hormone response.[3,6,7,39] During continuous exercise the slow internal milieu component is added to the fast nervous component in the activation of endocrine systems. Hormone responses are modulated by the impulses from receptors sensing temperature, intravascular volume, oxygen tension, and glucose availability.[3,6,7] The role of the slow internal milieu component is stressed by the theory of glucostatic control of hormonal responses to exercise.[124] In exercises with intensity over the anaerobic threshold, a significant stimulus for activation of the endocrine function may arise from metaboreceptors of skeletal muscles sensitive to the accumulation of anaerobic metabolism products.[6,7,64,66,106]

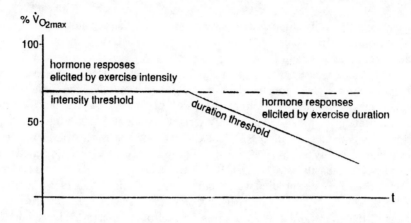

FIGURE 2-9. A scheme of threshold intensity and threshold duration of exercise for activation of endocrine responses. (From Viru, A., *Int. J. Sports Med.,* 13, 201, 1992. With permission.)

Consequently, during prolonged exercises the hormone response is determined both by the rate of the hormone response depending on exercise intensity and by changes in the organism. Decreasing availability of carbohydrates, dehydration, or changes in the electrolyte balance are examples of factors additionally influencing endocrine activities. The significance of these factors increases with exercise duration and, accordingly, the need for changes in the hormone ensemble rises with the duration of muscular activity. In some cases the need for hormone responses is revealed only after a certain amount of muscular work has been done. In this connection it is reasonable to establish a threshold duration of exercise to elicit the hormonal responses (Figure 2-9).

In exercises of under-threshold intensities the threshold duration is expressed by the onset of the hormone response. In this connection a long duration of the lag period of glucagon and calcitonin[125] responses, as well as in some cases the appearance of a rise in the corticotropin and cortisol levels only during the second hour of exercise[9,56] can be interpreted. In exercise the intensity of which is over the threshold, the achieved second threshold (threshold duration of exercise) is expressed by changes in the rate of the hormone response or in the appearance of a secondary activation of the endocrine function (Figure 2-10). In a 2-h exercise the most frequently observed variant of corticotropin and cortisol dynamics was a biphasic increase in their concentrations with peak values during the first 10 to 20 min and again at the end of exercise.[9] In regard to these two hormones it was established that the first rise in the levels is a short-term one and soon changes by a drop toward the initial values or below them. The secondary activation of the pituitary-adrenocortical system is characterized by stable high cortisol level that may be maintained for a very long time. An expression of this is the high cortisol levels after a marathon race,[29,32,68,71] triathlon,[69,126] 2-h skiing,[70] and 100 km running.[127] However, during a 1000-km run, the daily portion of 60 to 100 km did not elevate the cortisol level.[109] Only a very low running speed enabled this performance. Consequently, there exist minimal exercise intensity levels which will not lead to the activation of the pituitary-adrenocortical system even in an extreme duration of exercise.

TRAINING EFFECTS

The increase of cellular resources due to training reduces the necessity for overall mobilization of resources during vigorous exercise. In this connection the necessity for homeostatic reactions may also diminish to some extent. Together, both give a possibility for decreasing the exercise-induced hormonal responses or avoiding them altogether. A great amount of data has been published indicating that adrenocortical, adrenomedullary, and pancreatic α-cells secretion as well as somatotropin production is reduced during moderate exercise due to

FIGURE 2-10. Duration threshold for triggering hormone responses. Hormone dynamics in exercise of overthreshold intensity is indicated by solid lines, in exercises of underthreshold intensity by interrupted line. When threshold duration is reached, then in case of overthreshold intensities, either a further increase in hormonal response follows, or a new rise in hormone concentration appears in addition to the initial short-term increase. In case of underthreshold intensity, the hormone response may appear only after the threshold duration is reached.

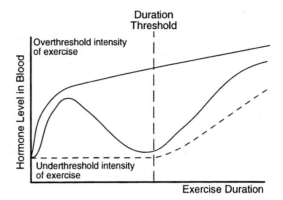

First of all, these alterations are related to the change in the threshold intensity of exercise for the activation of endocrine responses. After training, the threshold intensity of exercise, measured in units of power output, is shifted to a higher level.[129,130] Thereby exercises that used to be beyond the threshold, were under the threshold after training (Figure 2-11). More intensive exercises that exceed the new threshold level induce a pronounced hormonal response after the training period.[130] Pronounced hormonal responses to exercises of high intensity (in most cases to those exceeding the level of individual anaerobic threshold) are usual findings in highly qualified sportsmen.[9,10,29,89,101] When after training, the load of test exercise corresponded to approximately the same relative level (% VO_2max) as before the training period, the blood noradrenaline response proved to be approximately the same.[131] However, in one investigation a decrease in the responses of blood glucagon and adrenaline to exercise of the same relative intensity (62% VO_2max) was found after training.[132] Therefore, one must not exclude the alteration of threshold intensity in relation to VO_2max or a general reduction of activation of endocrine systems. In trained rats the increment in the blood corticosterone concentration was smaller than in untrained rats after injection of histamine, inhalation of ether, or surgery.[133]

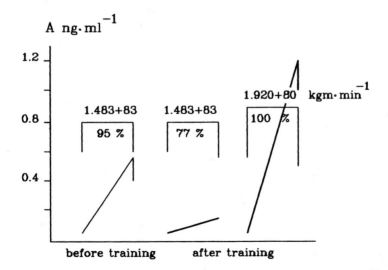

FIGURE 2-11. The effect of 5-min exercise on blood level of adrenaline before and after 7 weeks of training resulting in an increase of VO_2max from 3.46 ± 0.21 to 4.23 ± 0.13 l·min⁻¹. The relative (% VO_2max) and absolute (kg·min⁻¹) intensity of exercise is indicated on top of columns. Constructed by W.W. Winder et al.[130]

In regard to threshold by exercise duration, the training effect has not been established. In a study after a training period a delayed onset of corticotropin and cortisol responses was found during the 3-h exercise at 50% VO_2max. After training a delayed decrease in the blood glucose concentration was also observed.[134] When exercise intensity is below the threshold, a reasonably greater amount of exercise has to be performed to achieve the threshold by duration in a trained organism. However, some data suggest that in case of a biphasic increase in the hormone concentration (e.g. responses of corticotropin, cortisol, and β-endorphin to prolonged exercise), training promotes the appearance of a secondary activation of endocrine systems.[9,80] For explanation one must bear in mind that transition from the initial activation of hormone secretion to its inhibition may be connected with the need for time to speed up hormone biosynthesis. If this is so, the functional potential for hormone synthesis will determine the possible time for a secondary activation.

Training-induced adrenal hypertrophy is associated with an increased number of mitochondria, their vesicular cristae, elements of endoplasmic reticulum, and polysomes in adrenocorticocytes of the fascicular zone as well as with an elevated content of cytochrome a-a_3 in the adrenal cortex.[135] Mitochondria and endoplasmic reticulum are the main sites of biosynthesis of glucocorticoids. Consequently, the training-induced morphofunctional improvement has to be reflected in the augmented potential for hormone synthesis.

Adrenal hypertrophy is founded not only on the increase of the adrenal cortex but also the adrenal medulla.[128] Thus, a sports adrenal medulla develops.[6] The increased capacity of the adrenal medulla for hormone secretion is also founded on the augmented storage of adrenaline and noradrenaline,[39,136] as well as on the increased activity of tyrosine-hydroxylase and dopamine-β-hydroxylase[137] and improved noradrenaline methylation.[138] The training-induced increase in the capacity to secrete adrenaline was confirmed by the results about the effects of glucagon, acute hypobaric hypoxia and acute hypercapnia on the adrenaline concentration in the blood of endurance-trained athletes in comparison with sedentary males.[139] At the end of a prolonged exercise the adrenaline concentration in the plasma and the estimated adrenaline secretion were higher in athletes than in untrained subjects.[140]

An expression of the improved capacities of endocrine systems is the increased magnitude of blood catecholamine,[52,107,141] somatotropin,[52,142,143] corticotropin,[73] cortisol[52,143] and β-endorphin[73] responses to supramaximal exercise, and the enhanced plausibility for increase in the thyroxine level during exercise[92,144] in the trained organism. Consequently, in cases of maximal demand on the endocrine system, the hormonal responses are not reduced but magnified in athletes. Some data indicate that the differences in hormone responses may be partly connected with the various rates of responses in athletes and sedentary persons. After maximal cycling exercises until exhaustion the highest cortisol level occurred in endurance athletes just after exercise, but in untrained persons it occurred 15 min[145] or 1 h later.[146] In junior paddlers a 4-month training period augmented the cortisol response, but decreased the somatotropin, corticotropin and aldosterone response to all-out exercise of 4 min.[147]

Obviously, the actual training-induced changes in the hormone response to exercise depend on a combination of various alterations in the organism, including (a) an increase in the working capacity, resulting in a decrease in threshold intensities, (b) a specific adaptation to the training exercises, reducing the need for hormone responses, (c) an augmented lability of endocrine systems reflected in more rapid changes, and (d) an increased functional capacity of endocrine systems, allowing to achieve extremely pronounced and stable changes. In addition, a certain significance may belong to alteration in hormone metabolism. Data were obtained indicating that physical training increases the catecholamine turnover rate in rats.[148] In man this difference was not found in the resting state, but during exercise the adrenaline clearance seemed to be higher in trained persons.[140]

Training-induced changes may also occur on the control level. Endurance-trained men show alternated lutropin responses following stimulation by gonadoliberin.[149]

The training-induced alteration in responses of hormones that regulate the water and electrolyte balance (vasopressin, aldosterone) is not evident.[12,14,150] There are only some results indicating lower levels of plasma renin-angiotensin and vasopressin during exercises at equal intensities in trained individuals. In this study a greater absolute amount of fluid efflux to the interstitial space was formed in trained persons.[151] It is reasonable to suggest that these hormone responses depend more on homeostatic needs than on the improvement of physical working capacity and adaptation to exercises.

THE INTERPLAY BETWEEN SIGNIFICANCE OF EXERCISE DURATION AND THE FITNESS OF PERSONS

To evaluate the relative importance of exercise intensity and duration in hormone responses, the effects of two types of strenuous exercises were compared in qualified male rowers.[143] Both tests were performed on a rowing apparatus. One of them consisted of 7-min rowing at the highest possible rate. The other was 40-min rowing at the anaerobic threshold level, determined by lactate 4 mmol·l[-1]. The results indicated that with exercise duration an additional stimulus for cortisol and somatotropin responses arose, resulting in increases in the concentrations of these hormones to higher levels than those in 7-min very intensive exercise (Figure 2-12).

This experiment was repeated after a year of training. The increased performance capacity was associated with increases in somatotropin and cortisol concentrations to a higher level in the 7-min test and of cortisol in the 40-min test. Thus, training would appear to increase the capacity to secrete hormones. The functional capacity of the pituitary-adrenocortical system was capable of increasing the cortisol level even more, when rowers of national class repeated 2000 m rowing 8 times.

Consequently, in strenuous exercise cortisol and somatotropin concentration responses were determined by an integration of exercise intensity and duration, as well as the performance capacity of the subject. Responses were triggered, obviously, by exercise intensity. An additional stimulus arose from exercise duration. The actual magnitude of the response would seem to depend on the functional capacities of the endocrine systems.

HOMEOSTATIC NEEDS

The dependence of hormonal responses to exercise on homeostatic needs is obvious in regard to changes of hormones regulating water and electrolyte balances.

Vasopressin and the renin-angiotensin-aldosterone complex contribute to renal and sweat gland retention of fluids and electrolytes as well as to regulation of the peripheral vascular tone. Therefore, naturally, the responses of those hormones depend on water and salt supply and environmental t°. These conditions are the main determinants of water and electrolyte regulating hormone responses, rather than the modulating factors. A hyperhydration reduced vasopressin response to 15-min exercise at 70% VO_2max.[152] After salt loading, virtually no increase in plasma renin activity[49,153] and aldosterone concentration[49] was observed. During prolonged exercises in the heat, renin and angiotensin increases were significantly diminished by administration of sodium-potassium electrolyte solution, in amounts equivalent to the subjects' sweat loss.[154] After salt depletion the plasma renin activity roughly doubled during exercise.[155,156] The plasma volume loss and subsequent increase in the vasopressin and renin-angiotensin levels during 4 h of exercise were prevented by progressive rehydration.[157]

Hormonal control of euglycemia during exercise will be discussed in Chapter 3.

FACTORS MODULATING HORMONAL RESPONSES TO EXERCISE

During exercise the activity of endocrine systems is determined by the intensity and duration of muscular activity on the one hand, and by the adaptation of the organism to

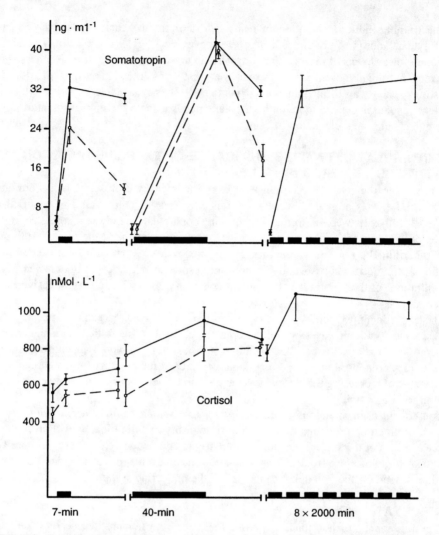

FIGURE 2-12. Somatotropin and cortisol concentrations before, immediately and 30 min after three rowing exercise tests: 7-min exercise on a rowing appratus performed at supramaximal intensity, 40-min exercise on a rowing apparatus performed at the intensity of anaerobic threshold, 8×2000 m rowing at 75 to 85% of the competition velocity (4-min rest periods between exercise periods). Mean and SEM are indicated. Open circles, interrupted lines — first experiment on promising junior rowers. Closed circles, solid lines — a year later, when the rowers had reached a performance level of national class. Asterisks denote significant difference ($P<0.05$) from the initial values of the group. (From Snegovskaya, V., and Viru, A., *Eur. J. Appl. Physiol.*, 67, 59, 1993. With permission.)

muscular activity, expressed in physical fitness indices, on the other hand. Besides these three main determinants there exist factors modulating the hormonal response to exercise (Figure 2-13). One of them is *emotional strain*. In a highly emotional situation the adrenocortical response was obtained in exercises of under-threshold intensity.[158] During a more intensive exercise the competitive situation caused a more pronounced increase in the noradrenaline[159] and 17-hydrocorticoid[160] concentration. The dependence of somatotropin response to exercise on emotional strain has also been suggested.[3] Subjects with high trait-anxiety exhibited both a higher pre-exercise adrenaline level and a higher noradrenaline response to exercise (cycling at the heart rate of 170 BPM) in comparison with subjects characterized by low trait-anxiety.[161] In another study of subjects with pronounced emotivity, the adrenaline but not the noradrenaline response to exercise at 80% VO_2max was exaggerated.[98] In persons with high trait-anxiety, serum testosterone and D_4-androstenedione levels were suppressed. An 80-min

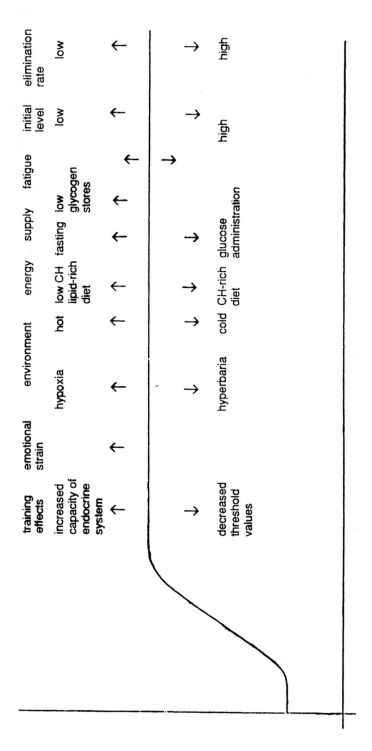

FIGURE 2-13. A scheme of influence of various factors on responses of hormones to mobilization of energy reserves. (From Viru, A., *Int. J. Sports Med.,* 13, 201, 1992. With permission.)

cycling at 80% VO_2max caused a pronounced increase in the blood androgens concentrations, but this response was less pronounced in high trait-anxiety persons than in low trait-anxiety persons. Lutropin was higher before, as well as during and after exercise in high trait-anxiety persons.[162]

Trained persons performed a 5-min supramaximal exercise twice: once alone in the laboratory, the other time in a competition situation, being stimulated to exhibit the best performance. In the competition situation the total amount of work was increased by 12 to 21%. The blood lactate level increased to 15.1 ± 0.8 mmol·l^{-1} instead of the 8.6 ± 0.6 mmol·l^{-1} of exercising alone. Catecholamine excretion was twice as high as after the exercise performed alone. Before competition exercise the blood insulin concentration was doubled, but the exercise-induced drop was significant only in the competition situation. In both situations the blood cortisol concentration increased by 18% immediately after exercise and by 20% 15 min after exercise.[163]

Hypoxic conditions enhance the hormone response to exercise [3,164,165] and induce the response in exercises of under-threshold intensity.[166] However, in hypoxic conditions the same absolute work level corresponds to an elevated relative exercise intensity. At the same relative intensities, noradrenaline, somatotropin, corticotropin, and cortisol responses were similar in hypoxic and normoxic conditions. Only the adrenaline response was exaggerated in trained but not in untrained men when they exercised in hypoxic conditions.[167] Hyperbaric conditions[3] as well as O_2 breathing[168] reduced the noradrenaline concentration during exercise.

During exercise the concentrations of noradrenaline, cortisol, somatotropin, and glucagon are higher when the environment is *hot*.[3] Fluid supplement abolished the exaggerated blood cortisol[153] and somatotropin[169] response to exercise in the hot environment. At 4 to 10°C catecholamine[170] and somatotropin [171,172] responses were inhibited.

The modulatory effect of *prior diet* on the hormone responses to exercise has been established in numerous studies. To a large extent, these modulations seem to be related to the differences in carbohydrate supply. A carbohydrate-rich diet[124, 173] as well as glucose administration[24,44,174-176] reduce the responses of hormones related to the mobilization of energy reserves (catecholamines,[124,173,174,176,177] glucagon,[24,44,174] somatotropin,[124,175] and cortisol[175]). In these cases an increase in the insulin level occurs instead of a drop.[24,25,44,174] The opposite effects were elicited by low carbohydrate and lipid-rich diets,[3,124,173] fasting,[3,178] and cases of decreased glycogen stores.[179,180] The results are in accordance with the view that the glucostatic mechanism plays an important role in determining the hormonal response to exercise.[124] Probably the main role belongs to the glucose-sensitive centers located in the brain.[3,177] It has been suggested that the responsiveness of these centers depends on insulin availability during the time preceding exercise. The exaggerated catecholamine and other hormone responses to exercise in states of insulin deficiency such as fasting, intake of a fat diet, and diabetes are considered to be proof of this view.[3]

There is some evidence that both *circadian and sessional rhythms* alter the hormone responses to exercise. In most cases when the pre-exercise level is high, the post-exercise level is also higher, but the magnitude of the response is lower than in cases of low pre-exercise level due to circadian and sessional rhythms.[181-183] Hormone responses to exercise are varied to some extent in various phases of the *ovarian-menstrual cycle*.[86,87,184] However, this influence is not reflected in all hormone responses.[185]

The activity of endocrine systems is controlled by feedback inhibition. It has been found that corticotropin-induced peaks, of the blood cortisol level depressed the subsequent meal-related peaks, the exercise-induced peaks, and augmented secretory episodes at the end of the night.[186] Intravenous administration of 10 mg dexamethasone 30 min prior to exercise eliminated the cortisol response at the 20th minute of exercise at 900 kpm.min^{-1}.[62] In dogs, in the absence of blood cortisol due to treatment with chloditan, the activation of the corticotropin function proceeded more intensively while standing with a load on the back; the reduction of the corticotropin concentration after its initial increment was less demonstrable as compared to that seen in the normal adrenal function.[187] According to these data, from the augmented pre-exercise level the blood cortisol concentration usually drops or does not elicit any change during exercise.[188, 189] There are also results suggesting that a high corticotropin level may suppress the activation of the pituitary function during exercise.[20]

In hormone responses of modest intensity the amplitude or even the direction of changes in the blood plasma hormone concentration depends to a considerable extent on the alteration of plasma volume,[190,191] or on hormone elimination rate.[114] It has been suggested that the elevated testosterone and estradiol concentrations in short-term exercises are mainly due to the decreased hormone elimination rate[192,193] or due to the decreased plasma volume[119] without actual changes in hormone secretion.

Special reviews have referred to many facts indicating the simultaneous occurrence of pronounced *fatigue* and of decreased activity symptoms of the sympatho-adrenal[128,148,194] and pituitary adrenocortical[128,194,195] systems both in men and test animals. Differently from other marathon runners, one subject who collapsed after running 15 km had very low testosterone and lutropin values. Instead of an increase in the cortisol level observed in other sportsmen, his cortisol concentration was unchanged.[71] In a group of middle- and long-distance runners a daily strenuous training regime caused first a pronounced elevation in the cortisol resting level in conjunction with unusually high responses of cortisol and somatotropin to training exercises. Afterwards a high resting level of blood cortisol was accompanied by a reversed cortisol response and a low somatotropin level after exercise.[196]

In conclusion, it must be stressed that hormone responses to exercise are determined and modulated by numerous factors. In regard to hormones controlling energy and protein metabolism, the main determinants of hormone responses to exercise are the intensity and duration of exercise and the organism's adaptation to exercise. The modulating factors are the emotivity of a person and the situation in which the exercise is performed, environmental conditions, previous diet, fatigue state, endogenous rhythms, initial level of hormones in the blood, and changes in the plasma volume and hormone elimination rate. The main determinants of hormones controlling the water and electrolyte balance are the shifts in the corresponding homeostatic parameters. Besides the above mentioned factors, pathological conditions as well as age differences may alter the endocrine functions during exercise.

When the exercise causes only moderate demands on endocrine systems, there is a pronounced inter-individual variability in hormone responses, and their dynamics express differences in individual tactics of adaptation: adjustments at the level of production of regulative molecules or adjustments at the level of reception of these molecules.

REFERENCES

1. **Derevenco, P.**, *Efortful si Sistemul Endocrin.*, Editora Dacia, Cluj-Napoca, 1976.
2. **Terjung, R.**, Endocrine responses to exercise, *Exerc. Sports Sci. Rev.*, 7, 153, 1979.
3. **Galbo, H.**, *Hormonal and Metabolic Adaptation to Exercise*, G. Thieme Verlag, Stuttgart, 1983.
4. **Fortherby, K., and Pal, S.B.**, Eds., *Exercise Endocrinology*, De Gruyter, Berlin-New York, 1985.
5. **Viru, A.**, *Hormones in Muscular Activity, Vol. 1, Hormonal Ensemble in Exercise*, CRC Press, Boca Raton, Fl., 1985.
6. **Galbo, H.**, Exercise physiology: humoral functions, *Sports Sci. Rev.*, 1, 65, 1992.
7. **Kjaer, M.**, Regulation of hormonal and metabolic responses during exercise in humans, *Exerc. Sport Sci. Rev.*, 20, 161, 1992.
8. **Viru, A.**, Plasma hormones and physical exercise, *Int. J. Sports Med.*, 13, 201, 1992.
9. **Viru, A., Karelson, K., and Smirnova, T.**, Stability and variability in hormone responses to prolonged exercise, *Int. J. Sports Med.*, 13, 230, 1992.

10. **Adlercreutz, H., Härkönen, M., Kuoppasalmi, K., Näveri, H., and Rehunen, S.**, Physical activity and hormones, *Adv. Cardiol.*, 18, 144, 1976.

11. **Costill, D.L., Branam, G., Fink, W., and Nelson, R.**, Exercise-induced sodium conservation: changes in plasma renin and aldosterone, *Med. Sci. Sports*, 8, 209, 1976.

12. **Geyssant, A., Geelen, G., Denis, C., Allevard, A.M., Vincent, M., Jarsaillor, E., Bizollon, C.A., Laceur, J.P., and Charib, C.**, Plasma vasopressin, renin activity, and aldosterone: effect of exercise and training, *Eur. J. Appl. Physiol.*, 46, 21, 1981.

13. **Kosunen, K., Pakarinen, A., Kuoppasalmi, K., Näveri, H., Rehunen, S., Stranderskjöld-Nordenstam, C.C., Härkönen, M., and Adlercreutz, H.**, Cardiovascular function and the renin-angiotensin-aldosterone system in long-distance runners during various training periods, *Scand. J. Clin. Lab. Invest.*, 40, 429, 1980.

14. **Melin, B., Eclache, J.B., Geelen, G., Annat, G., Allevard, A.M., Jarsaillon, E., Zebid, A., Legras, J.J., and Charab, C.**, Plasma AVP, neurophysin, renin activity, and aldosterone during submaximal exercise performed until exhaustion in trained and untrained man, *Eur. J. Appl. Physiol.*, 44, 141, 1980.

15. **Sundsfjord, J.A., Strömme, S.E., and Aakvaag, A.**, Plasma aldosterone (PA), plasma renin activity (PRA) and cortisol (F) during exercise, in *Metabolic Adaptation to Prolonged Physical Exercise*, Howald, H., Poortmans, J.P., Eds., Birkhäuser Verlag, Basel, 1975, 308.

16. **Buckler, J.M.**, Exercise as a screening test for growth hormone release, *Acta Endocrin*, 69, 219, 1972.

17. **Hartog, M., Havel, R.J., Copinschi, G., Earli, J.M., and Ritchie, B.C.**, The relationship between changes in serum levels of growth hormone and mobilization of fat during exercise in man, *Quart. J. Exp. Physiol.*, 52, 86, 1967.

18. **Hunter, W.M., Fonsenka, C.C., and Passmore, R.**, Growth hormone: important role in muscular exercise in adults, *Science*, 150, 1051, 1965.

19. **Sutton, J.R., and Lazarus, L.** Growth hormone in exercise: comparison of physiologic and pharmacologic stimuli, *J. Appl. Physiol.*, 41, 523, 1976.

20. **Viru, A., Smirnova, T., Tomson, K., and Matsin, T.**, Dynamics of blood levels of pituitary trophic hormones during prolonged exercise, in *Biochemistry of Exercise IV-B*, Poortmans, J., Niset, G., Eds., University Park Press, Baltimore, 1981, 100.

21. **Hartley, L.H., Mason, J.W., Hogan, R.P., Jones, L.G., Kotchen, T.A., Mougey, E.H., Wherry, F.E., Pennington, L.L., and Ricketts, P.T.**, Multiple hormonal responses to prolonged exercise in relation to physical training, *J. Appl. Physiol.*, 33, 607, 1972.

22. **Hilsted, J., Galbo, H., Somme, B., Schwartz, T., Fahrenkrug, J., Schaffalitzky de Muskadell, O.B., Lauristsen, K.B., and Trammer, B.**, Gastroenteropancreatic hormonal changes during exercise, *Am. J. Physiol.*, 239, G136, 1980.

23. **Hunter, W.M., and Sukkar, M.Y.**, Changes in plasma insulin levels during muscular exercise, *J. Physiol.*, 196, 110P, 1968.

24. **Luyckx, A.S., Pirnay, F., Krzentowski, G., and Lefebvre, P.**, Insulin and glucagon during muscular exercise in normal men, in *Biochemistry of Exercise IV-A*, Poortmans, J., Niset, J., Eds., University Park Press, Baltimore, 1981, 131.

25. **Pruett, E.D.R.**, Glucose and insulin during prolonged work stress in men living on different diets, *J. Appl. Physiol.*, 28, 199, 1970.

26. **Pruett, E.D.R.**, Plasma insulin concentration during prolonged work at near maximal oxygen uptake, *J. Appl. Physiol.*, 29, 155, 1970.

27. **Wirth, A., Diehm, C., Mayer, H., Mörl, H., Vogel, I., Björntrop, P., and Schlierf, G.**, Plasma C-peptide and insulin in trained and untrained subjects, *J. Appl. Physiol.*, 50, 71, 1981.

28. **Hermansen, L., Pruett, E.D.R., Osnes, J.B., and Giere, F.A.**, Blood glucose and plasma insulin response to maximal exercise and glucose infusion, *J. Appl. Physiol.*, 29, 13, 1970.

29. **Weicker, H., Rettenmeier, A., Ritthaler, F., Frank, H., Bieger, W.P., and Klett, G.**, Influence of anabolic and catabolic hormones on substrate concentration during various running distances, in *Biochemistry of Exercise IV-A*, Poortmans, J., Niset, G., Eds., University Park Press, Baltimore, 1981, 208.

30. **Dufaux, B., Assman, G., Order, U., Holderath, A., and Hollmann, W.**, Plasma lipoproteins, hormones and energy substrates during the first days after prolonged exercise, *Int. J. Sports Med.*, 2, 256, 1981.

31. **Dulac, S., Quirion, A., De Carufel, D., LeBlanc, J., Jobin, M., Côte, J., Brisson, G.R., Lavoie, J.M., and Diamand, P.**, Metabolic and hormonal responses to long-distance swimming in cold water, *Int. J. Sports Med.*, 8, 352, 1987.

32. **Dessypris, A., Wagar, G., Fyrquist, F., Makiren, T., Welin, M.G., and Lamber, B.A.**, Marathon run: effects on blood cortisol, ACTH, iodothyronines-TSH and vasopressin, *Acta Endocrin.*, 95, 151, 1980.

33. **Farrell, P.A.**, Adrenocorticotropin hormone and exercise, in *Exercise Endocrinology*, Fotherby, K., Pal, S.B., Eds., De Gruyter, Berlin, New York, 1985, 139.

34. **Elias, A.N., Wilson, A.F., Pandin, M.R., Chune, G., Utsumi, A., Kayaleth, R., and Stone, S.C.**, Corticotropin releasing hormone and gonadotropin secretion in physically active males after acute exercise, *Eur. J. Appl. Physiol.*, 62, 171, 1991.

35. **Galbo, H., Richter, E.A., Hilsted, J., Holst, J.J., Christensen, N.J., and Henrikson, J.,** Hormonal regulation during prolonged exercise, *Ann. N.Y. Acad. Sci.*, 301, 72, 1977.
36. **Häggendal, L., Hartley, L.H., and Saltin, B.,** Arterial noradrenaline concentration during exercise in relation to the relative work levels, *Scand. J. Clin. Lab. Invest.*, 26, 337, 1970.
37. **Hartley, L.H., Mason, J.W., Hogan, R.P., Jones, L.G., Kotchen, T.A., Mougey, E.H., Wherry, F.E., Penning, L.L., and Ricketts, P.T.,** Multiple hormonal responses to graded exercise in relation to physical training, *J. Appl. Physiol.*, 33, 602, 1972.
38. **Kindermann, W., Schnabel, A., Schmitt, W.M., Biro, G., Gassens, J., and Weber, F.,** Catecholamines, growth hormone, cortisol, insulin and sex hormones in aerobic and anaerobic exercise, *Eur. J. Appl. Physiol.*, 49, 389, 1982.
39. **Kjaer, M.,** Epinephrine and some other hormonal responses to exercise in man: With special reference to physical training, *Int. J. Sports Med.*, 10, 1, 1989.
40. **Lehmann, M., Keul, J., and DaPrada, M.,** Plasma catecholamines in trained and untrained volunteers during graduated exercises, *Int. J. Sports Med.*, 2, 143, 1981.
41. **Näveri, H., Kuoppasalmi, K., and Härkönen, M.,** Plasma glucagon and catecholamines during exhaustive short-term exercise, *Eur. J. Appl. Physiol.*, 53, 308, 1985.
42. **Péronnet, F., Blier, P., Brisson, G., Diamond, P., Ledoux, M., and Volle, M.,** Reproducibility of plasma catecholamine concentrations at rest and during exercise in man, *Eur. J. Appl. Physiol.*, 54, 555, 1986.
43. **Weicker, H.,** Ed., Sypathoadrenergic influence on hormonal, metabolic and cardiovascular functions during exercise, *Int. J. Sports Med.*, 9(Suppl. 2), 1988.
44. **Böttger, I., Schlein, E.M., Faloonia, J.F., Knochel, J.P., and Unger R.H.,** The effect of exercise on glucagon secretion, *J. Clin. Endocrin.*, 35, 117, 1972.
45. **Felig, P., Wahren, J., Hendler, R., and Ahlborg, G.,** Plasma glucagon levels in exercising man, *New Eng. J. Med.*, 287, 184, 1972.
46. **Convertino, V.A., Keil, L.C., Bernauer, E.M., and Greenlauf, J.E.,** Plasma volume, osmolality, vasopressin and renin activity during graded exercise in man, *J. Appl. Physiol.*, 50, 123, 1981.
47. **Wade, C.E. and Claybaugh, J.R.,** Plasma renin activity, vasopressin concentration and urinary excretion responses to exercise in man, *J. Appl. Physiol.*, 49, 930, 1980.
48. **Fasola, A.F., Martz, B.L., and Helmer, O.M.,** Renin activity during supine exercise in normotensives and hypertensives, *J. Appl. Physiol.*, 21, 1709, 1966.
49. **Cuneo, R.C., Espiner, E.A., Nichalls, M.G., and Yandle, T.G.,** Exercise induced increase in plasma natriuretic peptide and effect of sodium loading in normal man, *Horm. Metab. Res.*, 20, 115, 1988.
50. **Follenius, M., and Brandenberger, G.,** Increase in atrial natriuretic peptide in response to physical exercise, *Eur. J. Appl. Physiol.*, 57, 159, 1988.
51. **Kraemer, W.J., Armstrong, L.E., Hubbart, R.W., Marchitelli, L.J., Leva, N., Rock, P.B., and Dziadas, J.E.,** Response of plasma human atrial natriuretic factor to high intensity submaximal exercise in the heat, *Eur. J. Appl. Physiol.*, 57, 399, 1988.
52. **Bullen, B.A., Surinar, G.S., Beitins, I.Z., Carr, D.B., Reppert, S.M., Dotson, C.O., DeFencl, M., Gervino, E.V., and McArthur, J.W.,** Endurance training effects on plasma hormonal responsiveness and sex hormone excretion, *J. Appl. Physiol.*, 56, 1453, 1984.
53. **Theron, J.J., Corthkizen, J.M.C., and Rautenbach, M.M.,** Effect of physical exercise on plasma melatonin levels in normal volunteers, *S. Afr. Med. J.*, 66, 838, 1984.
54. **Davies, C.T.M., and Few, J.D.,** Effect of exercise on adrenocortical function, *J. Appl. Physiol.*, 35, 888, 1973.
55. **Janssen, G.M.E.,** *Marathon Running. Functional Changes in Male and Female Volunteers During Training and Contest*, Druknerij Alberts/Druko, Gulpen, 1986.
56. **Keibel, D.,** Nebennierenrinden-Hormone and Sportliche Leistung, *Med. u. Sport*, 14, 65, 1974.
57. **Kuoppasalmi, K., Näveri, H., Kosunen, K., Härkönen, M., and Adlercreutz, H.,** Plasma steroid levels in muscular exercise, in *Biochemistry of Exercise IV-B*, Poortmans, J., Niset, G., Eds., University Park Press, Baltimore, 1981, 149.
58. **Näveri, H.,** Blood hormone and metabolite levels during graded cycle ergometer exercise, *Scand. J. Clin. Lab. Invest.*, 45, 599, 1985.
59. **Staehelin, D., Labhart, A., Froesch, R., and Kägi, H.R.,** The effect of muscular exercise and hypoglycemia on the plasma level of 17-hydrosteroids in normal adults and in patients with the androgenital syndrome, *Acta Endocrin.*, 18, 521, 1955.
60. **Galbo, H., Hummer, L., Petersen, I.B., Christensen, N.J., and Bie, N.,** Thyroid and testicular hormonal responses to graded and prolonged exercise in man, *Eur. J. Appl. Physiol.*, 36, 101, 1977.
61. **Guglielmine, C., Paolini, A.R., and Conconi, F.,** Variations of serum testosterone concentration after physical exercises of different duration, *Int. J. Sports Med.*, 5, 246, 1984.
62. **Sutton, J.R., Coleman, M.J., Casey, J., and Lazarus, L.,** Androgen responses during physical exercise, *Br. Med. J.*, 1, 520, 1973.

63. **Webb, M.L., Wallace, J.P., Hamill, C., Hodgren, J.L., and Mashaly, M.M.**, Serum testosterone concentration during two hours of moderate intensity treadmill running in trained men and women, *Endocrine Res.*, 10, 27, 1984.

64. **Buono, M.J., Yeager, J.E., and Hodgden, J.A.**, Plasma adrenocorticotropin and cortisol responses to brief high-intensity exercise in humans, *J. Appl. Physiol.*, 61, 1337, 1986.

65. **Cumming, D.C., Brunsting, L.A., Strich, G., Ries, A.L., and Rebar, R.W.**, Reproductive hormone increases in response to acute exercise in man, *Med. Sci. Sports Exerc.*, 18, 369, 1986.

66. **Farrell, P.A., Gartwaite, T.L., and Gustafson, A.B.**, Plasma adrenocorticotropin and cortisol responses to submaximal and exhaustive exercise, *J. Appl. Physiol.*, 55, 1441, 1983.

67. **Vanhelder, W.P., Radomski, M.W., Goode, R.C., and Casey, K.**, Hormonal and metabolic response to three types of exercise of equal duration and external work output, *Eur. J. Appl. Physiol.*, 54, 337, 1985.

68. **Maron, M.B., Horwath, S.M., and Wilkerson, J.E.**, Acute blood biochemical alterations in response to marathon running, *Eur. J. Appl. Physiol.*, 34, 173, 1975.

69. **Rogers, G., Goodman, C., Mitchell, D., and Hattingh, J.**, The response of running to arduous triathlon competition, *Eur. J. Appl. Physiol.*, 55, 405, 1986.

70. **Zuliani, U., Novariani, A., Bonsetti, A., Astorri, E., Montani, G., Simoni, I., and Zappavigna, A.**, Endocrine modifications caused by sports activity. Effect in leisure-time cross-country skiers, *J. Sports Med. Phys. Fitness*, 24, 263, 1984.

71. **Dessypris, A., Kuoppasalmi, K., and Adlercreutz, H.**, Plasma cortisol, testosterone, androstenedione and lutenizing hormone (LH) in a noncompetitive marathon run, *J. Steroid Biochem.*, 7, 33, 1976.

72. **DeMerleir, K., Maektgeboren, N., Van Steirtegham, A., Gorus, F., Olbrecht, J., and Block, P.**, Beta-endorphin and ACTH levels in peripheral blood during and after aerobic and anaerobic exercise, *Eur. J. Appl. Physiol.*, 55, 5, 1986.

73. **Farrell, P.A., Kjaer, M., Bach, F.W., and Galbo, H.**, Beta-endorphin and adrenocorticotropin response to supramaximal treadmill exercise in trained and untrained males, *Acta Physiol. Scand.*, 130, 619, 1987.

74. **Fraioli, F., Moretti, C., Paolucci, D., Alicicco, E., Crescenzi, F., and Fortunio, G.**, Physical exercise stimulates marked concomitant release of β-endorphin and adrenocorticotropic hormone (ACTH) in peripheral blood in man, *Experimentia*, 36, 987, 1980.

75. **Rahkila, P., Hakala, E., Sahkinen, K., and Laatikainen, T.**, Response of plasma endorphins to running exercise in male and female endurance athletes, *Med. Sci. Sports Exerc.*, 19, 451, 1987.

76. **Colt, E.W.D., Wardlaw, S.L., and Frantz, A.G.**, The effect of running on plasma β-endorphin, *Life Sci.*, 28, 1637, 1981.

77. **Farrell, P., Gates, W., Maksud, M., and Morgan, W.**, Increases in plasma β-endorphin/β-lipotropin immunoreactivity after treadmill running in humans, *J. Appl. Physiol.*, 52, 1245, 1982.

78. **Langenfeld, M.E., Hart, L.S., and Kao, P.C.**, Plasma β-endorphin response to one-hour bicycling and running at 60% VO_2max, *Med. Sci. Sports Exerc.*, 19, 83, 1987.

79. **Dearman, J., and Francis, K.T.**, Plasma levels of catecholamines, cortisol and β-endorphins in male athletes after running 26.2, 6 and 2 miles, *J. Sports Med. Phys. Fitness*, 23, 30, 1983.

80. **Viru, A., Tendzegolskis, Z., and Smirnova, T.**, Changes of β-endorphin level in blood during prolonged exercise, *Endocrin. Exp.*, 24, 63, 1990.

81. **Kindermann, W. and Smith, W.M.**, Verhalten von Testosteron im Blutserum bei Körperarbeit unterschiedlicher Dauer and Intensität, *Deutsch. Z. Sportmed.*, 36, 99, 1985.

82. **Cumming, D.C., Wall, S.R., Quinney, H.A., and Belcastro, A.N.**, Decrease in serum testosterone levels with maximal intensity swimming exercise in trained male and female swimmers, *Endocrin. Res.*, 13, 31, 1982.

83. **Schmid, P., Wolf, W., Rainer, F., Schwaberger, G., and Pessenhofer, H.**, Progesteron and Prolaktinverhalter männlicher Sportler bei Kurzzeit- and Ausdauerbelastungen, in *Sport: Leistung and Gesundheit*, Heck, H., Hollmann, W., Liesen, H., Rost, R., Eds., Deutsche Ärzte Verlag, Köln, 1983, 199.

84. **Bonen, A., Ling, W.Y, MacIntyre, K.P., Neil, R., McGrail, J.C., and Belcastro, A.N.**, Effects of exercise on the serum concentrations of FSH, LH, progesterone and estradiol, *Eur. J. Appl. Physiol.*, 42, 15, 1979.

85. **Cumming, D.C., and Rebar, R.W.**, Hormonal changes with acute exercise and with training in women, *Seminar Reprod. Endocrin.*, 3, 55, 1985.

86. **Jurkowski, J.E., Jones, L.N, Walker, W.C., Younglai, E.V., and Sutton, J.R.**, Ovarian hormonal responses to exercise, *J. Appl. Physiol.*, 44, 109, 1978.

87. **Keizer, H.A., Kuipers, H., de Haan, J., Beckors, E., and Habets, L.**, Multiple hormonal responses to physical exercise in eumenorrheic trained and untrained women, *Int. J. Sports Med.*, 8(Suppl.3), 139, 1987.

88. **Bonen, A., and Keizer, H.A.**, Pituitary, ovarian, and adrenal hormone responses to marathon running, *Int. J. Sports Med.*, 8(Suppl.3), 161, 1987.

89. **Barreca, T., Reggiani, E., Franceschini, F., Bavastro, G., Messina, V., Menichetti, G., Odaglia, G., and Rolandi, E.**, Serum prolactin, growth hormone and cortisol in athletes and sedentary subjects after submaximal and exhaustive exercise, *J. Sports Med. Phys. Fitness*, 28, 89, 1988.

90. **MacConnie, S.E., Barkar, A., Lampman, R.M., Schork, M., and Anthony, B.I.Z.**, Decreased hypothalamic gonadotropin releasing hormone secretion in male marathon runners, *Horm. Reprod. Metab.*, 3(Suppl.), 2, 1986.

91. **Schmid, P., Push, H.H., Wolf, W., Pelger, E., Pessenhofer, H., Schwaberger, G., Pristautz, H., and Pürstner, P.**, Serum FSH, LH, and testosterone in humans after physical exercise, *Int. J. Sports Med.*, 3, 84, 1982.

92. **Caralis, D.G., Edwards, L., and Davis, P.J.**, Serum total and free thyroxine and triiodothyronine during dynamic muscular exercise in man, *Am. J. Physiol.*, 223, E115, 1977.

93. **O'Connell, M., Robbins, D.C., Horton, E.S., Sims, E.A.H., and Danforth, E.**, Changes in serum concentration of 3,3',5'-triiodothyronine and 3,5,3'-triiodothyronine during prolonged moderate exercise, *J. Clin. Endocrin.*, 49, 242, 1979.

94. **Refsum, H.E., and Strömme, S.B.**, Serum thyroxine, triiodothyronine and thyroid stimulating hormone after prolonged heavy exercise, *Scand. J. Clin. Lab. Invest.*, 39, 455, 1979.

95. **Terjung, R.L., and Tipton, C.M.**, Plasma thyroxine and thyroid-stimulating hormone levels during submaximal exercise in humans, *Am. J. Physiol.*, 200, 1840, 1971.

96. **Winder, W.W., and Premachandra, B.N.**, Thyroid hormones and muscular exercise, in *Biochemistry of Exercise IV-B.*, Poortmans, J., Niset, G., Eds., University Park Press, Baltimore, 1981, 131.

97. **Viru, A.**, Adaptive regulation of hormone interaction with receptor, *Exp. Clin. Endocrin.*, 97, 13, 1991.

98. **Pequignot, J.M., Peyrin, L., Favier, R., and Flandreis, R.**, Adrenergic response to emotivity and physical training, *Eur. J. Appl. Physiol.*, 40, 117, 1979.

99. **Kjaer, M., Secher, N.H., Bach, F.W., and Galbo, H.**, Role of motor center activity for hormonal changes and substrate mobilization in humans, *Am. J. Physiol.*, 253, R687, 1987.

100. **Leclercq, R., and Poortmans, J.R.**, Evolution of plasma cortisol during short-time exercise, in *3rd Int. Symp. on Biochemistry of Exercise*, Landry, F. and Orban, W.A.R., Eds., Symposia Specialists, Miami, 1978, 302.

101. **Petraglia, F., Barletta, C., Facchinetti, F., Sponazzola, F., Monzani, A., Scavo, D., and Genazzani, A.R.**, Response of circulating adrenocorticotropin, beta-endorphin, beta-lipotropin and cortisol to athletic competition, *Acta Endocrin.*, 118, 332, 1988.

102. **Fentem, P.H., Macdonald, I.A., Munoz, B., and Watson, S.A.**, Catecholamine responses to brief maximum exercise in man, *J. Physiol.*, 361, 80P, 1985.

103. **Kraemer, W.J., Patton, J.F., Knuttgen, H.G., Hannan, C.J., Kettler, T., Gordon, S.E., Dziados, J.E., Fry, A.C., Frykman, P.N., and Harman, E.A.**, Effects of high-intensity cycle exercise on sympathoadrenal-medulla response patterns, *J. Appl. Physiol.*, 70, 8–14, 1991.

104. **Schwarz, L., and Kindermann, W.**, β-endorphin, adrenocorticotropin hormone, cortisol and catecholamines during aerobic and anaerobic exercise, *Eur. J. Appl. Physiol.*, 61, 165, 1990.

105. **Galbo, H., Kjaer, M., and Secher, N.H.**, Cardiovascular, ventilatory and catecholamine responses to maximal exercise in partially curarized man, *J. Physiol.*, 389, 557, 1987.

106. **Kjaer, M., Secher, N.H., Bach, F.W., Sheikh, S., and Galbo, H.**, Hormonal and metabolic responses to exercise in humans: effect of sensory nervous blockade, *Am. J. Physiol.*, 257, E95, 1989.

107. **Vendsalu, A.**, Studies on adrenaline and noradrenaline in human plasma, *Acta Physiol. Scand.*, 49 (Suppl.173), 1960.

108. **Luger, A., Deuster, P.A., Kyle, S.B., Galleka, W.T., Montgomery, C.C., Gold, P.W., Loriaux, D.L., and Chrousas, P.G.**, Acute hypothalamic-pituitary-adrenal responses to the stress of treadmill exercise. Physiological adaptation to physical training, *N. Engl. J. Med.*, 316, 1309, 1987.

109. **Viru, A., Karelson, K., Smirnova, T., and Port, K.**, Activity of pituitary-adrenocortical system during various exercises, in *Advances in Exercise Physiology*, Nazar, K., Kaciuba-Uscilko, H., Terjung, R.L., Budohoski, L., Eds., Human Kinetics Publ., Champaign, 1990, 160.

110. **Port, K.**, Serum and saliva cortisol responses and blood lactate accumulation during incremental exercise testing, *Int. J. Sports Med.*, 12, 490, 1991.

111. **Rahkila, P., Hakala, E., Alén, M., Salminen, K., and Laatikainen, T.**, β-endorphin and corticotropin release is dependent on a threshold intensity of running exercise in male endurance athletes, *Life Sci.*, 43, 551, 1988.

112. **Mullin, J.P., and Howley, E.T.**, Dynamics of serum cortisol response to high intensity exercise in man, *Med. Sci. Sports*, 6, 72, 1974.

113. **Barwich, D., Rettenmeier, A., and Weicker, H.**, Serum levels of the so-called "stress hormones" in athletes after short-term consecutive exercise, *Int. J. Sport Med.*, 3 (Suppl. 22nd World Congress on Sports Medicine), 8, 1982.

114. **Few, J.D.**, Effect of exercise on the secretion and metabolism of cortisol in man, *J. Endocrin.*, 62, 341, 1974.

115. **Freund, B.J., Shizuru, E.M., Hashiro, G.M., and Claybaugh, J.R.**, Hormonal, electrolyte, and renal responses to exercise are intensity dependent, *J. Appl. Physiol.*, 70, 900, 1991.

116. **Galbo, H., Holst, J.J., and Christensen, N.J.**, Glucagon and plasma catecholamine response to graded and prolonged exercise in men, *J. Appl. Physiol.*, 38, 70, 1975.

117. **Karagiorgas, A., Garcia, J.F., and Brooks, G.A.**, Growth hormone response to continuous and intermittent exercise, *Med. Sci. Sports*, 11, 302, 1979.

118. **Deschnes, M.R., Krauner, W.J., Maresh, C.M., and Crivelle, J.F.**, Exercise-induced hormonal changes and their effects upon skeletal muscle tissue, *Sports Med.*, 12, 80, 1991.

119. **Wilkerson, J., Horvath, S. and Gutin, B.**, Plasma testosterone during treadmill exercise, *J. Appl. Physiol.*, 49, 249, 1980.

120. **Jezová, D., Vigas, M., Tatar, P., Kvetñansky, R., Nazar, K., Kaciuba-Uscilko, H., and Kozlowski, S.**, Plasma testosterone and catecholamine responses to physical exercise of different intensities in men, *Eur. J. Appl. Physiol.*, 54, 62, 1985.

121. **Buono, M.J., and Yeager, J.E.**, Increases in aldosterone precede those of cortisol during graded exercise, *J. Sports Med. Phys. Fitness*, 31, 48, 1991.

122. **Jürimäe, T., Karelson, K., Smirnova, T., and Viru, A.**, Alterations in blood hormone ensemble during exercises for improved endurance, *J. Phys. Educ. Sports Sci.*, 3, 7, 1991.

123. **Kuoppasalmi, K., Näveri, H., Härkönen, M., and Adlercreutz, H.**, Plasma cortisol, androstenedione, testosterone and luteinizing hormone in running exercises of different intensities, *Scand. J. Clin. Lab. Invest.*, 40, 403, 1980.

124. **Nazar, K.**, Glucostatic control of hormonal responses to physical exercise in man, in *Biochemistry of Exercise IV-A*, Poortmans, J., Niset, G., Eds., University Park Press, Baltimore, 1981, 188.

125. **Drzevetskaya, I.A., and Limanski, N.N.**, Thyrocalcitonin activity and calcium level in plasma during muscular activity, *Sechenov Physiol. J. USSR*, 64, 1498, 1978 (in Russian).

126. **Jürimäe, T., Viru, A., Karelson, K., and Smirnova, T.**, Biochemical changes in blood during the long and short triathlon competition, *J. Sports Med. Phys. Fitness*, 29, 305, 1989.

127. **Keul,. J., Kohler, B., Glutz, G., Luthi, U., Berg, A., and Howald, H.**, Biochemical changes in a 100 km run: carbohydrates, lipids, and hormones in serum, *Eur. J. Appl. Physiol.*, 47, 181, 1981.

128. **Viru, A.**, *Hormones in Muscular Activity*, Vol. II, Adaptive Effects of Hormones in Exercise, CRC Press, Boca Raton, 1985.

129. **Sutton, J.R.**, Hormonal and metabolic responses to exercise in subjects of high and low work capacities, *Med. Sci. Sports*, 10, 1, 1978.

130. **Winder, W.W., Hagberg, J.M., Hickson, R.C., Ehsani, A.A., and McLaine, J.A.** Time course of sympathoadrenal adaptation to endurance exercise training in man, *J. Appl. Physiol.*, 45, 370, 1978.

131. **Peronnet, F., Cléroux, J., Pernault, H., Counsineau, D., de Champlain, J., and Nadeau, R.**, Plasma noradrenaline response to exercise before and after training in humans, *J. Appl. Physiol.*, 51, 812, 1981.

132. **Winder, W.W., Hickson, R.C., Hagberg, J.M., Ehsani, A.A., and McLane, J.A.**, Training-induced changes in hormonal and metabolic responses to submaximal exercise, *J. Appl. Physiol.*, 46, 766, 1979.

133. **Frenkl, R.**, Pituitary-adrenal response to various stressors in trained and untrained organism, *Acta Physiol. Acad. Sci. Hung.*, 39, 41, 1971.

134. **Tabata, I., Atomi, Y., Mutoh, Y., and Miyashita, M.**, Effect of physical training on the responses of serum adrenocorticotropic hormone during prolonged exhausting exercise, *Eur. J. Appl. Physiol.*, 61, 188, 1990.

135. **Viru, A., and Seene, T.**, Peculiarities of adjustments in the adrenal cortex to various training regimes, *Biol. Sport*, 2, 90, 1985.

136. **Matlina, E.S., Pukhova, G.S., Galimov, S.D., Galentchik, A.I., and Almaeva, S.N.**, The catecholamines metabolism during adaptation to muscular activity, *Sechenov Physiol. J. USSR*, 62, 431, 1976 (in Russian).

137. **Parizkova, J., and Kvetñansky, R.**, Catecholamine metabolism and compositional growth in exercised and hypokinetic male rats, in *Catecholamines and Stress: Recent Advances*, Usdin, E., Kvetñansky, R., Kopin, I.J., Eds., Elsevier/North Holland, New York, 1980, 355.

138. **Bernet, F., et Denimal, J.**, Evolution de la response adrénosympatheque à l'exercise an cours de l'entrainement chez le rat, *Eur. J. Appl. Physiol.*, 33, 57, 1974.

139. **Kjaer, M., and Galbo, H.**, Effect of physical training on the capacity to secrete epinephrine, *J. Appl. Physiol.*, 64, 11, 1988.

140. **Kjaer, M., Christensen, N.J., Sonne, B., Richter, E.A., and Galbo, H.**, Effect of exercise on epinephrine turnover in trained and untrained subjects, *J. Appl. Physiol.*, 59, 1061, 1985.

141. **Kjaer, M., Farrell, P.A., Christensen, N.J., and Galbo, H.**, Increased epinephrine response and inaccurate glucoregulation in exercising athletes, *J. Appl. Physiol.*, 61, 1693, 1986.

142. **Bunt, J.C., Borleam, R.A., Bahr, J.M., and Nelson, R.A.**, Sex and training differences in human growth hormone levels during prolonged exercise, *J. Appl. Physiol.*, 61, 1796, 1986.

143. **Snegovskaya, V., and Viru, A.**, Steroid and pituitary hormone responses to rowing exercise: relative significance of exercise intensity and duration and performance level, *Eur. J. Appl. Physiol.*, 67, 59, 1993.

144. **Tomson, K.**, Effect of muscular activity on the thyroid homeostasis, *Acta Comment. Univ. Tartuensis*, 543, 93, 1980.

145. **Karelson, K., Jürimäe, T., and Smirnova, T.**, Action of intensive all-out exercises on hormone levels in blood, *Acta Comment. Univ. Tartuensis*, 922, 58, 1991 (in Russian).

146. **Mathur, D.H., Torida, A.L., and Dada, D.A.**, Serum cortisol and testosterone levels in conditioned male distance runners and nonathletes after maximal exercise, *J. Sports Med. Phys. Fitness*, 26, 245, 1986.

147. **Wisniewska, A., Wojczuk, J., Wojcieszak, I., Markowska, L., and Lukaszewska, J.**, Training-induced changes in hormonal responses to maximal arm exercise in top paddlers, *Biol. Sports*, 2, 183, 1985.

148. **Matlina, E.**, Effects of physical activity and other types of stress on catecholamine metabolism in various animal species, *J. Neurol. Transmis.*, 60, 11, 1984.

149. **Hackey, A., Sinning, W., and Bruot, B.**, Hypothalamic-pituitary-testicular axis function in endurance-trained males, *Int. J. Sports Med.*, 11, 298, 1990.

150. **Wade, C.E.**, Response, regulation and action of vasopressin during exercise: a review, *Med. Sci. Sports Exerc.*, 16, 506, 1984.

151. **Convertino, V.A., Keil, L.C., and Greenleaf, J.E.**, Plasma volume, renin, and vasopressin responses to graded exercise after training, *J. Appl. Physiol.*, 54, 508, 1983.

152. **Viinamäki, O.**, The effect of hydration status on plasma vasopressin release during physical exercise in man, *Acta Physiol. Scand.*, 139, 133, 1990.

153. **Francis, K.T.**, Effect of water and electrolyte replacement during exercise in the heat on biochemical indices of stress and performance, *Aviat. Space Environ. Med.*, 50, 125, 1979.

154. **Francis, K.T., and MacGregor, R.**, Effect of exercise in the heat on plasma renin and aldosterone with either water or a potassium-rich electrolyte solution, *Aviat. Space Environ. Med.*, 49, 461, 1978.

155. **Aurell, M., and Vikgren, P.**, Plasma renin activity in supine muscular exercise, *J. Appl. Physiol.*, 31, 839, 1971.

156. **Leenen, F.H.H., Boer, P., and Geyrkes, G.G.**, Sodium intake and the effects of isoprenol and exercise on plasma renin in man, *J. Appl. Physiol.*, 45, 870, 1978.

157. **Brandenberger, G., Candas, V., Follenius, M., Libert, J.P., and Kahn, J.M.**, Vascular fluid shifts and endocrine responses to exercise in the heat, *Eur. J. Appl. Physiol.*, 55, 123, 1986.

158. **Raymond, J.W., Code, J., and Tucci, J.R.**, Adrenocortical response to nonexhaustive muscular exercise, *Acta Endocrin.*, 70, 73, 1972.

159. **Stabrovski, J.M., Korovin, V.F., and Razumov, S.A.**, Activity of the sympatho-adrenal system during emotional and physical stress, caused by muscular activity, in *Endocrine Mechanisms of Regulation of Adaptation to Muscular Activity*, Viru, A., Ed., Vol. 2, Tartu, 1971, 217 (in Russian).

160. **Crabbé, J., Riondel, A., and Mach, E.**, Contribution a l'études des réactions corticosurrénaliennes, *Acta Endocrin.*, 22, 119, 1956.

161. **Péronnet, F., Blier, P., Brisson, G., Ledoux, M., Diamond, P., Volle, M., and de Carufel, D.**, Relationship between trait-anxiety and plasma catecholamine concentration at rest and during exercise, *Med. Sci. Sports Exerc.*, 14, 173, 1982.

162. **Diamard, P., Brison, G.R., Candas, B., and Peronnet, F.**, Trait anxiety, submaximal physical exercise and blood androgens, *Eur. J. Appl. Physiol.*, 58, 699, 1989.

163. **Smirnova, T., Vinnichuk, M., Karelson, K., and Viru, A.** Exercise-induced hormone response in competition situation, *Acta Physiol. Scand.*, 146 (Suppl. 608), 105, 1992.

164. **Davies, C.T.M., and Few, J.D.**, Effect of hypoxia on adrenocortical response to exercise, *J. Endocrin.*, 71, 157, 1976.

165. **Stock, M.J., Chapman, C., Stirling, J.L., and Campbell, I.T.**, Effects of exercise, altitude and food on blood hormone and metabolite levels, *J. Appl. Physiol.*, 45, 350, 1978.

166. **Sutton, J.R.**, Effect of acute hypoxia on the hormonal responses to exercise, *J. Appl. Physiol.*, 42, 587, 1977.

167. **Kjaer, M., Bangsbo, J., Lortie, G., and Galbo, H.**, Hormonal responses to exercise in humans: influence of hypoxia and physical training, *Am. J. Physiol.*, 254, R197, 1988.

168. **Hesse, B., Kemstrup, J.F., Halkjaer-Kristensen, J., and Petersen, F.B.**, Reduced noradrenaline response to dynamic exercise in man during O_2 breathing, *J. Appl. Physiol.*, 51, 176, 1981.

169. **Saini, J., Bothorel, B., Brandenberger, G., Candas V., and Follenius, M.**, Growth hormone and prolactin response to dehydration during exercise: effect of water and carbohydrate solution, *Eur. J. Appl. Physiol.*, 61, 61, 1990.

170. **Chin, A.K., Gledhill, W., and Fedchan, I.**, Sympatho-adrenal changes in athletes and nonathletes during graded exercise in a cold environment, in *Exercise Physiology*, Landry, F., Orban, W.A.A., Eds., Symposia Specialisms, Miami, 1978, 493.

171. **Buckler, J.M.**, The relationship between changes in plasma growth hormone levels and body temperature occurring with exercise in man, *Biomedicine*, 19, 193, 1973.

172. **Frewin, D.B., Frantz, A.G., and Downey, J.A.**, The effect of ambient temperature on the growth hormone and prolactin response to exercise, *Aust. J. Exp. Biol. Med.*, 54, 97, 1976.

173. **Jansson, E., Hjemdahl, P., and Kaijser, L.**, Diet-induced changes in sympatho-adrenal activity during submaximal exercise in relation to substrate utilization in men, *Acta Physiol. Scand.*, 114, 171, 1982.

174. **Ahlborg, G., and Felig, P.**, Influence of glucose ingestion on fuel-hormone response during prolonged exercise, *J. Appl. Physiol.*, 41, 683, 1976.

175. **Bonen, A., Belcastro, A.N., MacIntyre, K., and Gardner, J.**, Hormonal responses during rest and exercise with glucose, *Med. Sci. Sports*, 9, 64, 1977.
176. **Galbo, H., Christensen, N.J., and Holst, J.J.**, Glucose-induced decrease in glucagon and epinephrine responses to exercise in man, *J. Appl. Physiol.*, 42, 525, 1977.
177. **Kozlowski, S., Brzezinska, Z., Nazar, K., and Turlejska, E.**, Carbohydrate availability for the brain and muscles as a factor modifying sympathetic activity during exercise in dogs, in *Biochemistry of Exercise IV-B*, Poortmans, J., Niset, G., Eds., University Park Press, Baltimore, 1981, 54.
178. **Pequignot, J.M., Peyrin, L., and Péres, G.**, Catecholamine-fuel interrelationships during exercise in fasting men, *J. Appl. Physiol.*, 48, 109, 1980.
179. **Bonen, A., MacIntyre, K., Belcastro, A.N., and Piarce, G.**, Effect of reduced hepatic and glycogen depots on substrate and endocrine response during menstrual cycle of teenage athletes, *J. Appl. Physiol.*, 50, 545, 1981.
180. **Lavoie, J.-M., Consineau, D., Peronnet, F., and Provencher, P.J.**, Liver glycogen store and hypoglycemia during prolonged exercise in man, in *Biochemistry of Exercise*, Knuttgen, H.G., Vogel, J.A., Poortmans, J., Eds., Human Kinetics Publ., Champaign, 1983, 297.
181. **Blinova, N.G., Ksents, S.M., and Krasilova, J.I.**, Action of sessional periodicity of activity of pituitary-adrenocortical system on the dynamics of 11-hydroxycorticoids in blood of dogs during muscular activity, in *Mechanisms of Regulation of Physiologic Function in Extreme Conditions*, Tomsk State Univ., Tomsk, 1978, 22 (in Russian).
182. **Kolpakov, M.G., Kasin, E.M., Avdeyev, G.G., Blinova, N.G., and Vinogradova, N.N.**, Diurnal rhythm of corticosteroid response on ACTH and physical exercise, *Byull. Eksper. Biol. Med.*, 74, 15, 1972 (in Russian).
183. **Stephenson, L.A., Kolna, M.A., Francesconi, R., and Conzalez, R.R.**, Circadian variations in plasma renin activity, catecholamines and aldosterone during exercise in women, *Eur. J. Appl. Physiol.*, 58, 756, 1989.
184. **Bonen, A., and Belcastro, A.N.**, Effect of exercise and training on menstrual cycle hormones, *Austral. J. Sports Med.*, 10, 39, 1978.
185. **Viru, A., Smirnova, T., and Tomson, K.**, Alterations of blood cortisol content in female sportsmen during prolonged muscular work, *Acta Comment. Univ. Tartuensis*, 562, 54, 1981.
186. **Brandenberger, G., Follenius, M., Muzet, A., Simeoni, M., and Reinhardt, B.**, Interactions between spontaneous and provoked cortisol secretory episodes in man, *J. Clin. Endocrin.*, 59, 406, 1984.
187. **Shitov, L.A., and Viru, A.A.**, Interrelations between corticotropin and cortisol during static physical exercise, *Byull. Eksper. Biol. Med.*, 98, 391, 1984 (in Russian).
188. **Brandenberger, G., Follenius, M., Hietter, B., Reinhardt, B., and Simeoni, M.**, Feedback from meal-related peaks determines diurnal changes in cortisol response to exercise, *J. Clin. Endocrin.*, 54, 592, 1982.
189. **Few, J.D., Imms, F.J., and Weiner, J.S.**, Pituitary-adrenal response to static exercise in man, *Clin. Sci. Mol. Med.*, 49, 201, 1975.
190. **Imelik, O., and Kallikorm, A.**, The changes in the concentrations and total amounts of the hormones of adeno-hypophysis, suprarenal cortex and thyroid gland at muscular exercise, in *4th Int. Symp. on Biochemistry of Exercise*, Brussels, 1979, 11.
191. **Imelik, O., and Viru, A.**, Comparative investigation of changes in adrenocortical hormones in blood and urine in physical exercise, *Acta Comment. Univ. Tartuensis*, 606, 114, 1982.
192. **Keiser, A., Poortmans, J., and Bunnik, S.J.**, Influence of physical exercise on sex hormone metabolism, in *Biochemistry of Exercise IV-B*, Poortmans, J., Niset, G., Eds., University Park Press, Baltimore, 1981, 229.
193. **Sutton, J.R., Coleman, M.J., and Casey, J.H.**, Testosterone production rate during exercise, in *3rd Int. Sym. on Biochemistry of Exercise*, Landry, F., Orban, W.A., Eds., Symposia Specialists, Miami, 1978, 227.
194. **Kassil, G.N., Vainsfeldt, I.L., Matlina, E.S., and Schreiberg, O.L.**, *Humoral-Hormonal Mechanisms of Regulation of Function in Sports Activities*, Nauka, Moscow, 1978 (in Russian).
195. **Viru, A.**, *Functions of the Adrenal Cortex in Muscular Activity*, Medicina, Moscow, 1977 (in Russian).
196. **Viru, A., Kostina, L., and Zhurkina, L.**, Dynamics of cortisol and somatotropin content in blood of male and female sportsmen during their intensive training, *Fiziol. Zhurn.*, 34(4), 61, 1988 (in Russian).

Chapter 3

SIGNIFICANCE OF HORMONES IN REGULATION OF METABOLISM DURING EXERCISE

FACTORS DETERMINING THE HORMONE EFFECT

PRIVATE AND ATTENDING REGULATION

The main determinant of the tissue supply of hormones is the hormone concentration in the blood, depending on hormone inflow into the blood (intensity of hormone secretion by glands) as well as on hormone elimination from the blood. In the blood a greater part of the hormone is bound with specific plasma proteins. As in most cases, only a free unbound fraction of the hormone can penetrate through the capillary wall into the tissue, with the dynamic balance between bound and unbound fractions determining the actual hormone inflow into tissues. The capacity of hormone binding by plasma proteins is limited. Usually, intensive hormone secretion causes a hormone concentration exceeding the binding capacity, and therefore the concentration of free unbound fractions increases.

The quantity of hormones arriving at the tissues is divided between various sites (Figure 3-1). Most hormone molecules are bound by cellular proteins. There is a dynamic equilibrium between the free hormone content in the extracellular compartment and the hormone content bound by cellular proteins. A part of the arriving hormone content is bound by sites connecting the hormone with enzymes catalyzing its metabolic degradation. This represents a loss of hormone. The enzymes catalyzing the metabolic degradation of hormones are most active in the liver, but they are also found in many other tissues. Besides metabolic degradation, there are also biotransformations of hormones from more active forms into less active or inactive ones, or vice versa. Examples of these changes are biotransformations between cortisol and cortisone, thyroxine and triiodothyronine, and testosterone and 5α-hydroxytestosterone. The remainder of the active hormone content is divided into the fraction bound by specific cellular receptors of this hormone and the hormone content bound unspecifically by other proteins. The amount of hormone bound specifically by corresponding cellular receptors is the determinant of the hormone effect.

This determinant depends on two circumstances. On the one hand, when the hormone inflow into tissues increases, more active hormones reach the specific receptors, and therefore more hormones can be specifically bound by their own receptors. On the other hand, when the number of hormone receptors increases, the ratio between specific and unspecific binding sites is elevated. This means that an enhanced portion of hormone is bound specifically despite the unchanged hormone content in tissues. In this connection it is important to stress that the hormone effect is regulated both on the level of production and secretion of the signal molecules as well as on the level of their reception. Therefore, it is valid to discriminate between 'private regulation' and 'attending regulation' (Figure 3-2).

The most important part of attending regulation is the modulating regulation (Figure 3-3) that addresses its influences not only to the number of receptors and their state, but also to the postreceptory process (see Reference 1). Besides the modulating regulation, attending regulation

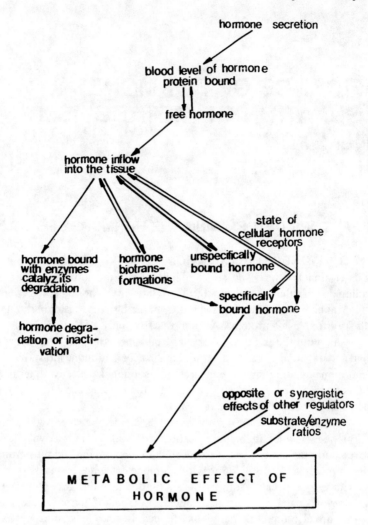

FIGURE 3-1. Factors determining the metabolic effect of hormones: (From Viru, A., *Hormones in Muscular Activity*, CRC Press, Boca Raton, 1985. With permission.)

may also be actualized through: (1) metabolic regulation, acting via the other receptors on cellular metabolism and thus changing the actualization of private regulation and (2) regulation of protein synthesis, acting on the synthesis of structure and enzyme proteins, participating in the actualization of private regulation. In case of additional synthesis of receptor proteins the modulating and protein-synthetic regulation are united into a common action.

Physiologically, the modulating regulation may be considered as (1) guaranteeing regulation for adjusting specific hormone receptors to the hormone concentration with the aim of maintaining the accordance between the number of binding sites and the acting signal molecules, (2) homeostatic regulation for decreasing the number of specific binding sites in cases of a chronically high hormone level in the blood or for increasing the number of binding sites in cases of chronic hormone deficiency with the aim of minimalizing or avoiding the harmful action of abnormal hormone levels, and (3) stress regulation to facilitate the regulatory effects through changes on receptor and postreceptor levels in addition to increased hormone secretion.[1]

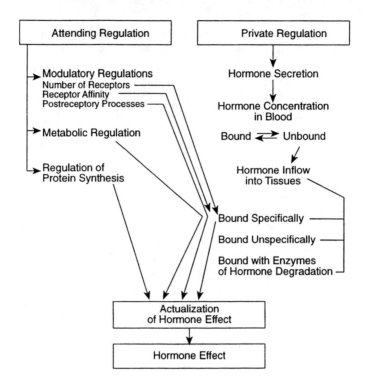

FIGURE 3-2. Private and attending regulation of the hormone effect. (From Viru, A., *Exp. Clin. Endocrin.*, 97, 13, 1991. With permission.)

EXERCISE-INDUCED EFFECTS AT THE LEVEL OF MODULATING REGULATION

Little is known about modulating regulation effects during and after acute exercise. Insulin binding to blood cells altered after exercise in both directions; some studies have pointed to an increased[2-5] while others to a decreased[2,3] binding after exercise. Both the increase and decrease were due to differences in the insulin-binding affinity without alterations in the total number of receptors per cell.[4-7] During a 3-h exercise at 40% VO_2max the specific binding of insulin to monocytes decreased in athletes[2] but increased in untrained men[8] and slightly in obese untrained subjects[3] and insulin-dependent diabetics.[9] The

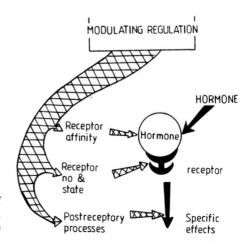

FIGURE 3-3. Modulating regulation of the levels of hormone receptors and postreceptory processes. (From Viru, A., *Exp. Clin. Endocrin.*, 97, 13, 1991. With permission.)

exercise-induced elevation as well as the reduction of insulin-binding could be reproduced by incubating the resting cells in serum obtained after exercise. Consequently, the exercise-induced serum factors can alter insulin-binding affinity. No effects of catecholamines, somatotropin, glucagon, and cortisol on insulin binding to blood cells could be detected by preincubation or direct incubation.[7] Somatostatin and prostaglandin β_1 were the only hormonal agents producing a small and reversible increase in monocyte insulin binding. Ketones were effective at concentrations unphysiologically high. Acidosis substantially diminished insulin binding to monocytes. Lactate (10 mmol·l^{-1}) induced a 28% drop in cellular insulin binding at low pH.[7]

In rats the insulin binding to the red and white parts of the gastocnemius muscle was depressed after exhaustive exercise in comparison with binding of the hormone to its receptors in unexercised animals.[10] In one investigation an increased insulin binding to rat muscles was found after exercise.[11] When the rats ran for 45 min, changes in insulin binding or in insulin receptor kinase activity were found in neither slow-twitch oxidative (SO) nor fast-twitch glycolytic (FG) fibers.[12] In humans, acute exercise either had no effect or might reduce insulin binding to muscle cells.[13] In another study during submaximal exercise insulin binding to skeletal muscles did not alter, but a decrease in the number of binding sites was observed after exhaustive exercise.[14] During 3 h of exercise insulin binding to adipocytes remained unchanged.[15]

There is also indirect evidence of modulating regulation effects on insulin action. In humans insulin-induced hypoglycemia is more pronounced after exercise.[16] However, this result may not be due to the modulating regulation, but simply to the decreased carbohydrate reserve and, therefore, to a less effective contraregulation. In the rat skeletal muscle the insulin effects on ^{14}C-glucose incorporation into glycogen were enhanced during the post-exercise period, particularly in deglycogenated muscles.[17] On the other hand, glucose tolerance and insulin sensitivity were not altered in the low muscle glycogen state induced by exhaustive exercise and fat diet.[16] In untrained subjects 1 h of moderate exercise increased sensitivity to the insulin effect on blood glucose uptake and oxidation.[19] V.A. Koivisto and H. Yki-Järvinen[15] have found an enhanced insulin-stimulated rise in glucose transport into adipose cells without alterations in insulin binding after exercise. Contrarily, R. Savari et al.[20] have observed a decreased insulin effect on glucose incorporation into triglycerides after cyclic exercise for 90 min.

In dogs, electrical stimulation of the gastrocnemius-plantaris muscle group increased the sensitivity of the muscles to the glycogenolytic effect of adrenaline.[21] There are various data in regard to the hyperglycemic effect of adrenaline. It is found that during exercise the hyperglycemic effect of adrenaline is more pronounced than at rest in both men[22] and rats.[23] In another study a diminished hyperglycemia effect of adrenaline was observed in exercising rats.[24] The sensitivity of the adipose tissue to respond *in vitro* to noradrenaline by release of glycerol was the same at rest and after a 30-min exercise in men.[25] The sensitivity of the heart in response to isoprotenol was decreased after exercise.[26] The β-adrenergic lipolytic or α_2-adrenergic antilipolytic responses of adipocytes changed with prolonged exercise in neither trained nor sedentary women.[27]

The binding affinity[8] and density of β-adrenoreceptors[29,30] increased in human blood cells after acute exercise. In human lymphocytes cycling exercise induced an increase in β_2-adrenoceptor density.[34] After exercise, isoprenaline caused a higher increase in cAMP production by these cells than before exercise.[30,31] Also, an exercise-induced fall in coupling of human β_2-adrenoreceptors is reported.[32] In rats 2 h of swimming lowered the sarcolemmal β_1- and β_2-adrenoreceptor density in the myocardium, and the ratio of β_1/β_2 receptors did not change.[33] In endurance-trained persons an exhaustive treadmill run changed neither the density nor affinity of α_2-adrenoreceptors in intact platelets.[34]

Possibilities of changes in steroid hormone receptor levels during exercise were also indicated. In rats the specific binding of androgens in the cytoplasma of the skeletal muscle steadily rose to the highest value 72 h after exercising.[35] Administration of the homologous hormone excluded the exercise-induced rise and caused a suppression in the binding.[36] Studies of the glucocorticoid receptor state in the heart cytosol showed that exhaustive swimming decreased the number of specific glucocorticoid binding sites as well as the ability to translocate receptor-steroid complexes into the cellular nucleus.[37] At the same time the amount of nonactivated receptors increased without changes in the amount of activated receptors.[38] A 90-min run at 23 m·min^{-1} did not inhibit or delay the appearance of activated glucocorticoid receptors from the unactivated state in skeletal muscles of various types after homologous hormone administration to adrenalectomized rats. Thus, the glucocorticoid receptor activation occurs at a rate that is independent of both fiber type and delivery of steroid to working muscles during exercise.[39]

The amount of available data is too small for drawing conclusions about the modulating regulation of hormone effects during exercise. Nevertheless, the results presented do not eliminate the possibility of such regulation.

TRAINING EFFECTS AT THE LEVEL OF MODULATING REGULATION

The role of modulating regulation is evidenced in regard to the training process. A number of indirect cases of altered sensitivity to catecholamines has been reported (see Reference 40). The data concerning cardiovascular functions give the impression that training induces a decreased sensitivity of α-adrenergic receptors in the heart and maybe also in the blood vessels. The sensitivity of β-adrenergic receptors in the heart does not actually change, but increases slightly in some cases.

S.H. Salzman et al.[41] found a decreased ^{3}H-adrenaline uptake by the heart ventricle per milligram of tissue in trained mice. They claimed that the decreased adrenaline uptake was the result of dilution of the cardiac binding sites for adrenaline associated with myocardial hypertrophy. In the myocardium of pigs no significant differences of β-adrenergic receptor concentrations were established between trained and untrained animals.[42] However, in the myocardium of trained rats, an increased number of β-adrenergic receptors,[43] or a decreased receptor number together with increased affinity[44] were found. Cardiac β-adrenoreceptor down-regulation was confirmed after endurance training without any shift in the percentage of the $β_1$- and $β_2$-adrenoreceptor subtypes.[33]

Various results were obtained in regard to training effects on blood cell adrenoreceptors. In athletes an increased number of β-receptor sites was found in blood granolocytes.[28,45] In polymorphonuclear leukocytes β-adrenergic receptor density was higher in marathon runners than in sedentary persons. Only in marathon runners did isoproterenol induce an increase in the cardiac stroke volume.[45] However, a comparison of seven elite marathoners and seven sedentary men did not reveal any effect of endurance training on the adrenergic receptor number and affinity in blood lymphocytes.[46] Training in swimming even decreased the density of β-adrenoreceptors in lymphocytes.[47] In long-distance runners and swimmers the β-adrenoreceptor density was lower than in weight-lifters, wrestlers, and untrained persons in conjunction with a decreased catecholamine level in the blood in a resting state as well as with reduced cAMP accumulation in lymphocytes after isoprenol administration.[48]

α-Adrenergic binding sites on intact platelets were decreased in endurance-trained subjects,[34] but increased in sportsmen using static strength exercises in training.[49] $α_2$-Adrenoreceptor density on platelets either did not differ between endurance-trained athletes and nonendurance-trained individuals[48] or was decreased in the first group.[50] The maximal binding and dissociation constants were significantly lower in endurance athletes.[34] In weight-lifters $α_2$-adrenoreceptor density was decreased.[48]

During the first days of training the number of β-adrenoreceptors decreased in various brain structures but not in the liver. After 2 weeks of training the number of β-adrenoreceptors was normalized in the midbrain and hypothalamus, but remained decreased in the hippocampus. In the liver the receptor density increased.[51]

In regard to metabolic effects the most common result is the increased lipolytic effect of adrenaline[52-55] but not that of noradrenaline.[56,57] Probably, this situation also reflects a more pronounced training effect on the β-adrenoreceptors than on the α-receptors. In active sportsmen the basal rate of lipolysis was about half of that in the untrained subjects, but after *in vitro* addition of adrenaline the lipolysis rate was highest in active sportsmen. No differences were found in lipolytic rates (either basal or adrenaline stimulated) in former sportsmen compared to untrained subjects.[58] The results obtained on human adipocytes were confirmed by studies on adipocytes of trained and sedentary rats.[59-62]

Training also enhanced the lipolytic action of dibutyl-cAMP in isolated lipolytes.[61] The same result was obtained by comparison of adipocytes from trained and sedentary women.[27] However, the total number of β-adrenoreceptors was unaffected by training in rats.[61] It was concluded that exercise training increases the lipolytic capacity of adipocytes at a metabolic step distal to stimulus recognition by adrenoreceptors.[27,61]

The first result of stimulation of β-adrenoreceptors is the activation of adenylate cyclase. The activity of this enzyme, catalyzing cAMP synthesis, has been found to be elevated in the muscular tissue of trained rats,[63] but not in hepatic cells[63] and adipocytes.[63-65] However, a more important result is the fact that in the presence of adrenaline, the rise in enzyme activity was substantially more pronounced in the muscle, liver, and adipose tissues of trained rats than in the tissues of untrained animals.[63] R.E. Shephard et al.[66] have found that after administration of isoprotenol the adenylate cyclase activity was lower in membrane preparations. Less pronounced was the cAMP accumulation in adipocytes. Nevertheless, the intensity of lipolysis was greater in adipocytes isolated from trained as compared to untrained rats. The reduced cAMP levels in adipocytes from trained rats might be attributed to the increased activity of cAMP-phosphodiesterase, obtained both in homogenate and particulate preparations.

The activity of cAMP-phosphodiesterase catalyzing the degradation of cAMP is found to be elevated in the skeletal muscles, liver,[63,67] adipose tissue,[63,64,67] and myocardium.[68] M.C. Thibault et al.[69] did not find any augmentation of cAMP-phosphodiesterase activity in the soleus, plantaris, and anterior tibial muscles of trained rats. Only in response to adrenaline did the enzyme activity reach a higher level in trained muscles. W.K. Palmer et al.[70] failed to confirm a training-induced increase in cAMP-phosphodiesterase activity in the adipose tissue of the rat. Training did not change the activity of phosphodiesterase with lower and higher k_m. According to N.N. Yakovlev,[63] after 1 month of training the enhanced adrenaline effect on adenylate cyclase was unchanged in the activity of cAMP-phosphodiesterase. This combination resulted in a rise in the sensitivity to adrenaline. During further training the enhanced adrenaline effect was counterbalanced by an augmented rate of cAMP degradation due to the increased cAMP-phosphodiesterase activity. Consequently, the well-trained organism possesses a labile and fine regulation of related metabolic processes.

In the mechanism of adrenaline action, the next step following cAMP accumulation is the activation of related protein kinases. In the adipose tissue, training did not induce increased activity of that enzyme.[64] A decreased level was observed in an investigation[71] together with elevated capacity for binding cAMP. M.I. Kalinski et al.[72] found an increased activity in isozymes I and II of cAMP-dependent protein kinase in the skeletal muscle due to training. In trained rats these activities remained high after prolonged exercise. In untrained rats the activity of cAMP-protein kinase decreased during prolonged exercise.[73] Endurance training increased the content of cAMP-protein kinase and of its thermostable protein inhibitor.[74] The latter exhibited approximately equal inhibitory effect in skeletal muscles of trained and untrained rats.[75]

A common effect of endurance training is the enhanced sensitivity to insulin. In trained persons glucose administration causes a less pronounced increase in insulin concentration, without a substantial change in glucose tolerance. Hence, tissue sensitivity to insulin action is enhanced.[76,77] Some data suggest that shifts in tissue sensitivity to insulin-induced glucose uptake may be related to an increased secretion of gastric-inhibiting polypeptide after training.[78] After 8 weeks of endurance training insulin sensitivity was improved together with increased activities of glycogen synthesis and hexokinase in muscles.[18] During insulin infusion, trained subjects also had higher responses to adrenaline, somatotropin, pancreatic polypeptide, and glycerol, and a lower glucagon response than untrained persons. Responses to C-peptide, noradrenaline, cortisol, lactate, free fatty acids, β-hydroxybutyrate, adrenaline, and blood pressure were similar.[79] Insulin-induced elevation of glucose oxidation was higher in endurance athletes than in untrained persons.[80] The euglycemic insulin-clamp technique provided confirmation that tissue sensitivity to physiologic hyperinsulinemia is higher in trained subjects: glucose uptake increased in athletes by 46% more than in untrained persons, and free fatty acid and glycerol levels in the blood decreased after 1 month of training to values 63 and 23% lower, respectively, than before training in previously untrained subjects.[81] Experiments with trained rats demonstrated an increased 2-deoxyglucose uptake into the soleus, red and white gastrocnemius, extensor digitorum longus, and diaphragm muscles.[82] In accordance, perfusion of the hindquarter with insulin enhanced glucose uptake and lactate oxidation in trained rats more than in untrained ones.[83] Increased sensitivity to insulin in the trained organism was demonstrated on isolated soleus muscle strips in regard to glycolysis and glycogen synthesis.[84]

In fat cells the rates of 2-deoxyglucose uptake and glucose oxidation,[60,85-87] as well as the lipogenetic effect of insulin,[58,61,88] are enhanced with training. An increase in the lipogenetic effect of insulin occurred in connection with the action of physical training on glucose transporters in fat-cell membranes.[89]

In comparison with active sportsmen, former sportsmen (4 to 8 years after finishing their participation in high-level competition) revealed an increased basal rate of lipolysis and reduced sensitivity to the lipogenic action of insulin. It was suggested that these changes may have significance for avoiding an augmentation of the adipose tissue after the drop in energy expenditure due to the change in physical activity.[58]

The insulin effect on glucose uptake by the liver is not enhanced in a trained organism.[90] Hence, elevated insulin sensitivity concerns the muscle and adipose tissues, but not that of the liver.

In trained rats, enhanced sensitivity to insulin was abolished after treatment with theophylline inhibiting the cAMP-phosphodiesterase activity. The sensitivity of this enzyme activity to the stimulatory action of insulin happened to be augmented in the muscles, the liver, and the adipose tissue.[91,92]

Increased insulin sensitivity is associated with changes in the specific binding of insulin. A training period of 6 months increased the specific binding of labeled insulin to the blood monocytes due to the augmented concentration of insulin receptors in conjunction with elevated maximal oxygen uptake and enhanced glucose uptake.[93] Accordingly, athletes surpass untrained persons by specific binding of ^{125}I-insulin to monocytes[2,94] as well as to erythrocytes.[95] A 6-week training induced together with elevated VO_2max an increased insulin binding to erythrocytes and increased exogenous glucose oxidation during exercise.[96] Increased insulin binding by skeletal muscles[97] and an elevated number of insulin receptors in this tissue[98] are the result of endurance training. Training did not alter the insulin receptor structure, but elevated the insulin receptor protein kinase activity.[98]

A. Wirth et al.[99] failed to find an increased number of insulin receptors in the adipocytes of trained rats. However, other studies demonstrated that a larger amount of insulin was specifically bound by the fat cells of trained rats.[86,87]

The effect of corticotropin on adrenocorticocytes as well as on lipolysis is mediated by the formation of cAMP. Therefore, one can also expect an altered sensitivity to corticotropin in training. Indeed, after training the lipolytic action of corticotropin is found to be increased in rats.[61] However, in another study training enhanced the stimulatory action of adrenaline on the adenylate cyclase, but that of corticotropin did not change.[100] There are different data about the training effect on the sensitivity of the adrenal cortex to corticotropin. Administration of corticotropin to athletes or trained rats, whose endogenous corticotropin function was suppressed by administration of dexamethasone, did not reveal differences in the adrenocortical response compared with the untrained control group.[101] N.N. Yakovlev[100] found an excessive rise in the blood corticosterone level in trained rats after administration of small doses of corticotropin (0.5 to 1.0 $mU \cdot 100 \ g^{-1}$), but not after a large dose (2.5 $mU \cdot 100 \ g^{-1}$). *In vitro* experiments gave evidence of both increased[102,103] and decreased[104] responsiveness to the addition of corticotropin to the incubation medium. Plotting these conflicting results against the duration of training showed that in cases of training for 2 to 4 weeks, the adrenocortical sensitivity to corticotropin increased, while after training for 6 to 8 weeks it appeared to be decreased in rats.[105]

The possibility of an altered sensitivity to steroid hormones arose from experiments indicating that systematic muscular activity makes skeletal muscles less sensitive to the catabolic effects of large doses of glucocorticoids.[106,107] However, the sensitization effect of training might be different in relation to physiological and nonphysiological hormone doses. Anyway, daily exercising, avoiding muscle wasting due to glucocorticoid treatment by 30%, did not reverse the glucocorticoid-induced suppression of the synthesis of myosin heavy chain. Exercising reduced glucocorticoid-induced myosin heavy chain degradation.[108]

Daily performance of intensive exercise during 10 days induced a decrease in the number of specific binding sites for glucocorticoids in the cytoplasm of myocardial cells. The affinity constant did not change. In adrenalectomized rats the change in the number of binding sites was not observed. The authors considered the change to be due to hypercorticism induced by daily exercise.[109] After more prolonged training periods no changes in cardiac androgen or glucocorticoid cytosol-specific binding concentration were observed.[110] In contrast, when training caused a dramatic cardiac enlargement (30%), the specific cytosol binding of glucocorticoids increased without a change in the binding of androgens.[111]

Swimming for 29 days induced an increase in the binding of labeled corticosterone to cytoplasmic proteins of skeletal muscles (1.9 times) and of the liver (2.7 times).[112] B.M. MacMannus and co-authors[113] did not find a greater testosterone uptake by the skeletal muscle in guinea pigs under the influence of training. Accordingly, R.C. Hickson et al.[114] did not detect changed androgen binding by cytosol of various muscles in rats after daily running during 8 weeks. However, B.J. Feldkoren[115] established an enhanced binding of testosterone to sarcoplasmic proteins of skeletal muscles due to 10-day swimming with an additional load of 6% body weight.

Training seems to sensitize the adipose tissue to the permissive action of glucocorticoids. In isolated adipocytes dexamethasone results in a stimulation of lipolysis through the permissive action on the adrenaline lipolytic effect. This action appears after a 2-h or longer incubation of isolated adipocytes with the glucocorticoid.[116] Accordingly, the potentiation of adrenaline lipolytic effect by dexamethasone was not observed in the case of a 30-min incubation of adipocytes isolated from untrained men or rats. However, addition of a small dose of dexamethasone (20 $\mu g \cdot l^{-1}$) to the incubation medium of isolated adipocytes, obtained from well-trained endurance athletes as well as from trained rats, resulted in an enhanced lipolytic effect of adrenaline. A small dose of insulin, which did not block the lipolytic effect of adrenaline, eliminated the cortisol-induced increase in adrenaline action on adipocytes from a trained organism.[62] Hence, the potentiation of adrenaline effect by cortisol was actualized through a locus sensitive to the opposite action of insulin.

A comparison of alterations in plasma osmolality and vasopressin concentration during exercise led to a suggestion about the enhanced sensitivity to vasopressin action in trained persons.[117]

In conclusion, the results presented suggest that training may alter the hormone reception and/or the post-receptory processes. Therefore, the same hormone level in the blood does not mean an equal metabolic effect in the trained and the untrained organism.

MOBILIZATION OF ENERGY RESERVES

ACTIVATION OF GLYCOGENOLYSIS IN SKELETAL MUSCLES

As early as 1938, experiments on isolated muscles suggested that adrenaline is a stimulator of anaerobic glycolysis in the muscles.[118] Ionic shifts and release of acetylcholine concomitant with initiating muscular contraction are capable of stimulating glycogen breakdown in muscles. However, the stimulatory actions are insufficient to maintain glycogenolysis at the required level during exercise. An additional stimulation by adrenaline is necessary. An increasing body of experimental data support the essential role of adrenaline in mobilization of energy reserves.[119]

The effect of adrenaline on glycogen phosphorylase is mediated by β-adrenergic receptors.[120] Experiments on humans,[121] dogs,[122] and rats[123,124] have proved that β-adrenergic blockade diminished the use of muscle glycogen during exercise, as well as the release of lactate.[122,124,125] The same effect was obtained with a selective β_2-adrenergic blockade.[126] In humans propranolol infusion eliminated the increase in muscle cAMP content during dynamic exercise and reduced the phosphorylase activation.[127] There are also alternative results indicating the ineffectiveness of β-blockade in eliminating muscle glycogenolysis during exercise.[128-130] Evidently, there must be another pathway for stimulating glycogenolysis, probably with the aid of an increased activity of phosphorylase due to changes in muscle concentrations of ATP, AMP, and inorganic phosphate.[131]

Differences in the results may be partly due to the various types of muscles studied. Propranolol (a β-blocker) excluded the decrease in glycogen content in fast-twitch oxidative-glycolytic and slow-twitch oxidative muscles in the course of running and swimming. In the fast-twitch glycolytic muscles glycogenolysis was blocked after running for 30 min at 12 m·min⁻¹, but was almost normal after running to exhaustion at the same speed.[124] Therefore, in the fast-twitch glycolytic muscles the absence of the adrenaline effect is compensated for by another action stimulating glycogenolysis. When adrenaline was injected subcutaneously before running for 60 min, a cumulative effect of the hormone and exercise on the glycogen drop occurred in the glycolytic muscle. In the oxidative and oxidative-glycolytic muscles the glycogen depletion rate, caused by endogenous adrenaline and other exercise-induced factors, was sufficiently rapid and no additional effect of exogenous adrenaline was observed.[24]

Surgical or chemical sympathectomy could not prevent muscle glycogenolysis during exercise in rats.[63,132] In sympathectomized rats, electrical stimulation of muscles led to a more pronounced glycogen phosphorylase activation in the gastrocnemius than in normal rats. The differences in lactate accumulation were negligible. In the soleus reduced increases in lactate concentration and phosphorylase activity were observed.[133] A reduced noradrenaline release from sympathetic nerve endings due to the postganglionic blockade led to an even more pronounced glycogen depletion in fast-twitch muscles. Glycogen utilization was not modified in a slow-twitch muscle.[134] Consequently, sympathetic innervation either is not essential for muscle glycogenolysis or its action is effectively compensated for by adrenomedullary hormones. In any case, the mediator of sympathetic nerve endings, noradrenaline, is not a potent stimulator of muscular glycogenolysis.[135]

In trained rats a drop in the muscle glycogen content occurred during running to exhaustion in spite of the elimination of the response of catecholamines by adrenaldemedullation as well as by combining adrenaldemedullation with the β-adrenergic blockade and/or hypophysectomy.[128] When running at 25.5 m·min⁻¹ for a mean of 53 min, the glycogen content decreased in the skeletal muscles in spite of chemical sympathectomy, adrenaldemedullation, or a combination of these treatments. However, the glycogen concentrations in the soleus and in the red portion of the gastrocnemius muscles of adrenaldemedullated and adrenaldemedullated-sympathectomized rats were 3.8 and 2.5 times higher after exercise than those of the normal, exercised rats. The extent of glycogen depletion in the white portion of the gastrocnemius muscle was similar for all exercise groups.[136]

In most studies the adrenaldemedullation substantially aggravated glycogen depletion during exercise or excluded this process in oxidative muscles almost completely.[137,138] In conjunction with this, the activity of phosphorylase (a + b) decreased in the muscles of adrenaldemedullated animals.[139] Infusion of adrenaline, which simulated endogenous hormone secretion, completely restored glycogenolysis during exercise in adrenaldemedullated rats.[140]

In normal men the quadriceps muscles of both legs were intermittently stimulated for 30 min. Adrenaline infusion from the 15th to 30th minute of muscle stimulation doubled the mole fraction of phosphorylase a and glycogenolysis.[141]

Most striking evidence of the essential role of adrenaline in muscle glycogenolysis has been obtained in experiments on isolated muscle preparation. In contracting isolated rat muscles the intensity of glycogenolysis initially rose promptly. However, this rise was only transient. A more prolonged increase in the rate of glycogenolysis, together with increased mechanical work, was obtained following the administration of either adrenaline or noradrenaline. These effects were prevented by β-adrenergic but not by α-adrenergic blockade.[142] Conversion of phosphorylase b to a, as well as glycogenolysis, is also transient in muscles during their contraction;[143] both of these processes are reactivated by adrenaline.[144] In agreement with these data are the results of E.A. Richter and co-authors.[145] In the isolated, perfused rat hindquarter it has been found that contractions, per se, stimulate glycogenolysis only for a brief period, and that a direct effect of adrenaline is needed for continued glycogenolysis during exercise. The adrenaline effect was associated with increased cAMP production, phosphorylase activation, and glycogen synthesis inactivation. Adrenaline also increased oxygen uptake and muscle performance. Propranolol abolished the effects of adrenaline except for an increased oxygen uptake. Phentolamine (α-adrenergic blocker) abolished the effect of adrenaline on oxygen uptake and muscle performance and lessened the adrenaline-induced increase in glycogenolysis but did not reduce cAMP production, phosphorylase activation, or glycogen synthesis inactivation. Consequently, some of the adrenaline effects on the contracting muscle are elicited by stimulating α-adrenoreceptors besides the main metabolic effects through the stimulation of β-receptors.[146]

Consequently, adrenaline can be considered an essential tool in the activation of glycogenolysis in exercising muscles (Figure 3-4). However, the adrenergic stimulation of phosphorylase activity proved to be reversed by contractile activity.[147] It was concluded that muscle glycogenolysis is regulated both by the degree of muscular activity and the available adrenaline.[148] Adrenal hormones enhance glycogenolysis also in nonexercising muscles during exercise.[149]

Experiments on rats with adrenocortical or thyroid insufficiencies pointed to some significance of corresponding hormones. During prolonged exercise the blood plasma levels of glucose and lactate, as well as the liver and muscle glycogen contents, were lower in adrenalectomized rats than in adrenalectomized rats treated with cortisone.[123,150] During running to exhaustion (duration of running 197 ± 25 min), a reduced glycogen use was observed in the soleus but not in the quadriceps femoris in adrenalectomized rats.[152] After swimming for 4 h a less pronounced drop in glycogen reserves was established both in red and white portions of quadriceps muscles of adrenalectomized rats than in the intact animals.[151] It

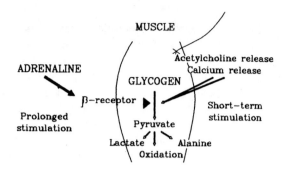

FIGURE 3-4. Triggering of glycogenolysis in skeletal muscle during exercise.

can be speculated that the aggravated glycogen utilization in skeletal muscles of adrenalectomized rats during exercise is due to the lack of permissive action of glucocorticoids on the glycogenolytic effect of adrenaline.

In hypothyroid rats the muscle glycogen consumption was exaggerated during 40 min of running. Since in thyroid-deficient rats pyruvate, and particularly palmitade, oxidation by the muscle tissue decreased *in vitro*, it was suggested that the reduced capacity for utilizing free fatty acids enhances glycogen consumption in the skeletal muscles of those rats.[153]

GLYCOGENOLYSIS IN THE MYOCARDIUM

Treadmill running that caused an elevation in the plasma adrenaline and noradrenaline levels resulted in a twofold increase in the myocardial cAMP level in conjunction with 50% activation of phosphorylase to its a-form and depletion of glycogen.[154] However, chemical sympathectomy, adrenaldemedullation, or a combination of these treatments did not aggravate glycogen depletion in the myocardium.[132,134] On the other hand, the blockade of β-adrenergic receptors prevented heart glycogen and triglyceride mobilization during exercise.[155] The regulation of glycogenolysis in the myocardium is more complicated than in the skeletal muscles and the consumption of cardiac glycogen can be readily avoided by using other energy substrates. This seems to be the reason why it is difficult to establish the role of catecholamines in exercise-induced glycogenolysis in the myocardium.

Administration of thyroxine before exercise enhanced the decrease in the cardiac glycogen content in rats.[156] Estradiol is capable of a sparing effect in regard to the myocardial glycogen during exercise.[157]

REGULATION OF GLYCOGENOLYSIS IN THE LIVER

According to contemporary knowledge, hepatic glycogenolysis is controlled by various hormones, including catecholamines, glycagin, angiotensin II, vasopressin, oxitocin, parathormone, and vasoactive intestinal peptide as stimulators, insulin as an inhibitor, and glucocorticoids as a permissive factor.[158] In addition, direct sympathic and parasympathic nervous influences are demonstrated.[159] In such situations it is almost impossible to convincingly establish the significance of any single factor. Also, the significance of direct nervous factors during exercise remains poorly established. A blockade of noradrenergic nervous pathways excludes hyperglycemia induced by an intensive short-term exercise.[160] In contrast, postganglionic blockade, reducing noradrenaline release from sympathetic nerve endings, did not modify liver glycogen utilization.[134]

There are various results about the effect of catecholamines on liver glycolysis in the expression of blood glucose values or in the depletion of hepatic glycogen stores. In dogs, total sympathectomy did not change the blood glucose dynamics during exercise.[161] In chemically sympathectomized rats the blood glucose level was even higher than in normal animals at the end of running to exhaustion; however, treated rats were able to run for only one third of the duration that normal animals ran.[132]

In rats the depletion of hepatic glycogen reserves during various exercises was not prevented by either lack of adrenomedullar hormones (adrenalectomized rats treated with cortisol), adrenaldemedullation in combination with ganglionic blockade with hexamethonium, β-adrenrgic blockade with propranolol, hypophysectomy, or hypophysectomy in combination with β-blockade.[128] During running, liver glycogen decreased at similar rates and hepatic cAMP increased to the same extent in adrenaldemedullated and sham-operated rats.[138] β-Adrenergic blockade has been shown to diminish hepatic glycogen depletion in swimming[162] but not in running[163] rats. In dogs β-adrenergic blockade failed to impair the liver glycogen drop and hepatic glucose production rate.[130] The lack of β-adrenergic receptor contribution in hepatic glycogenolysis was confirmed by the fact that exercise-induced glycogen depletion occurred in the absence of a rise in the cAMP concentration.[164] Moreover, D.A. Arnall et al.[165] did not find a rise in the hepatic glycogen depletion during exercise due to simultaneous adrenaline infusion despite an increase in the blood plasma level of adrenaline up to 4.3 ng·ml⁻¹.

Consequently, adrenaline is unessential for stimulating liver glycogenolysis during exercise.

A potent stimulus to the hepatic glycogenolysis approach arises from the increased blood level of glucagon. During exercises, glucagon concentration increases after a prolonged lagperiod (see above), and the role of glucagon seems to be important only in the last stage of prolonged exercises. However, in the presence of a decreased insulin concentration in the plasma, the liver becomes more sensitive to glucagon. Therefore, even if glucagon concentration does not change during exercise, its effect can still become apparent.[166] The increase in the hepatic glucose production rate in pancreatectomized dogs[166] speaks against the main role of glucagon in the hepatic glycogen mobilization.

Acute inhibition of glucagon secretion by administration of somatostatin is accompanied by a transient reduction of glucose in blood.[167,168] In exercising humans the hepatic glucose production was suppressed during hypoglucagonemia due to somatostatin administration.[169] Administration of glucagon antiserum reduced the depletion of liver glycogen during exercises.[168,170] The general conclusion drawn from these experiments is that the basal level of glucagon normally accounts for a certain hepatic glucose production at rest and during exercise. However, the basal glucagon level need not be essential for an exercise-induced rise in the hepatic glucose output.[171] J. Wahren and O. Björkman[172] assume that hyperglucagonemia, as well as hypoinsulinemia, have a permissive rather than regulatory influence on exercise-induced changes in the hepatic glucose output.

M. Vranic et al.[173] affirm that glucose production by the liver is regulated mainly by the glucagon-insulin ratio. The liver is highly sensitive to small changes in the insulin concentration. Hence, it is to be expected that a decrease in the insulin level in the blood during exercise will result in stimulation of hepatic glycogenolysis and gluconeogenesis.[174] Indeed, during exercise a further acute depression of the already decreased insulin concentration by infusion of mannoheptulose caused a sudden rise in glucose production that was avoided by simultaneous insulin infusion.[175] When the concentrations of insulin, glucagon, and glucose in the plasma are maintained at a basal level during exercise by means of intravenous glucose infusion, the normal two- to three-fold increase in the hepatic glucose production is not affected.[176] With the aid of insulin administration the increase in hepatic glycogenolysis was avoided during exercise in one study.[177] In other studies the maintenance of hyperinsulinemia by insulin infusion did not inhibit exercise-induced stimulation of the hepatic glucose output.[178,179]

Experiments on dogs indicated that during swimming for 150 min the decrease in the blood insulin level accounts for 80% of the hepatic glucose production by direct influence on the liver and by indirect influence on glucagon secretion.[180]

Administration of estradiol to female sterilized rats delayed glycogen mobilization from the liver during the first hour of swimming. Hypoglycemia developing at the end of the fifth hour of swimming was less pronounced in estradiol-treated rats. These data suggested that estradiol exerts a sparing effect on carbohydrate reserves in rats during exercise.[181]

GLUCONEOGENESIS

Approximately 70 to 75% of the hepatic glucose output is derived from glycogenolysis and the remainder from gluconeogenesis.[174] The precursor substrates available for conversion to glucose are lactate, pyruvate, glycerol, and the glucogenic amino acids. Among the amino acids, alanine makes the largest contribution, accounting for some 5 to 8% of the total glucose output and 20 to 25% of the gluconeogenic components.[175,182] During prolonged mild exercise that increases the hepatic glucose output twofold, the relative contribution of gluconeogenesis to the overall hepatic output increases from 25 to 45% (Figure 3-5), indicating a three-fold rise in the absolute rate of gluconeogenesis.[172]

Among the hormones responsible for a rise in gluconeogenesis one must take into account adrenaline, glucagon, glucocorticoids, and insulin. These hormones can act either directly on the gluconeogenic enzymes or on the mobilization of precursors necessary for gluconeogenesis.

As was mentioned above, in adrenalectomized rats muscle glycogen depletion is aggravated. On the other hand, a drop in the hepatic glycogen store as well as hypoglycemia are very pronounced at the end of prolonged exercise.[152] After administration of adrenocortical extract to normal rats, the decrease in their liver glycogen content was less pronounced during a prolonged period of muscular contractions.[183] These results can be interpreted as a decreased rate of gluconeogenesis in adrenalectomized rats and as an elevated rate of this process in rats treated with glucocorticoids.

In normal rats a prompt decrease in the liver glycogen content was observed during the first 4 h of swimming. From the fifth to twelfth hours of swimming the hepatic glycogen content did not increase significantly (Figure 3-6). This was possibly due to the predominance of lipid oxidation and intensive gluconeogenesis. The liver glycogen content dropped again during the last 4 h of swimming (from the thirteenth to sixteenth hours of swimming). The concentration of corticosterone in the blood plasma increased substantially at the beginning of exercise and persisted at a high level until the eighth hour of swimming. By the twelfth hour of swimming the corticosterone level was insignificantly higher and at the end of 16-h exercise it was below the initial level. It was suggested that the secondary drop in the liver glycogen content was related to the decrease in the rate of gluconeogenesis resulting from a decrease in the glucocorticoid level.[151]

Insulin decreases the supply of gluconeogenic processes by substrates and inhibits the glucose-alanine cycle.[182] Thus, the exercise-induced hypoinsulinemia is a promoting factor in gluconeogenesis. In accordance with this, in diabetics during exercise the rate of uptake of precursors of gluconeogenesis by abdominal organs was higher than in normal persons.[184] During exercise the rate of the glucose – glucose-6-phosphate cycle was three times higher in diabetic dogs. Treatment of diabetic dogs with glucocorticoids increased the rate of the cycle up to 15 times as compared to normal dogs.[185]

There are no available data strictly providing the gluconeogenic effect of the increased glucagon level during exercise. Indirect evidence of the role of glucagon arises from the data that show that during exercise, administration of glucagon enhances hyperalaninemia.[186]

UTILIZATION OF BLOOD GLUCOSE

Insulin as well as muscular contractions stimulate the uptake of glucose by muscle cells. Both of them induce a twofold increase in the number of glucose transporters in plasma membranes of the rat hindlimb muscles.[187] Insulin and contractile effects on glucose uptake are additives suggesting that these stimuli mobilize different pools of glucose transporters.[148] Results were obtained showing that in the absence of insulin the glucose uptake by rat hindquarters, isolated immediately after a 45-min run, was on the same level as in nonexercised

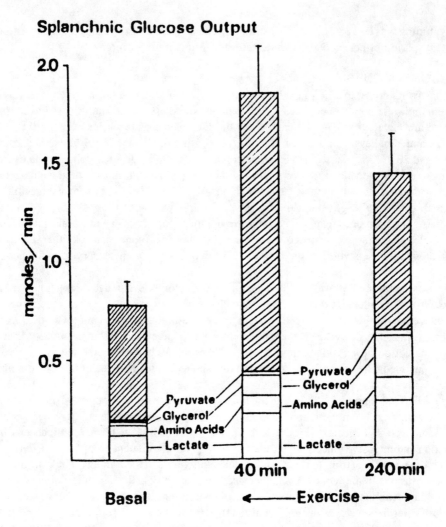

FIGURE 3-5. Liver glucose output during 4-h exercise in man. (From Wahren, J., and Björkman, O., *Biochemistry of Exercise IV-A*, Poortmans, J., and Niset, G., Eds., University Park Press, Baltimore, 1981, 149. With permission.)

controls; addition of insulin increased the glucose uptake.[17] When prior swimming increased the glucose uptake by the perfused rat hindquarter, the addition of insulin into the perfusate did not further increase the glucose uptake.[188] There are also data indicating that muscular contractions caused a seven-fold increase in glucose uptake by the perfused muscle from a diabetic rat despite the lack of insulin in the perfusate.[189]

Insulin increases glucose clearance in exercising dogs.[175] In pancreatectomized dogs exercise did not increase the elimination rate of glucose from the blood plasma.[190] In these dogs infusion of minimal amounts of insulin (necessary for maintaining the glucose level in the blood during exercise) did increase the glucose elimination rate during a strenuous but not a moderate exercise.[166]

In the exercising human forearm the glucose uptake was augmented due to administration of insulin.[191] In normal subjects the use of glucose during exercise can be elevated by hyperinsulinemia after glucose administration.[192] However, the peripheral glucose utilization increases in exercise, although there is a reduction in the circulating insulin level.[174]

On the basis of all these results taken together, the following conclusions were drawn: (1) insulin is an essential hormone for regulating the flux of glucose during exercise;[193] (2) additional insulin availability does not significantly change the increment in glucose uptake

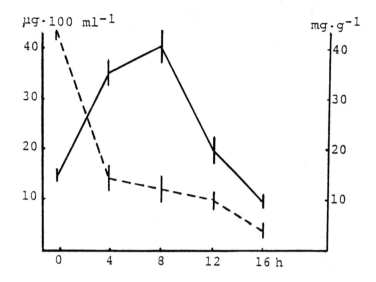

FIGURE 3-6. Blood corticosterone (µg/100 ml plasma) and liver glycogen (mg/g of wet tissue) in normal rats after swimming for 4, 8, 12 and 16 h. Solid line — blood corticosterone, interrupted line — liver glycogen. (From Viru, M., Litvinova, L., Smirnova, T., and Viru, A., *J. Sports Med. Phys. Fitness*, 1994. With permission.)

caused by exercise;[17,179] (3) the presence of a low concentration of insulin exerts a permissive effect on the glucose uptake by the contracting muscle.[174]

As a general conclusion it was suggested that the presence of insulin is not essential for a small exercise-induced increase in the muscle glucose uptake, but an amount of insulin is required for the full response.[173]

Adrenaline inhibits glucose uptake by the skeletal muscle.[194] Adrenaline suppresses the insulin-stimulated level of glucose uptake as well.[195] In this connection one may explain the hypoglycemia in man[121] and dogs[122,130] during exercise after β-adrenergic blockade. The same result was obtained in rats after adrenaldemedullation.[140] M. Berger et al.[177] suggested that the increased glucose utilization is balanced by the combined action of a decreased level of insulin and increased levels of adrenaline, cortisol, and glucagon in the blood. However, the diminished hyperglycemic effect of adrenaline during exercise[24] suggests that the inhibitory effect of adrenaline on glucose uptake by muscles is completely counteracted by the stimulatory effect of the contractions and insulin.

In dogs adrenaline infusion substantially decreased the metabolism of labeled glucose and amplified peripheral glycogenolysis during exercise.[196] Adrenaldemedullation abolished the exercise-induced hyperglycemia seen in sham-operated animals.[138] This fact has to be explained by the lack of decrease in blood glucose clearance due to the increased level of adrenaline seen in the normal organism.

The inhibitory effect may be exerted also by somatotropin. In patients with hypopituitarism a moderate exercise of 30 min did not elevate the somatotropin level in the blood as was observed in normal subjects. The blood glucose and pyruvate levels were higher in patients during this exercise and also after 90 min of running.[197] In rats the development of hypoglycemia during exhaustive running was avoided by ganglionic blockade but not by adrenaldemedullation, β-adrenergic blockade, and hypophysectomy.[128]

Thus, among factors controlling blood glucose utilization during exercise, the main role belongs to an essential, critical level of insulin.

BLOOD GLUCOSE HOMEOSTASIS DURING EXERCISE

During the first 60 min of light exercise (30 to 40% VO_2max) the normal glucose level in the blood plasma is maintained by an increase in the hepatic glucose output that balances the increase in glucose utilization by working muscles and other tissues.[198,199] The regulative role of insulin and glucagon in these changes was considered to be minimal, since no change in their levels was detected over the first 60 min of light exercise.[198] In another study these changes were also detected in 60-min exercises at 40% VO_2max.[199] During a more strenuous or more prolonged exercise these changes are pronounced. Even in these circumstances, the precise role of the mentioned hormonal changes in glucose homeostasis is not clear. A study of pancreatectomized dogs led to the suggestion that changes in insulin and glucagon concentraions were not necessary for the regulation of blood glucose concentration in exercise.[193] In contrast, the use of various combinations of somatostatin and glucagon infusion during exercise indicated that the ratio of glucagon to insulin was directly correlated with glucose production.[168] The importance of the glucagon response in stimulating glucose production in exercising dogs has been confirmed in a more recent study.[200]

When changes in insulin and glucagon were prevented with the aid of simultaneous infusion of somatostatin, insulin, and glucagon, the plasma glucose concentration fell during 1 h of exercise at 40% VO_2max. The fall was particularly pronounced if a high level of insulin (approximately 20 $\mu mol \cdot ml^{-1}$) was maintained during exercise. In this case the glucose uptake increased to a greater extent than in the normal situation, and glucose production did not increase sufficiently to compensate for the increase in glucose uptake associated with an elevated rate of glucose oxidation. It was concluded that during prolonged exercise there must be a reduction in insulin concentration and/or an increase in glucagon concentration if euglycemia is to be maintained. If such changes do not occur, hypoglycemia follows.[199] During the experiment of somatostatin, insulin, and glucagon infusion, adrenaline and noradrenaline levels were elevated more than in normal conditions. Despite that, hypoglycemia occurred.[199]

MOBILIZATION OF LIPID RESOURCES

The main link in the mobilization of lipid resources is the activation of lipases. Hormone-sensitive lipase is the rate-limiting enzyme in the lipolytic process. For its activation human adipocytes possess stimulatory β-adrenoreceptors besides inhibitory α-receptors. The activation of the enzyme is effected through reversible phosphorylation catalyzed by cAMP (see Reference 201).

In the activation of lipases, a number of hormones participate (Figure 3-7). Their role during exercise was well demonstrated by P.D. Gollnick and co-workers.[128] They found that exercise-induced lipolysis was depressed by hypophysectomy or by β-adrenergic blockade in rats. The combination of hypophysectomy and β-blockade completely abolished the exercise-induced rise in the adipose and plasma levels of free fatty acids. The β-adrenergic blockade excluded the lipolytic action of catecholamines and impaired the increased secretion of glucagon. Hypophysectomy aggravated the activation of the pituitary-thyroid and pituitary-adrenocortical systems and eliminated the direct actions of somatotropin, thyrotropin, and corticotropin. In another experiment the increase in the plasma level of free fatty acids induced by a 1-h swim was abolished by adrenalectomy, hypophysectomy, or thyroidectomy; β-adrenergic blockade or adrenaldemedullation did not prevent free fatty acid release.[202]

A large body of experimental data has been collected about the significance of the lipolytic action of catecholamines during exercise. In rats the exercise-induced release of free fatty acids was impaired after adrenaldemedullation[123] as well as after chemical sympathectomy.[132] In adrenaldemedullated rats the free fatty acid response to exercise was normalized by adrenaline administration. In untrained rats the β-blockade was effective, but not in trained ones.[203] Effective β-blockade was shown in exercising dogs[130] and men[163] in regard to the release of free fatty acids. The results of a study suggest that the catecholamine-induced increase of lipolysis is mainly mediated via beta-1-adrenoreceptors.[204] Total blockade of β-receptors by propranolol fully prevented the reduction of the triglyceride level both in the

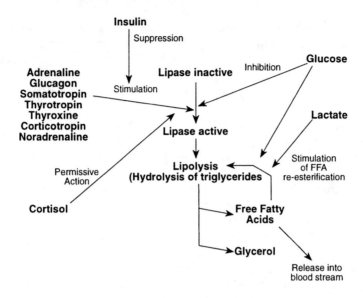

FIGURE 3-7. Hormonal control of lipolysis during exercise.

red muscle[205] and in the myocardium[155] during swimming for 3 h with an additional load of 1% body weight.

There is no convincing evidence as to the special role of glucagon in exercise-induced lipolysis. H. Galbo[171] suggests that the role of glucagon in this process is not indispensable.

During exercise the increase in the blood level of somatotropin is usually accompanied by an elevated concentration of free fatty acids. Both responses are eliminated by glucose administration.[206] The role of pituitary hormones in exercise-induced lipolysis is emphasized by data about the depression of a rise in the free fatty acid level due to hypophysectomy.[128,202] Nevertheless, in patients with hypopituitarism, a moderate exercise for 30 min did not elevate the somatotropin level in the blood, as was observed in normal subjects, but the increase in the blood concentration of glycerol, free fatty acids, and ketone bodies was even more pronounced.[197] When patients with Cushing's disease were both adrenalectomized and hypophysectomized, the rise in free fatty acids and glycerol persisted during exercise.[207] In normal men a prior somatotropin administration elevated its level but not the free fatty acids response during exercise.[208] The lipolytic effect of somatotropin, unlike that of other lipolytic hormones, required a lag period of at least 1 h.[116] Hence, the presence or absence of simultaneous and comparable changes in the blood levels of somatotropin and free fatty acids does not have any physiological meaning. Thus, no convincing evidence of the decisive role of pituitary hormones in lipolysis in humans during exercise is as yet available.

There is some evidence of the participation of thyroid hormones in the mobilization of lipid resources during exercise. In dogs, administration of thyroxine or triiodothyronine enhanced the rise in the free fatty acids level during runs of 15, 30, and 60 min.[209] In hyperthyroid patients, exercise-induced increase in the free fatty acids concentration was more pronounced than in normal persons.[210] In exercising thyroidectomized dogs, the plasma free fatty acids level[211,212] and free fatty acids turnover rate[211] were far below those found in normal dogs during exercise. Accordingly, both at rest and during exercise, normal rats maintained higher plasma levels of glycerol and free fatty acids than thyroid-deficient animals.[211] Thyroid hormones have also been implicated in the lipoprotein changes induced by physical exercise.[213]

Adrenalectomy decreased the rise in the free fatty acids level in the blood plasma during prolonged exercise.[123,150,152] Cortisone treatment reversed this change.[123] However, in adrenalectomized patients with Cushing's disease the exercise-induced rise in the plasma levels of free fatty acids and glycerol were more pronounced than in normal persons, in spite of the higher level of insulin.[207] This can be attributed to the effect of the higher levels of corticotropin, noradrenaline, and glucagon in those patients. The glucocorticoid action on lipolysis is not a direct effect, but rather a permissive influence on adrenaline and other hormone actions.[214]

Insulin possesses a direct antilipolytic action.[215] This effect is related to the decrease in the cAMP content[216] and increased cAMP-phosphodiesterase activity[217] as well as to conversion of the hormone-sensitive lipase from the phosphorylated to the dephosphorylated state.[218] It was suggested that during prolonged exercise the decrease in the blood insulin level was a tool for the transition from utilization of carbohydrates to lipid oxidation.[190,219] This standpoint was confirmed by reciprocal changes in insulin and free fatty acids concentrations during prolonged exercise,[220] as well as by the exaggerated free fatty acids and glycerol responses and fatty acids oxidations to exercise both in diabetic animals[211,221] and diabetic patients.[222] Insulin treatment tended to normalize these responses to exercise.[222] In insulin-deficient diabetics fat oxidation accounts for a selectively larger portion of total fuel utilization by the exercising muscle than is observed in healthy persons.[222] Lipolysis was also higher during exercise when the subjects were made hypoinsulinemic by prolonged fasting.[171] Furthermore, enhancement of the exercise-induced depression of the plasma insulin concentration by infusion of somatostatin was accompanied by accelerated lipolysis.[223] The exercise-induced decrease in the muscle triglyceride content and their oxidation is higher in pancreatectomized than in normal dogs.[224]

In conclusion, adrenaline is the main hormonal factor inducing intensive glycogenolysis in exercising muscles as well as lipolysis in the adipose tissue. These effects of adrenaline are supported by the permissive action of glucocorticoids. Besides adrenaline, the lipolytic action also belongs to glucagon, somatotropin, thyroxine, and some other hormones. One cannot exclude their participation. However, there is no convincing evidence of their decisive role. Adrenaline is not responsible for the increase in hepatic glucose output. In this process the main significance belongs to hypoinsulinemia and probably also to direct nervous influences. Hypoinsulinemia does not exclude glucose transport to muscle cells. Some results suggest the participation of somatotropin in the control of glucose utilization during exercise. Hypoinsulinemia is a decisive factor in the mobilization of lipid resources. The lipolytic action of various hormones can be actualized only after the decrease in the insulin level in the blood.

MOBILIZATION OF PROTEIN RESOURCES

Typical responses to acute exercise are suppressed protein synthesis and elevated protein degradation.[225,226] Comparison of these responses in muscles containing various types of fibers indicated that the rate of protein synthesis was suppressed and the rate of protein degradation was elevated mainly in muscles less active during exercise.[227] Thus, the less active muscles, but not those that fulfill the main task during exercise performance, are used as a reservoir for mobilization of protein resources. The exercise-induced catabolism is not extended to contractile proteins.[227,228] During exercise the catabolic response is extended to the smooth muscle of the gastrointestinal tract, lymphoid tissue, liver, and kidney (see Reference 226).

Both the antianabolic and catabolic effects have to be considered as tools for mobilization of protein resources during a stressful situation (Figure 3-8). As a result, an increased pool of available free amino acids is created. Due to the suppressed protein synthesis, the free amino acids pool is used for supplying the necessary protein synthesis by 'building materials' only to a minor extent. The amino acids are mainly used for additional energy supply to contracting muscles. There are at least three pathways connecting free amino acids with energy processes. One of these consists in the oxidation of branched-chain amino acids. The main site of this

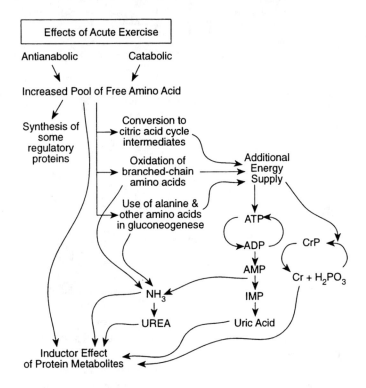

FIGURE 3-8.   Creation and utilization of the pool of free amino acids during exercise.

pathway is the contracting muscle. An increased oxidation of leucine during exercise was established in human[229,230] as well as in animal[231,232] studies. The metabolism of several amino acids leads to the formation of metabolites of the citric cycle, which also has a beneficial effect on muscle metabolism by increasing the capacity of the citric cycle for oxidizing the acetyl-CoA units generated from pyruvate and free fatty acids.[225] A pathway goes through alanine (and glutamine) formation in the muscles from pyruvate and amino groups reversed in the oxidation of branched-chain amino acids (Figure 3-8). Alanine is transported by the blood to the liver where the nitrogen-free products of its deamination are used in gluconeogenesis.[182] A by-product of amino acid use is urea formation at the expense of the released amino groups.

Many of the alterations in the hormonal ensemble during exercise favor (or even constitute the main cause of) protein and amino acid mobilization. First, attention must be paid to the action of glucocorticoids. The general catabolic action of glucocorticoids has long ago been documented by the negative nitrogen balance. Regarding muscular tissue, it has been shown that glucocorticoids cause a suppression of protein synthesis, augmented release of amino acids, elevated protein degradation rate, enhanced activity of myofibrillar proteases, and increased excretion of 3-methylhistidine.[226,233]

All these changes are undoubtedly subjected to many control factors and the similarity of responses caused both by glucocorticoids and exercise does not prove the single role of glucocorticoids. For example, in adrenalectomized rats the dynamics of 3-methylhistidine excretion during and after daily moderate exercise was found to be the same as in normal animals.[234]

The many factors involved in the control of protein and amino acid mobilization during exercise (Figure 3-9) are emphasized by studies that indicate that muscular activity exerts a protective effect against the catabolic action of glucocorticoids on the muscular tissue.[106,107] This effect probably rules out the possible harmful action of a high level of glucocorticoids. Muscular activity inhibits the stimulating effect of glucocorticoids on myofibrillar alkaline proteases.[107] Here a substantial role may be played by the opposite action of testosterone.

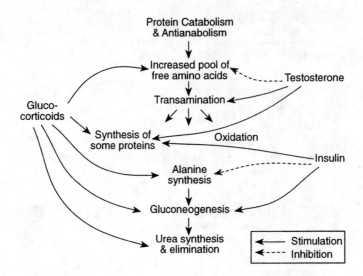

FIGURE 3-9. Hormonal control of amino acid metabolism during exercise.

Systematic muscular activity did not stimulate the alkaline proteolytic activity of the skeletal muscle if testosterone was administered simultaneously.[235] Accordingly, G.L. Dohm and T.M. Louis[236] found that decreased testosterone concentrations during muscular activity might promote the apparently increased protein catabolism evidenced by elevated urea excretion. Besides testosterone, the inhibitory action of adrenaline and cAMP on muscle protein degradation may have some significance as well.[237,238] However, in rats after administration of sympatholyte the increase in the urea concentrations in the blood, muscle, and liver was less pronounced than in the control experiment.[239] The significance of the inhibitory action of insulin on proteolysis[240] is questionable because of its decrease during exercise.

It was mentioned above that the site of the catabolic response to exercise is within the inactive but not the active muscles. Therefore, at least during acute exercise, the protective effects against the general catabolic action of glucocorticoids may arise directly from the contracting muscles. This question still waits for an answer.

Calcium (Ca^{++}) is a factor stimulating proteolysis in the skeletal muscle[238] (see also p. 206). Therefore, the influence on protein degradation may begin with the release of calcium ions from the sarcoplasmic reticulum during the excitation of the muscle cell. The action of hormones obviously either amplifies or modulates the response primarily induced by Ca^{++}. However, it is not impossible that the *in vivo* accumulation of calcium ions up to the level of stimulating proteolysis is related to the alterations in the function of the calcium pump.

The increased level of glucocorticoids in the blood and hypoinsulinemia common to vigorous exercise provide a stimulus for increased alanine production. Thyroxine may provide an additional stimulus here. The significance of glucocorticoids during exercise has been confirmed in adrenalectomized patients with Cushing's disease. Exercise caused a less pronounced increase in the blood plasma alanine concentration in these patients than it did in normal persons.[207]

J.B. Critz and T.J. Withrow[241] established an increased transaminase activity in the skeletal and heart muscles after swimming. In rats, after adrenalectomy or pharmacological blockade of adrenocortical activity, no increase in transaminase activity was found. Hence, the process of enhanced transamination of amino acids, including alanine formation, is dependent on the adrenocortical activity.

Studies *in vitro* have shown that adrenaline or cAMP application inhibits alanine release from the skeletal muscle. Adrenaline also reduces alanine formation in the muscles obtained

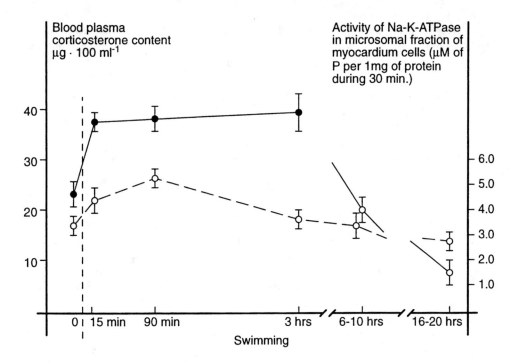

FIGURE 3-10. Dynamics of blood corticosterone level (solid line) and activity of Na,K-ATPase in myocardium during prolonged swimming at 33 to 34°C. From Kôrge, P. Roosson, S., and Oks, M., *Acta Cardiol.*, 29, 303, 1974. With permission.)

from diabetic rats or animals treated with thyroxine or cortisone. However, alanine and glutamine formation from precursor amino acids is unaffected by adrenaline or cAMP application.[242] It seems reasonable to assume that in the exercising normal organism these effects of adrenaline are negligible, as alanine production still rises despite hyperadrenalinemia.

Hypertestosteronemia due to testosterone infusion caused a diminished alanine level during exercise.[243] Therefore, changes in the blood testosterone level may modify the alanine response to exercise. Glucagon or prostaglandin E₁ application did not interfere with alanine and glutamine release by the isolated skeletal muscles.[242]

Besides gluconeogenesis, amino acids may also be used for protein synthesis in the liver during exercise. A decreased incorporation of labeled amino acids into liver proteins was observed in rats sacrificed immediately after swimming for 90 min, while the level of free amino acids in the liver decreased by 43%. Such a combination suggests that the main use of amino acids is probably for gluconeogenesis. Immediately after swimming for 12 h protein synthesis continued to be depressed in the muscle, but returned to normal in the liver tissue. The level of free amino acids remained below normal (by 57%). In this situation the hepatic free amino acid pool was, obviously, also used for protein synthesis to a remarkable extent. In this series in female rats an increased blood corticosterone level was observed only after swimming for 12 h. It was suggested that the augmented adrenocortical activity might be of importance for the restoration of the protein synthesis rate in the liver in conditions of enhanced energy demands.[244] The stimulation of protein synthesis in the liver, amino acid transport into hepatocytes, and gluconeogenesis by glucocorticoids are well established phenomena.

The role of glucocorticoids in the use of free amino acids by the liver during exercise was demonstrated in studies after swimming for 3 h. This exercise caused an increase in the blood corticosterone level, accompanied by a decreased free amino acid level and an augmented alanine aminotransferase activity in the liver of sham-operated rats. In adrenalectomized rats these changes were not observed, but they appeared again when corticosterone was administered to adrenalectomized rats before swimming. While swimming induced a trend to a decreased amino acid level in the muscles of sham-operated rats, in adrenalectomized rats the opposite trend was observed.[244]

Differently from normal rats, adrenal insufficiency excluded the exercise-induced rise in the alanine levels of blood plasma, oxidative muscle, and liver. While in normal rats elevated alanine contents were associated with an increased activity of alanine-aminotransferase in oxidative fibers, in adrenalectomized rats the enzyme activity did not change in muscles and decreased in the hepatic tissue during exercise. The dependence of exercise-induced changes on corticosteroids was confirmed by the increase of the enzyme activity after exercise in adrenalectomized rats treated with 125 µg of corticosterone. In normal rats, training excluded both the rise of blood corticosterone and activation of hepatic alanine-aminotransferase during exercise. Thus, the stimulation of the glucose-alanine cycle by glucocorticoids promotes the alanine supply and utilization in the liver during exercise. In adrenalectomized rats, arginase activity decreased during exercise in conjunction with a lack of further elevation of urea levels in the blood, liver, and skeletal muscles. Consequently, the use of alanine and other amino acids for urea formation depends on glucocorticoids.[245]

Evidence of the dependence of tryptophan oxygenase activity on the induction of enzyme synthesis by glucocorticoids was obtained in experiments with adrenalectomized rats. Hepatic tryptophan oxygenase activity in rats after prolonged swimming was suppressed by adrenalectomy and elevated by administration of cortisol for 5 days prior to adrenalectomized rats. When the RNA synthesis was blocked by treatment with actinomycin D, cortisol did not elevate the enzyme activity.[246] Thus, the change in tryptophan oxygenase activity was founded on the enzyme induction by glucocorticoids.

Despite the general suppression of protein synthesis in skeletal muscles during exercise, the intensified synthesis of some particular proteins during exercise cannot be excluded. For example, during exercise the ^{14}C-leucine incorporation into both myosin heavy chain and actin decreased, but increased into the myosin light chain.[247] Reasonably, there may be an increased synthesis of some regulatory proteins as well.

Swimming caused an elevation of the activity of Na^+,K^+-ATPase. A period of swimming for 90 min was required to detect a statistically significant increase in the enzyme activity in the microsomal fraction of the myocardial cells of untrained rats (Figure 3-10). Further continuation of exercise up to 6 to 10 h was accompanied by the return of the enzyme activity to the initial level. After an extreme duration of exercise (more than 16 h) the Na^+,K^+-ATPase activity decreased significantly. The dynamics of plasma corticosterone concentrations and the activity of myocardial Na^+,K^+-ATPase were approximately parallel during these exercises.[248] In the skeletal muscle with predominantly white fibers the Na^+,K^+-ATPase activity was increased immediately after swimming for 90 min and dropped to the initial level after swimming until exhaustion. In the muscle with predominantly red fibers no significant changes were found. In previously trained rats swimming for 1.5 h did not increase either the plasma level of corticosterone or the myocardial $Na^{+\cdot}K^+$-ATPase activity. After an extreme duration of swimming (18 to 20 h) corticosterone in the blood of trained rats remained at an elevated level and the Na^+,K^+-ATPase activity did not differ from the initial levels.[249] Rats exhausted by a 1-week hard training regimen, exibited a decreased level of corticosterone in the blood and a diminished Na^+,K^+-ATPase activity in the skeletal muscle.[250]

Swimming with an additional load of 3% body weight until exhaustion (mean duration 201 min) caused a substantial increase in the Na^+,K^+-ATPase activity in the myocardial cells of normal rats. In adrenalectomized rats the lowered enzyme activity persisted after the exercise.[251]

These studies led to the suggestion that during prolonged exercises an additional synthesis of Na^+,K^+-ATPase is necessary for maintaining an adequate function of the Na^+,K^+-pump. The induction of this synthesis obviously required a sufficient supply of glucocorticoids.

In conclusion, mobilization of protein resources is the function of the pituitary-adrenocortical system. However, as everywhere in the organism, this function is actualized in complicated cooperation with other regulatory factors. The co-action of various hormones obviously excludes a dangerous exaggeration of the glucocorticoid catabolic action.

HOMEOSTATIC REGULATION OF WATER-ELECTROLYTE BALANCE DURING EXERCISE

During exercise perspiration is called forth to avoid overheating of the body. Water losses by perspiration make it necessary to inhibit diuresis with the aim of preventing dehydration. When total body water declines during work, the level of plasma water is relatively well maintained because there is a rapid exchange of water between the plasma and extravascular sources.[252] Thus, water losses are, in great part, made up from intracellular water. The result is intracellular dehydration, which may impair cellular metabolism. A loss of water of more than 2 to 4% of body mass disturbs the cardiovascular function and causes a decrease in the working capacity in humans.[253] The inhibition of diuresis by stimulating water resorption in the tubulus of nephrons is the function of vasopressin. However, the antidiuretic action of the elevated level of vasopressin can be opposed by the influences of other factors. The main result of vasopressin at the kidney level — the increased tubular resorption of water — is not always revealed during exercise. B. Melin et al.[254] found that during all-out exercise at 80% VO_2max the vasopressin concentration in the plasma increased 4.8 times but the decrease in the urine flow was not statistically significant.

The water content of body fluid compartments depends on osmolality. To check water diuresis independent of plasma and urine osmolality, the free water clearance is calculated. During exercise the free water clearance tended to become positive in humans. This change was in combination with the increased vasopressin concentration in the plasma.[254] During repeated exercises the increases in the vasopressin level and plasma osmolality were simultaneous.[255] Prostaglandins may block the action of vasopressin. Nevertheless, in men an inhibition of prostaglandin synthesis was evoked by aspirin administration for 3 days prior to exercise. This procedure, however, did not influence the alterations in creatine clearance, urine volume, osmolar clearance, and electrolyte excretion.[256]

During exercise the water balance is influenced not only by water losses due to perspiration, diuresis, and exhaled water vapor, but also by the production of water in glycogen breakdown and oxidation processes.[257] It is calculated that during endurance exercises the combustion of glycogen leads to a release of intracellular water that can amount to 1.5 l or more in a well-trained 65-kg athlete.[258] Nevertheless, in humans water losses usually exceed the intracellular water output.

The sweat excreted by humans during exercise is hypotonic, thereby preserving the salt stores.[259] Of all the chemicals lost with sweat, sodium and chlorine make up by far the most. At the same time, these ions are primarily responsible for maintaining the water content of the extracellular compartment.[259] In spite of the fact that in sweat the concentration of sodium and chlorine are roughly one third of that found in the plasma,[259] the total loss of 4.1 l (5.8% reduction in body weight) resulted in Na^+ and Cl^- losses of 155 and 137 mM, respectively, in comparison with K^+ and Mg^{++} losses of 16 and 13 mM. These sweat losses produced a deficit in the body sodium and chlorine of 5 and 7%, respectively. At the same time the total body K^+ and Mg^{++} decreased less than 1.2%.[260]

Therefore, prolonged exercises cause, above all, the loss of ions that are mainly extracellular. In connection with the loss of Na^+ the question arises as how does it act on the transmembrane ion shift that initiates the process of excitation with the cell type-specific physiological response, including the contraction act in the muscle cell? It must be noted that a more pronounced water loss helps to maintain an adequate sodium concentration in the exctracellular compartment and, thereby, avoids the decrease in the ionic gradient for sodium. Usually, during prolonged exercise the sodium concentration in the plasma does not decrease, or it may even increase a little.[259] B. Melin et al.[254] found a significant increase in plasma osmolality during exercise at 80% VO_2max in well-trained sportsmen. In less-trained sportsmen and untrained persons plasma osmolality did not change. However, a critical decrease in the sodium concentration in the extracellular compartment is possible if during exercise sweat losses are replaced by water without any addition of salt.

The renin-angiotensin-aldosterone system controls the sodium level in the extracellular compartment. The main effect of this system is an increased Na^+ resorption with the aim of conserving sodium in the organism. The occurrence of this effect of aldosterone during prolonged exercise has been demonstrated by D.L. Costill et al.[260] This is evidenced also by the decreased sodium concentration and Na/K ratio in the urine as well as by the increased potassium excretion during exercise.[259] The latter is some compensation for the release of potassium from the muscles as a result of glycogen and protein breakdown.[261,262]

V.A. Convertino et al.[263] found a pronounced increase in the plasma volume together with elevated plasma osmolality and albumin content during 8 days of repetitive 2-h cycling at 65% VO_2max. They associate the plasma hypervolaemia with the rise in plasma vasopressin as well as renin concentration that stimulate aldosterone production through conversion of angiotensin I to angiotensin II. Additionally, the rise in albumin concentration provided increased water-binding capacity for the blood. During a 500-km road race that extended over 20 days, ordinary flow rates, creatinine clearance, osmotic clearance, and free water clearance as well as urinary excretion of vasopressin showed no significant change in the runners. Plasma osmolality and urinary aldosterone excretion increased. As a result of aldosterone action, the urinary sodium concentration and the percentage of filtered sodium excreted were significantly lowered on the days of running.

The distribution of water and electrolytes between the extra- and intracellular compartments and the rate of related transmembrane shifts depends on the Na,K-pump function. The energy for the Na,K-pump activity is provided by hydrolysis of ATP. The activity of Na,K-ATPase catalyzing this process depends on shifts in sodium and potassium concentrations between the extra- and intracellular compartments. At the same time, hormones also exert their action on the enzyme.

Studies of the Na,K-pump function in exercise gave two main results. First, after a very prolonged period of exercise the efficiency of the Na,K-pump decreased in the myocardial and skeletomuscular cells in association with the reduced Na,K-ATPase activity. As a consequence, sodium ions are not eliminated from the muscle cells and their concentration increases.[248,249] The resultant increase in the osmotic pressure of the intracellular compartment causes the accumulation of water inside the cells. The second main result was the relation of these changes to the decreased adrenocortical activity (see above). Later the activation of the Na,K-pump function by exercise was confirmed.[264] Under resting conditions *in vitro* less than 10% of the total population of Na,K-pumps in skeletal muscles is utilized.[264] Hence, there is a considerable spare capacity for active Na,K-transport to be used during exercise. Nevertheless, the muscle contains too few Na,K-pumps to maintain its K^+ content when assuming full activation of all the available Na,K-pumps. These estimates are in keeping with the observation that during contractile activity, muscles undergo a net loss of K^+.[265] Therefore, the concentration of Na,K-pumps in skeletal muscle is rate limiting for the K^+ homeostasis during exercise.[264] A wide variety of studies have shown that adrenaline and noradrenaline at

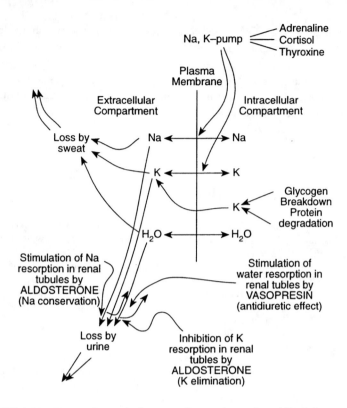

FIGURE 3-11. Hormonal control of water, sodium, and potassium shifts during exercise.

physiological concentrations stimulate active Na^+,K^+-transport in muscle fibers by up to 100% within a few minutes.[266,267] The regulative significance of the exercise-induced increase in catecholamine levels is indicated by the fact that hyperkalaemia caused by exercise is exaggerated when the β-adrenoreceptors are blocked.[264] Activation of the Na,K-pump is induced also by insulin.[264] However, the drop of insulin secretion during exercise makes this regulatory influence doubtful during acute exercise.

Training produces an increase in the Na,K-ATPase activity in the sarcolemma[268] as well as the total concentration of [^{3}H]-ouabain binding sites (Na,K-pumps) in muscle biopsies.[269,270] This effect may be related to the thyroid hormone-induced up-regulation of Na,K-pump concentration.[264,271] Figure 3-11 sums up the role of hormones in control of the water-electrolyte balance.

FIGURE 3-12. Dynamics of calcium (interrupted line) and calcitonin (solid line) levels in blood plasma during prolonged exercise. (From Drzevetskaya, I. A., and Limanskii, N. N., *Sechenov Physiol. J. USSR*, 64, 1498, 1978. With permission.)

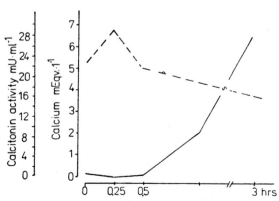

Powerful regulators of calcium metabolism are calcitonin and parathormone. Data were presented that showed that during prolonged exercise[272] the dynamics of calcium concentration in the blood plasma was reciprocal to the increase in the plasma calcitonin activity, obviously reflecting the effect of the hormone (Figure 3-12). At the end of a 20-min exercise increased levels of total and ionized calcium were observed in association with the increase in calcitonin and the decrease in parathormone levels.[273]

REFERENCES

1. **Viru, A.**, Adaptive regulation of hormone interaction with receptor, *Exp. Clin. Endocrin.*, 97, 13, 1991.
2. **Koivisto, V.A., Soman, V., Conrad, P., Hendler, R., Nadel, E., and Felig, P.**, Insulin binding to monocytes in trained athletes, *J. Clin. Invest.*, 64, 1011, 1979.
3. **Koivisto, V.A., Soman, V., and Felig, P.**, Effects of acute exercise on insulin binding to monocytes in obesity, *Metabolism*, 29, 168, 1980.
4. **Bieger, W.P., Weiss, M., and Weicker, H.**, Insulin affinity and hormone-dependent activity of human circulating monocytes after exercise, in *Biochemistry of Exercise IV-A*, Poortmans, J. and Niset, G., Eds., University Park Press, Baltimore, 1981, 163.
5. **Okuno, J., Fujii, S., Okada, K., Tabota, T., Tanaka, S., and Wada, M.**, Effects of acute exercise on insulin binding to erythrocytes in normal man, *Horm. Metab. Res.*, 15, 366, 1983.
6. **Michel, G., Vocke, T., Fiehn, W., Weicker, H., Schwarz, W., and Bieger, W.P.**, Bidirectional alteration of insulin receptor affinity by different forms of physical exercise, *Am. J. Physiol.*, 246, E156, 1984.
7. **Michel, G., Schwarz, W., and Bieger, W.P.**, Exercise-induced regulation of insulin receptor affinity: role of circulating metabolites, *Int. J. Sports Med.*, 6, 100, 1985.
8. **Soman, V.R., Koivisto, V.A., Grantham, P., and Felig, P.**, Increased insulin binding to monocytes after exercise in normal man, *J. Clin. Endocrin.*, 47, 216, 1978.
9. **Pedersen, O., Beck-Nielsen, H., and Heding, L.**, Increased insulin receptors after exercise in patients with insulin-dependent diabetes mellitus, *N. Engl. J. Med.*, 301, 886, 1980.
10. **Clune, P., Bonen, A., Sopper, M.M., Hood, D., and Tan, M.H.**, Insulin binding to rodent skeletal muscle after exhaustive exercise, *Med. Sci. Sports*, 14, 150, 1982.
11. **Webster, B.A., Vigna, S.R., and Paquette, T.**, Acute exercise, epinephrine and diabetes enhance insulin binding to skeletal muscle, *Am. J. Physiol.*, 250, E186, 1986.
12. **Treadway, J.L., James, D.E., Burcel, E., and Ruderman, N.B.**, Effect of exercise on insulin receptor binding and kinase activity in skeletal muscle, *Am. J. Physiol.*, 256, E138, 1989.
13. **Bonen, A., Tan, M.H., Clune, P., and Kirby, R.L.**, Effects of exercise on insulin binding to human muscle, *Am. J. Physiol.*, 248, E403, 1985.
14. **Pedersen, O., and Bak, J.**, Effect of acute exercise and physical training on insulin receptor and insulin action, in *Biochemistry of Exercise VI*, Saltin, B., Ed., Human Kinetics, Champaign, 1986, 87.
15. **Koivisto, V.A., and Yki-Järvinen, H.**, Effect of exercise on insulin binding and glucose transport in adipocytes of normal humans, *J. Appl. Physiol.*, 63, 1319, 1987.
16. **Sendrail, M., and Blancardi, C.**, Action du travail musculaire sur la sensibilite a l'insuline, *C.R. Soc. Biol.*, 110, 1190, 1932.
17. **Richter, E.A., Garetto, L.P., Goodman, M.N., and Ruderman, N.B.**, Muscle metabolism following exercise in rat. Increased sensitivity to insulin, *J. Clin. Invest.*, 69, 785, 1982.
18. **Ivy, J.L., Sherman, W.M., Miller, W., Farrell, S., and Frishberg, B.**, Glycogen synthesis: effect of diet and training, in *Biochemistry of Exercise*, Knuttgen, H.G., Vogel, J.A., and Poortmans, K., Eds., Human Kinetics, Champaign, 1983, 291.
19. **Mikenes, K.J., Sonne, B., Farrell, P.A., Tronier, B., and Galbo, H.**, Effect of physical exercise on sensitivity and responsiveness to insulin in humans, *Am. J. Physiol.*, 254, E248, 1988.
20. **Savard, R., Després, J.-P., Marcotte, M., Thériault, G., Tremblay, A., and Bouchard, C.**, Acute effects of endurance exercise on human adipose tissue metabolism, *Metabolism*, 36, 480, 1987.
21. **Chapler, C.K.**, Effects of propranol and epinephrine infusion on glycogenolysis in dog skeletal muscle in situ, *Can. J. Physiol. Pharmacol.*, 50, 471, 1971.
22. **Dill, D.B., Edwards, H.T., and deMeio, R.H.**, Effect of adrenaline injection in moderate work, *Am. J. Physiol.*, 111, 9, 1935.
23. **Yakovlev, N.N.**, Dependence of carbohydrate-phosphorus metabolism in working muscles on the state of central nervous system, *Ukr. Biokhim. Zh.*, 27, 444, 1955.

24. **Gorski, J.**, Exercise-induced changes of reactivity of different types of muscle on glycogenolytic effect of adrenaline, *Pflügers Arch. Ges. Physiol.*, 373, 1, 1978.

25. **Koivisto, V., Akerblom, H.K., and Nikkilä, E.A.**, Carbohydrate and lipid metabolism during exercise in experimental diabetes, *Acta Endocrin.*, 32 (Suppl. 203), 3, 1976.

26. **Friedman, D.B., Ordway, G.A., and Williams, R.S.**, Exercise-induced functional desensitization of canine cardiac β-adrenergic receptors, *J. Appl. Physiol.*, 62, 1721, 1987.

27. **Crampes, F., Beauville, M., Riviere, D., Garrigues, M., and Lafontan, M.**, Lack of desensitization of catecholamine-induced lipolysis in fat cells from trained and sedentary women after physical exercise, *J. Clin. Endocrin.*, 67, 1011, 1988.

28. **Bieger, W., Zittel, R., Zappe, H., and Weicker, H.**, Einfluß körperlicher Aktivität auf du Katecholaminrezeptor-Regulation, in *Sport: Leistung and Gesundheit*, Heck, H., Holmann, W., Liesen, H., and Rost, R., Eds., Deutch Arzte Verlag, Köln, 1983, 271.

29. **Landmann, R., Portenier, M., Staehelin, M., Wesp, M., and Box, R.**, Changes in β-adrenoreceptors and leucocyte subpopulation after physical exercise in normal subjects, *Naunyn-Schmiedeberg's Arch. Pharmacol.*, 337, 261, 1988.

30. **Mäki, T.**, Density and functioning of human lyphocytic β-adrenergic receptors during prolonged physical exercise, *Acta Physiol. Scand.*, 136, 569, 1989.

31. **Graafsma, S.J., Van Tits, L.J.H., Willems, R.H.G.M., Hectors, M.D.C., Rodrigues de Miranda, J.F., De Point, J.J.H.H.M., and Thien, T.**, β₂-adrenoceptor up-regulation in regulation to cAMP production in human lymphocytes after physical exercise, *Br. J. Clin. Pharmacol.*, 30 (Suppl. 1), 142, 1990.

32. **Davies, A.D.**, Exercise-induced fall in coupling of human β₂-adrenergic receptors, *Metabolism*, 37, 916, 1988.

33. **Werle, E.O., Strobel, G., and Weicker, H.**, Decrease in rat cardiac beta₁- and beta₂-adrenoreceptors by training and endurance exercise, *Life Sci.*, 46, 9, 1990.

34. **Lehmann, M., Hasler, K., Bergdolt, E., and Keul, J.**, Alpha 2-adrenoreceptor density on intact platelets and adrenaline-induced platelet aggregation in endurance and nonendurance trained subjects, *Int. J. Sports Med.*, 7, 172, 1986.

35. **Tchaikovsky, V.S., Astratenkova, I.V., and Basharina, O.B.**, The effect of exercise on the content and receptor of the steroid hormones in rat skeletal muscles, *J. Steroid Biochem.*, 24, 251, 1986.

36. **Tchaikovsky, V.S., Rogozkin, V.A., and Ivanova, E.M.**, Influence of anabolic steroids on testosterone contents and reception during physical exercise, in *16th Meet. FEBS. Abstr.*, Moscow, 1984, 426.

37. **Kôrge, P., and Medijainen, L.**, The effect of isoprenaline and physical exertion to exhaustion on the mechanism of glucocorticoid action in the rat heart, *J. Mol. Cell. Cardiol.*, 18. 557, 1986.

38. **Kôrge, P., Vigel, E., and Timpmann, S.**, The effect of physical exertions on the content of nonactivated glucocorticoid receptor in the heart cytosol: a finding supporting the nuclear localization of free receptor, *Clin. Physiol.*, 5 (Suppl. 4), 30, 1985.

39. **Czerwinski, S.M., and Hickson, R.C.**, Glucocorticoid receptor activation during exercise in muscle, *J. Appl. Physiol.*, 68, 1615, 1990.

40. **Viru, A. and Toode, K.**, Modulierende Regulation von Hormoneffekten bei Muskulärer Aktivität, in *Sportmedizinische Forschung*, Weiss, M. and Rieder, H., Eds., Springer-Verlag, Berlin, 1991, 83.

41. **Salzman, S.H., Hirsch, E.Z., Hellerstein, H.K., and Bruell, J.H.**, Adaptation to muscular exercise: myo-cardial epinephrine ³H-uptake, *J. Appl. Physiol.*, 29, 92, 1970.

42. **Chase, J.M., Hamilin, R.L., Fox, E.L., and Bartels, R.L.**, Intrinsic heart rate and beta-adrenergic receptor number in trained and untrained swine, *Med. Sci. Sports Exerc.*, 13, 129, 1981.

43. **Moore, R.L., Riedy, M., and Gollnick, P.D.**, Effect of training on β-adrenergic receptor number in rat heart, *J. Appl. Physiol.*, 52, 1133, 1982.

44. **Takeda, N., Daniniak, P., Turck, D., Rupp, H., and Jacov, K.**, The influence of endurance training on catecholamine responsiveness, β-adrenoreceptor density and myosin isozyme pattern of rat ventricular myocardium, *Basic Res. Cardiol.*, 80, 88, 1985.

45. **Lehmann, M., Dickhuth, H.H., Schmid, P., Porzig, H., and Keul, J.**, Plasma catecholamines, β-adrenergic receptors, and isoproterenol sensitivity in endurance trained and nonendurance trained volunteers, *Eur. J. Appl. Physiol.*, 52, 362, 1984.

46. **Williams, R.S., Eden, R.S., Moll, M.E., Lester, R.M., and Wallance, A.G.**, Autonomic mechanism of training bradycardia: β-adrenergic receptors in humans, *J. Appl. Physiol.*, 51, 1232, 1981.

47. **Butler, J., Brien, M.O., Malley, K.O., and Kelly, J.G.**, Relationship of β-adrenoreceptor density to fitness in athletes, *Nature (London)*, 298, 60, 1982.

48. **Jost, J., Weiss, M., and Weicker, H.**, Comparison of sympathoadrenergic regulation at rest and of the adrenoceptor system in swimmers, long-distance runners, weight-lifters, wrestlers and untrained men, *Eur. J. Appl. Physiol.*, 58, 596, 1989.

49. **Lehmann, M., Schmid, P., Bergdalt, E., Jacob, E., Spöri, U., and Keul, J.**, Ist die Alpha-Adrenorezeptorendichte an intakten Trombozyten bei statisch strainierten Athleters erhöht?, *Klin. Wochenchr.*, 62, 992, 1984.

50. **Lackette, W., McCurdy, R., Smith, S., and Carreto, O.**, Endurance training and human α_2-adrenergic receptors on platelets, *Med. Sci. Sports Exerc.*, 19, 7, 1987.

51. **Nakamura, T., Kitayama, I., and Nomura, N.**, Effect of forced-running stress on β-adrenergic receptors in rat brain and liver, *Neurosci. Res. Suppl.*, 9, 151, 1989.

52. **Després, J.P., Savard, R., Tremblay, A., and Bouchard, C.**, Adipocyte diameter and lipolytic activity in marathon runners. Relationship to body fatness, *Eur. J. Appl. Physiol.*, 51, 223, 1989.

53. **Després, J.P., Bouchard, C., Savard, R., Tremblay, A., Marcotte, M., and Theriault, M.**, Effects of exercise-training and detraining on fat cell lipolysis in men and women, *Eur. J. Appl. Physiol.*, 53, 25, 1984.

54. **Crampes, F., Beauville, M., Riviere, D., and Garrigues, M.**, Effect of physical training in humans on the response of isolated fat cells to epinephrine, *J. Appl. Physiol.*, 61, 25, 1986.

55. **Crampes,, F., Riviere, D., Beauville, M., Marceron, M., and Garrigues, M.**, Lipolytic response of adipocytes to epinephrine in sedentary and exercise-trained subjects: sex-related differences, *Eur. J. Appl. Physiol.*, 59, 249, 1989.

56. **LeBlanc, J., Boulay, M., Dulac, S., Jobin, M., Labrie, A., and Rousseau-Migneron, S.**, Metabolic and cardiovascular responses to norepinephrine in trained and nontrained human subjects, *J. Appl. Physiol.*, 42, 166, 1977.

57. **Valliers, J., and Thibault, M.C.**, Norepinephrine mobilization of free fatty acids in endurance trained rats, *Med. Sci. Sports Exerc.*, 12, 133, 1980.

58. **Viru, A., Toode, K., and Eller, A.**, Adipocyte responses to adrenaline and insulin in active and former sportsmen, *Eur. J. Appl. Physiol.*, 64, 345, 1992.

59. **Askew, E.W., Dohm, G.L., Huston, R.L., Sneed, T.W., and Dowdy, R.R.**, Response of rat tissue lipases to physical training and exercise, *Proc. Soc. Exp. Biol. Med.*, 141, 123, 1972.

60. **Owens, J.L., Tullet, E.O., Nutter, D.O., and Girolamo, M.**, Influence of moderate exercise on adipocyte metabolism and hormonal responsiveness, *J. Appl. Physiol.*, 43, 425, 1977.

61. **Bukowiecki, L., Lupien, J., Collea, N., Paradis, A., Richard, D., and LeBlanc, J.**, Mechanism of enhanced lipolysis in adipose tissue of exercise-trained rats, *Am. J. Physiol.*, 239, E422, 1980.

62. **Toode, K., Viru, A., and Eller, A.**, Lipolytic action of hormones on adipocytes in exercise-trained organism, *Jpn. J. Physiol.*, 43, 253, 1993.

63. **Yakovlev, N.N.**, The role of sympathetic nervous system in the adaptation of skeletal muscle to increased activity, in *Metabolic Adaptation to Prolonged Physical Exercise*, Howald, H. and Poortmans, J.R., Eds., Birkhäuser Verlag, Basel, 1975, 293.

64. **Shephard, R.E., Semberowich, W.L., Green, H.E., and Gollnick, P.D.**, Effect of physical training on control mechanisms of lipolysis in rat fat cell ghosts, *J. Appl. Physiol.*, 42, 884, 1977.

65. **Askew, E.W., Hecker, A.L., Coppes, V.G., and Stifel, F.B.**, Cyclic AMP metabolism in adipose tissue of exercise-trained rats, *J. Lipid Res.*, 19, 729, 1978.

66. **Shephard, R.E., Noble, E.G., Klug, G.A., and Gollnick, P.D.**, Lipolysis and cAMP accumulation in adipocytes in response to physical training, *J. Appl. Physiol.*, 50, 143, 1981.

67. **Niyazmukhamedov, M.B., and Yakovlev, N.N.**, Changes of 3′,5′-AMP-phosphodiesterase activity and inactivation of insulin during muscular exercise, *Sechenov Physiol. J. USSR*, 62, 768, 1976 (in Russian).

68. **Palmer, W.K.**, Effect of exercise on cardiac cyclic AMP, *Med. Sci. Sports Exerc.*, 20, 525, 1988.

69. **Thibault, M.C., Côté, C., Valliers, J., LeBlanc, J., and Bukowiecki, L.**, cAMP phosphodiesterase and phosphorylase in rats following endurance training, isoproterenol treatment and cold exposure, *Med. Sci. Sports*, 10. 41, 1978.

70. **Palmer, W.K., Kalina, C.A., Studney, T.A., and Oscai, L.B.**, Exercises and the cAMP system in rat adipose tissue. II. Nucleotide catabolism, *J. Appl. Physiol.*, 50, 255, 1981.

71. **Oscai, L.B., Caruso, R.A., Wergeles, A.C., and Palmer, W.K.**, Exercise and the cAMP system in rat adipose tissue. I. Lipid mobilization, *J. Appl. Physiol.*, 50, 250, 1981.

72. **Kalinski, M.I., Kurski, M.D., Zemtsova, I.L., and Ossipenko, A.A.**, Alterations of some properties of cAMP-dependent proteinkinases of skeletal muscles in training with physical exercises, *Biochimia*, 46, 120, 1981 (in Russian).

73. **Kurskij, M.D., Ossipenko, A.A., Kalinski, M.I., and Kondratjuk, T.P.**, Some properties of rat skeletal muscle adenosine-3′,5′-monophosphate-dependent protein kinase at normal state and after long-term physical loading up to fatigue, *Biochimia*, 43, 1676, 1978 (in Russian).

74. **Kalinski, M.J., Zemtsova, I.I., Kurskij, M.P., and Ossipenko, A.A.**, Action of training and exercise on 3′,5′-AMP content and activity of enzymes of its metabolism in rat muscles, *Ukr. Biokhim. Zh.*, 52, 611, 1980 (in Russian).

75. **Zemtsova, I.I., Kalinski, M.I., Kurski, M.D., and Ossipenko, A.A.**, Action of termostabile protein inhibitor on activity of 3′,5′-AMP-depednent proteinkinase of skeletal muscles during training with prolonged physical exercise, *Dokl. Akad. Nauk. Ukrain SSR*, 5(2), 72, 1981 (in Russian).

76. **Björntrop, P.K., deJounge, K.S., Sjöstrand, L., and Sullivan, L.**, The effect of physical training on insulin production in obesity, *Metabolism*, 19, 631, 1970.

77. **Johansen, K., and Munck, O.**, The relationship between maximal oxygen uptake and glucose tolerance/ insulin response ratio in normal young men, *Horm. Metab. Res.*, 11, 424, 1979.
78. **Kahle, E.B., O'Dorisio, T.M., Walker, R.B., Eisenman, P.A., Reiser, S., Cataland, S., and Zipf, W.B.**, Exercise adaptation responses for gastric inhibitory polypeptide (GIP) and insulin in obese children. Possible extra-pancreatic effects, *Diabetes*, 35, 579, 1986.
79. **Kjaer, M., Mikenes, K.J., Christensen, N.J., Tronier, B., Vinten, J., Sonne, B., Richter, E.A., and Galbo, H.**, Glucose turnover and hormonal changes during insulin-induced hypoglycemia in trained humans, *J. Appl. Physiol.*, 57, 21, 1984.
80. **Mikenes, K.J., Sonne, B., Farrell, P.A., Tronier, B., and Galbo, H.**, Effect of training on the dose-response relationship for insulin action in man, *J. Appl. Physiol.*, 66, 695, 1989.
81. **Sato, Y., Hayamizu, S., Yamamoto, C., Okhuwa, Y., Yamanouchi, K., and Sakamoto, N.**, Improved insulin sensitivity in carbohydrate and lipid metabolism after physical training, *Int. J. Sports Med.*, 7, 307, 1986.
82. **James, D.E., Burleigh, K.M., Kraegen, E.W., and Chisholm, D.J.**, Effect of acute exercise and prolonged training on insulin response to intravenous glucose *in vivo* in rat, *J. Appl. Physiol.*, 55, 1660, 1983.
83. **Kemmer, F.W., Berger, M., Herberg, L., and Gries, F.-D.**, Effects of physical training on glucose tolerance and on glucose metabolism of isolated muscle in normal rats, *Diabetologia*, 13, 407, 1977.
84. **Espinal, J., Dohm, G.L., and Newsholme, E.A.**, Sensitivity to insulin of glycolysis and glycogen synthesis of isolated soleus-muscle strips from sedentary exercised and exercise-trained rats, *Biochem. J.*, 212, 453, 1983.
85. **Kral, J.G., Jacobsson, B., Smith, U., and Björntrop, P.**, The effects of physical exercise on fat cell metabolism in the rat, *Acta Physiol. Scand.*, 90, 664, 1974.
86. **Craig, B.W., Hammons, G.T., Garthwaite, S.M., Jarett, L., and Holloszy, J.O.**, Adaptation of fat cells to exercise: response of glucose uptake and oxidation to insulin, *J. Appl. Physiol.*, 51, 1500, 1981.
87. **Vinter, J., and Galbo, H.**, Effect of physical training on transport and metabolism of glucose in adipocytes, *Am. J. Physiol.*, 244, E129, 1983.
88. **Savard, R., Després, J.P., Deshaies, Y., Marcotte, M., and Bouchard, C.**, Adipose tissue lipid accumulation pathways in marathon runners, *Int. J. Sports Med.*, 6, 287, 1985.
89. **Vinten, J., Norgaard-Petersen, L., Sonne, B., and Galbo, H.**, Effect of physical training on glucose transporters in fat cell fractions, *Biochim. Biophys. Acta*, 841, 223, 1985.
90. **Mondon, C.E., Dolkas, C.B., and Reaven, G.M.**, Site of enhanced insulin sensitivity in exercise trained rats at rest, *Am. J. Physiol.*, 239, E169, 1980.
91. **Niyazmukhammedov, M.B.**, On the analysis of increased sensitivity to insulin, *Sechenov Physiol. J. USSR*, 62, 626, 1976 (in Russian).
92. **Niyazmukhammedov, M.B., and Yakovlev, N.N.**, Changes of 3',5'-AMP phosphodiesterase activity and inactivation of insulin during muscular activity, *Sechenov Physiol. J. USSR*, 62, 768, 1976 (in Russian).
93. **Soman, V.R., Koivisto, V.A., Deibert, D., Felig, P., and De Franzo, R.A.**, Increased insulin sensitivity and insulin binding to monocytes after physical training, *N. Engl. J. Med.*, 301, 1200, 1979.
94. **LeBlanc, J., Nadeau, A., Boulay, M., and Rousseau-Migneron, S.**, Effects of physical training and adiposity on glucose metabolism and ^{125}J-insulin binding, *J. Appl. Physiol.*, 46, 235, 1979.
95. **Burnstein, R., Polychronakos, C., Toews, C.J., MacDoughall, J.D., Guyda, H.J., and Posner, B.I.**, Acute reversal of the enhanced insulin action in trained athletes. Association with insulin receptor changes, *Diabetes*, 34, 756, 1985.
96. **Krzentowski, G., Pirnay, F., Luyckx, A., Lacroix, M., Mosara, F., and Lefebvre, P.**, Effects of training on glucose oxidation, *Int. J. Sports Med.*, 3 (Abstractservice), 1982.
97. **Tan, M.H., and Bonen, A.**, Physical training enhances insulin binding and glucose uptake by skeletal muscle, *Clin. Invest. Med.*, 5, 39B, 1982.
98. **Dohm, G.L., Sinha, M.K., and Caro, J.F.**, Insulin receptor binding and protein kinase activity in muscles of trained rats, *Am. J. Physiol.*, 252, E170, 1987.
99. **Wirth, A., Holm, G., Nilsson, B., Smith, U., and Björntrop, P.**, Insulin kinetics and insulin binding to adipocytes in physically trained and foot-restricted rats, *Am. J. Physiol.*, 238, E108, 1980.
100. **Yakovlev, N.N.**, Changes of the organism's sensitivity to adrenocorticotropin elicited by the adaptation to increased muscular activity, *Sechenov Physiol. J. USSR*, 63, 320, 1977 (in Russian).
101. **Frenkl, R., Csalay, L., Csákváry, G., and Lángfy, G.**, Untersuchung der ACTH-Wirkung auf den Steroidspiegel des Plasmas in trainierten and im untrainierten Organismus, *Med. Sport*, 10, 122, 1970.
102. **Frenkl, R., and Csálay, L.**, The effect of regular muscular activity on adrenocortical function in rats, *J. Sports Med. Phys. Fitness*, 2, 207, 1962.
103. **Frenkl, R., Csálay, L., and Csákváry, G.**, Further experimental results concerning the relationship of muscular exercise and adrenal function, *Endokrinologie*, 66, 285, 1975.
104. **Tharp, G.D., and Buuck, R.**, Adrenal adaptation to chronic exercise, *J. Appl. Physiol.*, 37, 720, 1974.
105. **Viru, A.**, *Hormones in Muscular Activity*, Vol. II, CRC Press, Boca Raton, FL, 1985.

106. **Hickson, R.C., and Davis, J.R.**, Partial prevention of glucocorticoid-induced muscle atrophy by endurance training, *Am. J. Physiol.*, 241, E226, 1981.

107. **Seene, T., and Viru, A.**, The catabolic effect of glucocorticoid on different types of skeletal muscle fibers and its dependence upon muscle activity and interaction with anabolic steroids, *J. Steroid Biochem.*, 16, 349, 1982.

108. **Czerwinski, S.M., Zak, R., Kurowski, T.T., Falduto, M.T., and Hickson, R.C.**, Myosin heavy chain turnover and glucocorticoid deterrence by exercise in muscle, *J. Appl. Physiol.*, 67, 2311, 1989.

109. **Eller, A., Nyskas, C., Szabo, G., and Endröczi, E.**, Corticosterone binding in myocardial tissue of rats after chronic stress and adrenalectomy, *Acta Physiol. Acad. Sci. Hung.*, 53, 205, 1981.

110. **Kurowski, T.T., Chatterton, R.T., and Hickson, R.C.**, Glucocorticoid-induced cardiac hypertrophy: additive effects of exercise, *J. Appl. Physiol.*, 57, 514, 1984.

111. **Hickson, R.C., Calassi, T.M., Kurowski, T.T., Daniels, D.G., and Chatterton, R.T.**, Androgen and glucocorticoid mechanisms in exercise-induced cardiac hypertrophy, *Am. J. Physiol.*, 246, H761, 1984.

112. **Feldkoren, B.J., and Kosedub, T.N.**, Effect of anabolic steroids on content of corticosterone in adrenals during systematic physical exercise, *Acta Comment. Univ. Tartuensis*, 562, 114, 1982 (in Russian).

113. **McMannus, B.M., Lamb, D.R., Judis, J.J., and Scala, J.**, Skeletal muscle leucine incorporation and testosterone uptake in exercised guinea pigs, *Eur. J. Appl. Physiol.*, 34, 149, 1975.

114. **Hickson, R.C., Kurowski, T.T., Capaccio, J.A., and Chatterton, R.T.**, Androgen cytosol binding in exercise-induced sparing of muscle atrophy, *Am. J. Physiol.*, 247, E597, 1984.

115. **Feldkoren, B.J.**, The effect of retabolil and training on synthesis of ribosomal RNA in skeletal muscle, in *Medicine and Sport*, Rogozkin, V., Litvinova, V., and Hakina, J., Eds., Leningrad, Research Institute of Physical Culture, 1979, 124.

116. **Fain, J.N., Kovacev, V.P., and Scow, R.O.**, Effect of growth hormone and dexamethasone on lipolysis and metabolism in isolated fat cells of the rat, *J. Biol. Chem.*, 240, 3522, 1965.

117. **Freund, B.J., Claynaugh, J.R., Dice, M.S., and Mashiro, G.M.**, Hormonal and vascular fluid response to maximal exercise in trained and untrained males, *J. Appl. Physiol.*, 63, 669, 1987.

118. **Yakovlev, N.N.**, The role of insulin and adrenalin in the anaerobious phase of carbohydrate metabolism in the muscles, *Bull. Inst. Sci. Lesshaft.*, 21(3), 65, 1938.

119. **Yakovlev, N.N., and Viru, A.**, Adrenergic regulation of adaptation to muscular activity, *Int. J. Sports Med.*, 6, 255, 1985.

120. **Dietz, M.R., Chilasson, J.-L., Soderling, T.R., and Exton, J.H.**, Epinephrine regulation of skeletal muscle glycogen metabolism, *J. Biol. Chem.*, 255, 2301, 1980.

121. **Uusitupa, M., Siitonen, O., Härkönen, M., Arv, A., Hermaa, R., and Gordin, A.**, The metabolic and hormonal effects of selective and non-selective beta-blockade during physical exercise, *Acta Endocrin.*, 94 (Suppl. 237), 84, 1980.

122. **Issekutz, B.**, Role of beta-adrenergic receptors in mobilization of energy sources in exercising dogs, *J. Appl. Physiol.*, 44, 869, 1978.

123. **Malig, H., Stern, D., Altland, P., Highman, B., and Brode, B.**, The physiologic role of the sympathetic nervous system in exercise, *J. Pharmacol. Exp. Ther.*, 154, 35, 1966.

124. **Górski, J., and Pietrzyk, K.**, The effect of beta-adrenergic receptor blockade on intramuscular glycogen mobilization during exercise, *Eur. J. Appl. Physiol.*, 48, 201, 1982.

125. **Juhlin-Dannfelt, A., and Aström, H.**, Influence of β-adrenoceptor blockade on leg blood flow and lactate release in man, *Scand. J. Clin. Lab. Invest.*, 39, 179, 1979.

126. **Trudeau, F., Péronnet, F., Béliveau, L., and Brisson, G.**, Metabolic and endocrine responses to prolonged exercise in rats under β_2-adrenergic blockade, *Can. J. Physiol. Pharmacol.*, 67, 192, 1989.

127. **Chasiotis, D., Brandt, R., Harris, R.C., and Hultman, E.**, Effects of β-blockade on glycogen metabolism in human subjects during exercise, *Am. J. Physiol.*, 245, E166, 1983.

128. **Gollnick, P.D., Soule, R.G., Taylor, A.W., Williams, C., and Ianuzzo, C.D.**, Exercise-induced glycogenolysis and lipolysis in the rat: hormonal influence, *Am. J. Physiol.*, 219, 729, 1970.

129. **Kaisser, P.**, Physical performance and muscle metabolism during β-adrenergic blockade in man, *Acta Physiol. Scand., Suppl.*, 536, 1984.

130. **Nazar, K., Brzerzinska, Z., and Kozlowski, S.**, Sympathetic activity during prolonged physical exercise in dogs: control of energy substrate utilization, in *Metabolic Adaptation to Prolonged Physical Exercise*, Howald, H., and Poortmans, J.R., Eds., Birkhäuser Verlag, Basel, 1975, 204.

131. **Gollnick, P.D., Karlson, J., Piehl, K., and Saltin, B.**, Phosphorylase a in human skeletal muscle during exercise and electrical stimultion, *J. Appl. Physiol.*, 45, 852, 1978.

132. **Péronnet, F., and Imbach, A.**, Endurance and metabolic adjustments to exercise in sympathectomized (6-OHDA) rats, in *Biochemistry of Exercise*, Knuttgen, H.G., Vogel, J.A., and Poortmans, J., Eds., Human Kinetics, Champaign, 1983, 762.

133. **Cartier, L.-J., and Gollnick, P.D.**, Sympathoadrenal system and activation of glycogenolysis during muscular activity, *J. Appl. Physiol.*, 58, 1122, 1985.

134. **Trudeau, F., Péronnet, F., Béliveau, L., and Brisson, B.**, Sympatho-endocrine and metabolic responses to exercise under post-ganglionic blockade in rats, *Horm. Metab. Res.*, 20, 546, 1988.
135. **Bloom, W.L., and Russel, J.A.**, Effects of epinephrine and norepinephrine on carbohydrate metabolism in rats, *Am. J. Physiol.*, 183, 356, 1955.
136. **Hashimoto, I., Knudson, M.B., Noble, E.G., Klug, G.A., and Gollnick, P.D.**, Exercise-induced glycogen mobilization in sympthectomized rats, *Med. Sci. Sports*, 11, 75, 1979.
137. **Richter, E.A., Galbo, H., and Christensen, N.J.**, Control of exercise-induced muscular glycogenolysis by adrenal medullary hormones in rats, *J. Appl. Physiol.*, 50, 21, 1981.
138. **Marker, J.C., Arnall, D.A., Conlee, R.K., and Winder, W.W.**, Effect of adrenodemedullation in metabolic responses to high-intensity exercise, *Am. J. Physiol.*, 251, R552, 1986.
139. **Galbo, H., Richter, E., Christensen, N.J., and Holst, J.J.**, Sympathetic control of metabolic and hormonal response to exercise in rats, *Acta Physiol. Scand.*, 102, 441, 1978.
140. **Richter, E.A., Galbo, H., Sonne, B., Holst, J.J., and Christensen, N.J.**, Adrenal medullary control of muscular and hepatic glycogenolysis and of pancreatic hormonal secretion in exercising rats, *Acta Physiol. Scand.*, 108, 235, 1980.
141. **Spriet, L.L., Ren, J.M., and Hultman, E.**, Epinephrine infusion enhances muscle glycogenolysis during prolonged electrical stimulation, *J. Appl. Physiol.*, 64, 1439, 1988.
142. **Nesher, R., Karl, I.E., and Kipnis, D.M.**, Epitrochlearis muscle. II. Metabolic effects of contraction and catecholamines, *Am. J. Physiol.*, 239, E461, 180.
143. **Conlee, R.K., McLane, J.A., Rennie, M.J., Winder, W.W., and Holloszy, J.O.**, Reversal of phosphorylase activation in muscle despite continued contractile activity, *Am. J. Physiol.*, 237, R291, 1979.
144. **Fell, R.D., Holloszy, J.O., Ivy, J.L., and Rennie, M.J.**, Adrenaline reactivates muscle phosphorylase after reversal of activity with repeated contraction, *J. Physiol.*, 317, 21P, 1981.
145. **Richter, E.A., Ruderman, N.B., Gavras, H., Belur, E.R., and Galbo, H.**, Muscle glycogenolysis during exercise: dual control by epinephrine and contractions, *Am. J. Physiol.*, 242, E25, 1982.
146. **Richter, E.A., Ruderman, N.B., and Galbo, H.**, Alpha- and beta-adrenergic effects on muscle metabolism in contracting, perfused muscle, in *Biochemistry of Exercise*, Knuttgen, H.G., Vogel, J.A., and Poortmans, J., Eds., Human Kinetics, Champaign, 1983, 766.
147. **Hostmark, A.T., Gronnerod, O., and Horn, R.S.**, Muscle contractions inhibit adrenergic effects on glycogen enzymes, *Horm. Metab. Res.*, 10, 81, 1978.
148. **Bonen, A., McDermott, J.C., and Huther, C.A.**, Carbohydrate metabolism in skeletal muscle: an update of current concepts, *Int. J. Sports Med.*, 10, 385, 1989.
149. **McDermott, J.G., Elder, G.C., and Bonen, A.**, Adrenal hormones enhance glycogenolysis in nonexercising muscle during exercise, *J. Appl. Physiol.*, 63, 1275, 1987.
150. **Struck, P.J., and Tipton, C.M.**, Effect of acute exercise on glycogen levels in adrenalectomized rats, *Endocrinology*, 95, 1385, 1974.
151. **Viru, M., Litvinova, L., Smirnova, T., and Viru, A.**, Glucocorticoids in metabolic control during exercise: glycogen metabolism, *J. Sports Med. Phys. Fitness*, 1994 (accepted for publication).
152. **Gorski, J., Nowacka, M., Namiot, Z., and Kiryluk, T.**, Effect of exercise on energy substrates metabolism in tissues of adrenalectomized rats, *Acta Physiol. Pol.*, 38, 331, 1987.
153. **Baldwin, K.M., Hooker, A.M., Herrick, R., and Schrader, L.**, Muscle respiratory capacity and glycogen consumption in thyroid deficient (T_x) rats, *Med. Sci. Sports*, 10, 45, 1978.
154. **Goldfarb, A.H., and Kandrick, Z.V.**, Effect of an exercise run to exhaustion on cAMP in the rat heart, *J. Appl. Physiol.*, 51, 1539, 1981.
155. **Stankiewicz-Choraszucha, B., and Górski, J.**, Effect of substrate supply and beta-adrenergic blockade on heart glycogen and triglyceride utilization during exercise in the rat, *Eur. J. Appl. Physiol.*, 43, 11, 1980.
156. **Mach, Z., and Grabowska-Maslanka, H.**, Wplyw wysilku fizicnego u szczurow z hypertyroksynemia na przemiane weglowdanova w miesniu sercowyn, *Folia Med. Cracow*, 19, 519, 1977.
157. **Kendrick, Z.V., Steffen, C.A., Rumsey, W.L., and Goldberg, D.I.**, Effect of estradiol on tissue glycogen metabolism in exercised oophorectomized rats, *J. Appl. Physiol.*, 63, 492, 1987.
158. **Hems, D.A., and Whitton, P.D.**, Control of hepatic glycogenolysis, *Physiol. Rev.*, 60, 1, 1980.
159. **Shimazu, T.**, Neural regulation of hepatic glucose metabolism in mammals, *Diab. Metab. Rev.*, 3, 185, 1987.
160. **Smythe, G.A., Pascoe, W.S., and Storlien, L.H.**, Hypothalamic noradrenergic and sympathoadrenal control of glycemia after stress, *Am. J. Physiol.*, 256, 231, 1989.
161. **Brouha, L., Cannon, W., and Dill, D.B.**, Blood-sugar variations in normal and in sympathectomized dogs, *J. Physiol.*, 95, 431, 1939.
162. **Kindler, J., Clasing, D., Alfes, H., and Schulz, V.**, Der Effekt von β-Rezepteren-blockern auf den Glykogenstoffwechsel der Rattenleber unter körperlicher Belastung, *Arzeim. Forsch. Drug. Res.*, 28, 1376, 1978.
163. **Juhlin-Dannfelt, A.C., Terblanche, S.E., Fell, R.D., Young, J.C., and Holloszy, J.O.**, Effect of beta-adrenergic receptor blockade on glycogenolysis during exercises, *J. Appl. Physiol.*, 40, 840, 1976.

164. **Winder, W.W., Boullier, J., and Fell, R.D.,** Liver glycogenolysis during exercise without a significant increase in cAMP, *Am. J. Physiol.,* 237, R147, 1979.

165. **Arnall, D.A., Marker, J.C., Conlee, R.K., and Winder, W.W.,** Effect of infusing epinephrine on liver and muscle glycogenolysis during exercise in rats, *Am. J. Physiol.,* 250, E641, 1986.

166. **Vranic, M., Kawamori, R., and Wranshall, G.A.,** The role of insulin and glucagon in regulating glucose turnover in dogs during exercise, *Med. Sci. Sports,* 7, 27, 1975.

167. **Sherwin, R.S., Hendler, R., DeFronzo, R., Wahren, J., and Felig, P.,** Glucose homeostasis during prolonged suppression of glucagon and insulin secretion by somatostatin, *Proc. Natl. Acad. Sci. U.S.A.,* 74, 348, 1977.

168. **Issekutz, B., and Vranic, M.,** Role of glucagon in regulation of glucose production in exercising dogs, *Am. J. Physiol.,* 28, E13, 1980.

169. **Björkman, O., Felig, P., Hagenfeldt, L., and Wahren, J.,** Influence of hypoglucagonemia on splanchnic glucose output during leg exercise in man, *Clin. Physiol.,* 1, 43, 1981.

170. **Richter, E.A., Galbo, H., Holst, J.J., and Sonne, B.,** Significance of glucagon for insulin secretion and hepatic glycogenolysis during exercise in rats, *Horm. Metab. Res.,* 13, 323, 1981.

171. **Galbo, H.,** *Hormonal and Metabolic Adaptation to Exercise,* Georg Thieme Verlag, Stuttgart, 1983.

172. **Wahren, J., and Björkman, O.,** Hormones, exercise, and regulation of splanchnic glucose output in normal men, in *Biochemistry of Exercise IV-A,* Poortmans, J., and Niset, G., Eds., University Park Press, Baltimore, 1981, 149.

173. **Vranic, M., Lickley, H.L.A., Björkman, O., and Wasserman, D.,** Regulation of glucose production and utilization in exercise: physiology and diabetes, *Can. J. Sports Sci.,* 12 (Suppl. 1), 120S, 1987.

174. **Wahren, J.,** Metabolic adaptation to physical exercise in man, in *Endocrinology,* Vol. 3, DeGroot, L.J. et al., Eds., Grune & Stratton, San Francisco, 1979, 1911.

175. **Issekutz, B.,** The role of hypoinsulinemia in exercise metabolism, *Diabetes,* 29, 629, 1980.

176. **Felig, P., and Wahren, J.,** Fuel homeostasis in exercise, *N. Engl. J. Med.,* 293, 1078, 1975.

177. **Berger, M., Assel, J.-P., and Jorgens, V.,** Effects endocriniens et métaboliques de l'exercise musculaire chez l'homme, *Diabete Metab.,* 6, 59, 1980.

178. **Kawamori, R., and Vranic, M.,** Mechanism of exercise-induced hypoglycemia in depancreatized dogs maintained on long-lasting insulin, *J. Clin. Invest.,* 59, 331, 1977.

179. **Felig, P., and Wahren, J.,** Role of insulin and glucagon in the regulation of hepatic glucose production during exercise, *Diabetes,* 28 (Suppl. 1), 71, 1979.

180. **Wasserman, D.H., Williams, P.E., Brooks, L.D., Goldstein, R.E., and Cherrington, A.D.,** Exercise-induced fall in insulin and hepatic carbohydrate metabolism during muscular work, *Am. J. Physiol.,* 256, E500, 1989.

181. **Górski, J., Stankiewicz, B., Brycka, R., and Kiezka, K.,** The effect of estradiol on carbohydrate utilization during prolonged exercise in rats, *Acta Physiol. Pol.,* 27, 361, 1976.

182. **Felig, P.,** The glucose-alanine cycle, *Metabolism,* 22, 179. 1973.

183. **Ingle, D.J., Nezymis, J.E., and Jeffries, J.W.,** Work performance of normal rats given continuous injections of adrenal cortex extracts, *Am. J. Physiol.,* 157, 99, 1949.

184. **Sestaff, L., Trap-Jensen, J., Lyngsoe, J., Claussen, J.P., Holst, J.J., Nielsen, S.L., Rehfeldt, J.P., and Scheffalitzky de Muckadell, O.,** Regulation of gluconeogenesis and ketogenesis during rest and exercise in diabetic subjects and normal men, *Clin. Sci. Mol. Med.,* 55, 411, 1977.

185. **Shaw, W.A.S., Issekutz, T.B., and Issekutz, B.,** Gluconeogenesis from glycerol at rest and during exercise in normal, diabetic, and methylprednisolone-treated dogs, *Metabolism,* 25, 329, 1976.

186. **Broden, V., Kuhn, E., and Andel, M.,** Glukagon a metabolismus pri intenszin fyzické zátézi, *Cas. Lek. Cesk.,* 115, 892, 1976.

187. **Douen, A.G., Ramlai, T., Klip, A., Young, D.A., Cartee, G.D., and Holloszy, J.O.,** Exercise-induced increase in glucose transporters in plasma membranes of rat skeletal muscle, *Endocrinology,* 124, 449, 1989.

188. **Ivy, J.L., and Holloszy, J.O.,** Persistent increase in glucose uptake by rat skeletal muscle following exercise, *Am. J. Physiol.,* 241, C200, 1981.

189. **Wallberg-Henriksson, H., and Holloszy, J.O.,** Insulin is not necessary for the stimulation of muscle glucose uptake by contractile activity, *Acta Endocrinol.,* 106 (Suppl. 263), 264, 1984.

190. **Issekutz, B., Paul, B., and Miller, H.J.,** Metabolism in normal and pancreatomized dogs during steady-state exercise, *Am. J. Physiol.,* 213, 857, 1967.

191. **Trap-Jensen, J., Dahl-Hansen, A.B., Kühl, C., and Moer, J.,** Effect of insulin on glucose uptake in the exercising human forearm, *Acta Endocrinol.,* 82 (Suppl. 203), 2, 1976.

192. **Ahlborg, G., and Felig, P.,** Substrate utilization during prolonged exercise preceded by ingestion of glucose, *Am. J. Physiol.,* 233, E188, 1977.

193. **Vranic, M., Kawamori, R., Pek, S., Kovacevic, N., and Wrenshall, G.A.,** The essentiality of insulin and the role of glucagon in regulating glucose utilization and production during strenuous exercise in dogs, *J. Clin. Invest.,* 57, 245, 1976.

194. **Himms-Hagen, J.,** Sympathetic regulation of metabolism, *Pharmacol. Rev.,* 19, 367, 1967.

195. **Chiasson, J.L., Shikama, H., Chu, D.T.W., and Exton, J.H.**, Inhibitory effect of epinephrine on insulin-stimulated glucose uptake by rat skeletal muscle, *J. Clin. Invest.*, 68, 706, 1981.
196. **Issekutz, B.**, Effect of epinephrine on carbohydrate metabolism in exercising dogs, *Metabolism*, 34, 457, 1985.
197. **Johnson, R.A., Rennie, M.J., Walton, J.L., and Webster, M.H.C.**, The effect of moderate exercise on blood metabolites in patients with hypopituitarism, *Clin. Sci.*, 40, 127, 1971.
198. **Ahlborg, G., Felig, P., Hagenfeldt, L., Hendler, R., and Wahren, J.**, Substrate turnover during prolonged exercise in man, Splanchnic and leg metabolism of glucose, free fatty acids and amino acids, *J. Clin. Invest.*, 53, 1080, 1974.
199. **Wolfe, R.R., Nadel, E.R., Show, J.H.F., Stephenson, L.A., and Wolfe, M.H.**, Role of changes in insulin and glucagon in glucose homeostasis in exercise, *J. Clin. Invest.*, 77, 900, 1986.
200. **Wasserman, D.H., Lichley, H.L.A., and Vranic, M.**, Interactions between glucagon and other counterregulatory hormones during normoglycemia and hypoglycemia exercise in dogs, *J. Clin. Invest.*, 74, 1404, 1984.
201. **Bülow, J.**, Lipid mobilization and utilization, in *Principles of Exercise Biochemistry*, J.R. Poortmans, Ed., Karger, Basel, 1988, 140.
202. **Faderspil, G., Lefebvre, P., Luyckx, A., and DePale, A.**, Endocrine mechanisms of exercise induced fatty acids mobilization in rats, in *Metabolic Adaptation to Prolonged Physical Exercise*, Howald, H., and Poortmans, J.R., Eds., Birkhäuser Verlag, Basel, 1975, 301.
203. **Gollnick, P.D.**, Exercise, adrenergic blockade and free fatty acid mobilization, *Am. J. Physiol.*, 213, 734, 1967.
204. **Franz, J.W., Lohman, F.W., Koch, G., and Quable, H.J.**, Aspects of hormonal regulation of lipolysis during exercise: effects of chronic β-receptor blockade, *Int. J. Sports Med.*, 4, 14, 1983.
205. **Stankiewicz-Choraszucha, B., and Górski, J.**, Effect of beta-adrenergic blockade on intramuscular triglyceride mobilization during exercise, *Experimentia*, 34, 357, 1978.
206. **Hunter, W.M., Fonsenka, C.C., and Passmore, R.**, Growth hormone: important role in muscular exercise in adults, *Science*, 150, 1051, 1965.
207. **Barwich, D., Hägele, H., Weiss, M., and Weicker, H.**, Hormonal and metabolic adjustment in patients with central Cushing's disease after adrenalectomy, *Int. J. Sports Med.*, 2, 220, 1981.
208. **Toode, K., Smirnova, T., Tendzegolskis, Z., and Viru, A.**, Growth hormone action on blood glucose, lipids and insulin during exercise, *Biol. Sport*, 10, 99, 1993.
209. **Kaciuba-Uśćilko, H., Greenleaf, J.E., Kozlowski, S., Brzezinska, Z., Nazar, K., and Ziemba, A.**, Thyroid hormone-induced changes in body temperature and metabolism during exercise in dogs, *Am. J. Physiol.*, 229, 260, 1975.
210. **Nazar, K., Chwabinska-Moneta, J., Machalla, J., and Kaciuba-Uśćilko, H.**, Metabolic and body temperature changes during exercise in hyperthyroid patients, *Clin. Sci. Mol. Med.*, 54, 323, 1978.
211. **Paul, P.**, Effects of long lasting physical exercise and training on lipid metabolism, in *Metabolic Adaptation to Prolonged Exercise*, Howald, H., and Poortmans, J., Eds., Birkhäuser Verlag, Basel, 1975, 156.
212. **Kaciuba-Uśćilko, H., Brzezinska, Z., and Kobryn, A.**, Metabolic and temperature responses to physical exercise in thyroidectomized dog, *Eur. J. Appl. Physiol.*, 40, 219, 1979.
213. **Story, J.A., and Griffith, D.R.**, Effects of thyroxine and exercise on serum and hepatic cholesterol in mature rats, *Horm. Metab. Res.*, 4, 380, 1972.
214. **Fain, J.N.**, Inhibition of glucose transport in fat cells and activation of lipolysis by glucocorticoids, in *Glucocorticoid Hormone Action*, Baxter, J.D., and Rousseau, G.G., Eds., Springer-Verlag, Berlin, 1979, 547.
215. **Fain, J.N., Kovacev, V.P., and Scow, R.O.**, Antilipolytic effect on insulin in isolated fat cells of the rat, *Endocrinology*, 78, 773, 1966.
216. **Butcher, R.W., Sneyd, J.G.T., Park, C.R., and Sutherland, E.W.**, Effect of insulin on adenosine 3′,5′-monophosphate in the rat epididymal fat pad, *J. Biol. Chem.*, 24, 1651, 1966.
217. **Senft, G., Schultz, G., Munske, K., and Hoffman, M.**, Influence of insulin on cyclic 3′,5′-AMP phosphodiesterase activity in liver, skeletal muscle, adipose tissue, and kidney, *Diabetologia*, 4, 322, 1988.
218. **Nilsson, N.Ö., Strolfors, P., Fredrikson, G., and Belfrage, P.**, Regulation of adipose tissue lipolysis: effects of noradrenaline and insulin on phosphorylation of hormone-sensitive lipase and on lipolysis in intact rat adipocyte, *FEBS Lett.*, 111, 125, 1980.
219. **Hunter, W.M., and Sukkar, M.Y.**, Changes in plasma insulin levels during muscular exercise, *J. Physiol.*, 196, 110P, 1968.
220. **Wahren, J., Felig, P., Hagenfeldt, L., Hendler, R., and Ahlborg, G.**, Splanchnic and leg metabolism of glucose, free fatty acids and amino acids during prolonged exercise in man, in *Metabolic Adaptation to Prolonged Exercise*, Howald, H., and Poortmans, J., Eds., Birkhäuser Verlag, Basel, 1975, 144.
221. **Issekutz, B., Miller, H.J., and Rodahl, K.**, Effect of exercise on FFA metabolism of pancreatomized dogs, *Am. J. Physiol.*, 205, 645, 1963.
222. **Wahren, J., Felig, P., and Hagenfeldt, L.**, Physical exercise and fuel homeostasis in diabetes mellitus, *Diabetologia*, 14, 213, 1978.

223. **Brockman, R.P.**, Effect of somatostatin on plasma glucagon and insulin and glucose turnover in exercising sheep, *J. Appl. Physiol.*, 47, 273, 1979.

224. **Issekutz, B., and Paul, P.**, Intramuscular energy sources in exercising normal and pancreatomized dog, *Am. J. Physiol.*, 215, 197, 1968.

225. **Dohm, G.L., Kasperek, G.J., Tapscott, E.B., and Barakat, H.A.**, Protein metabolism during endurance exercise, *Fed. Proc.*, 44, 348, 1875.

226. **Viru, A.**, Mobilization of structural proteins during exercise, *Sports Med.*, 4, 95, 1987.

227. **Varrik, E., Viru, A., Ööpik, V., and Viru, M.**, Exercise-induced catabolic responses in various muscle fibers, *Can. J. Sports Sci.*, 17, 125, 1992.

228. **Dohm, L.G., Tapscott, E.B., and Kasperek, G.J.**, Protein degradation during endurance exercise and recovery, *Med. Sci. Sports Exerc.*, 19 (Suppl.), S166, 1987.

229. **Millward, D.J., Davies, C.T.M., Halliday, D., Wolman, S.L., Matthews, D.M., and Rennie, M.J.**, Effect of exercise on protein metabolism in humans as explored with stable isotopes, *Fed. Proc.*, 41, 2686, 1982.

230. **Wolfe, R.R., Goodennough, R.D., Wolfe, M.H., Royl, G.T., and Nadel, E.R.**, Isotopic analysis of leucine and urea metabolism in exercising humans, *J. Appl. Physiol.*, 52, 458, 1982.

231. **White, T.P., and Brooks, G.A.**, U-^{14}C-glucose, -alanine, and -leucine oxidation in rats at rest and two intensities of running, *Am. J. Physiol.*, 240, E155, 1981.

232. **Lemon, P.W.R., Nagle, F.J., Mullin, J.P., and Benevenga, N.J.**, *In vitro* leucine oxidation at rest and during two intensities of exercise, *J. Appl. Physiol.*, 56, 947, 1982.

233. **Mayer, M., and Rosen, F.**, Interaction of glucocorticoids and androgens with skeletal muscle, *Metabolism*, 26, 937, 1977.

234. **Varrik, E., Seene, T., and Viru, A.**, 3-Methylhistidine excretion during training exercises in adrenalectomized animals, *Acta Comment. Univ. Tartuensis*, 670, 83, 1984 (in Russian).

235. **Dahlmann, B., Widjoja, A., and Reinauer, H.**, Antagonistic effects of endurance training and testosterone on alkaline proteolytic activity in rat skeletal muscle, *Eur. J. Appl. Physiol.*, 46, 229, 1981.

236. **Dohm, G.L., and Louis, T.M.**, Changes in androstenedione, testosterone and protein metabolism as a result of exercise, *Proc. Soc. Exp. Biol. Med.*, 158, 622, 1978.

237. **Li, J.B., and Jefferson, L.S.**, Effect of isoproterenol on amino acid levels and protein turnover in skeletal muscle, *Am. J. Phys.*, 232, E243, 1977.

238. **Etlinger, J.D., and Matsumato, K.**, Interaction of calcium, cyclic AMP, and tension in the regulation of protein degradation in muscle, in *Metabolism and Functional Changes during Exercise*, Semiginovsky, B. and Tucek, S., Eds., Charles University, Prague, 1982, 57.

239. **Lenkova, P.I., Usik. S.V., and Yakovlev, N.N.**, Changes of urea content in blood and tissues in muscular activity in dependence of the adaptation of the organism, *Sechenov Physiol. J. USSR*, 59, 1097, 1973 (in Russian).

240. **Fulks, R.M., Li, J.B., and Goldberg, A.L.**, Effect of insulin, glucose and amino acids on protein turnover in rat diaphragm, *J. Biol. Chem.*, 250, 290, 1975.

241. **Critz, J.B., and Withrow, T.J.**, Adrenocortical blockade and the transaminase response to exercise, *Steroids*, 5, 719, 1965.

242. **Garber, A.J., Karl, J.E., and Kipnis, D.M.**, Alanine and glutamine synthesis and release from skeletal muscle. IV. β-Adrenergic inhibition of amino acid release, *J. Biol. Chem.*, 251, 851, 1976.

243. **Guezennec, G.Y., Ferre, P., Serrurier, B., Merino, D., Amonad, M., and Pesquires, P.C.**, Metabolic effects of testosterone during prolonged physical exercise and fasting, *Eur. J. Appl. Physiol.*, 52, 300, 1984.

244. **Viru, A., and Eller, A.**, Adrenocortical regulation of protein metabolism during prolonged physical exertions, *Byull. Eksp. Biol. Med.*, 82, 1436, 1976 (in Russian).

245. **Viru, A., Litvinova, L., Viru, M., and Smirnova, T.**, Glucocorticoids in metabolic control during exercise: alanine metabolism, *J. Appl. Physiol.*, 76, 801, 1994.

246. **Viru, A., and Smirnova, T.**, Involvement of protein synthesis in action of glucocorticoids on working capacity of adrenalectomized rats, *Int. J. Sports Med.*, 6, 225, 1985.

247. **Seene, T., Alev, K., and Pehme, A.**, Effect of muscular activity on the turnover rate of actin and myosin heavy and light chains in different types of skeletal muscle, *Int. J. Sports Med.*, 7, 287, 1986.

248. **Kôrge, P., Roosson, S., and Oks, M.**, Heart adaptation to physical exertion in relation to work duration, *Acta Cardiol.*, 29, 303, 1974.

249. **Kôrge, P., Masso, R., and Roosson, S.**, The effect of physical conditioning on cardiac response to acute exercise, *Can. J. Physiol. Pharmacol.*, 52, 745, 1974.

250. **Kôrge, P., Viru, A., and Roosson, S.**, The effect of chronic physical overload on skeletal muscle metabolism and adrenocortical activity, *Acta Physiol. Acad. Sci. Hung.*, 45, 41, 1974.

251. **Kôrge, P., and Roosson, S.**, The importance of adrenal glands in the improved adaptation of trained animals to physical exertion, *Endokrinologie*, 64, 232, 1975.

252. **Kozlowski, S., and Saltin, B.**, Effect of sweat loss on body fluids, *J. Appl. Physiol.*, 19, 1119, 1964.

253. **Saltin, B., and Costill, D.**, Fluid and electrolyte balance during prolonged exercise, in *Exercise, Nutrition and Energy Metabolism*, Horton, E.S., and Terjung, R.L., Eds., Macmillan, New York, 1988, 150.

254. **Melin, B., Eclache, J.B., Geelen, G., Annert, G., Allevard, A.M., Jersaillon, E., Zelid, A., Legras, J.J., and Charab, C.,** Plasma AVP, neurophysin, renin activity and aldosterone during submaximal exercise performed until exhaustion in trained and untrained man, *Eur. J. Appl. Physiol.,* 44, 141, 1980.

255. **Barwich, D., Keilholz, U., Merkt, J., and Weicker, H.,** Serum kinetic des antidiuretischen Hormons (ADH) and Säure-Basen-Henshalts bei fahrradenergometrischer Ausbelastung, in *Sport: Leistung and Gesundheit,* Heck, H., Hollmann, W., Liegen, H., and Rost, R., Eds., Deutsch Ärzte Verlag, Köln, 1983, 221.

256. **Zambraski, E., Rofrano, T., and Ciccone, C.,** Effect of aspirin treatment on kidney function in exercising man, *Med. Sci. Sports Exerc.,* 14, 419, 1982.

257. **Olsson, K.E., and Saltin, B.,** Variations in total body water with muscle glycogen changes in man, *Acta Physiol. Scand.,* 80, 11, 1970.

258. **Saltin, B.,** Aerobic work capacity and circulation at exercise in man. With special reference to the effect of prolonged exercise and /or heat exposure, *Acta Physiol. Scand.,* 62 (Suppl. 230), 1964.

259. **Costill, D.L., and Miller, J.M.,** Nutrition for endurance sport: carbohydrate and fluid balance, *Int. J. Sports Med.,* 1, 2, 1980.

260. **Costill, D.L., Branam, G., Fink, W., and Nelson, R.,** Exercise-induced sodium concentration changes in plasma renin and aldosterone, *Med. Sci. Sports,* 8, 209, 1976.

261. **Fenn, W.O.,** Electrolytes in muscle, *Physiol. Rev.,* 16, 450, 1936.

262. **Bergström, J., Gaurnieri, G., and Hultmann, E.,** Changes in muscle water and electrolytes during exercise, in *Limiting Factors of Physical Performance,* Keul, J., Ed., Georg Thieme Verlag, Stuttgart, 1973, 173.

263. **Convertino, V.A., Keil, L.C., and Greenleaf, J.E.,** Plasma volume, renin, and vasopressin responses to graded exercise after training, *J. Appl. Physiol.,* 54, 508, 1983.

264. **Clausen, T.,** Regulation of active Na^+-K^+ transport in skeletal muscle, *Physiol. Rev.,* 66, 542, 1986.

265. **Sjøgaard, G., Adams, R.P., and Saltin, B.,** Water and ion shifts in skeletal muscle of humans with intense dynamic knee extension, *Am. J. Physiol.,* 248, R190, 1985.

266. **Clausen, T., and Flatman, J.A.,** The effect of catecholamines on Na,K transport and membrane potential in rat soleus muscle, *J. Physiol.,* 270, 383, 1977.

267. **Clausen, T., and Flatman, J.A.,** Effects of insulin and epinephrine on Na^+-K^+ and glucose transport in soleus muscle, *Am. J. Physiol.,* 252, E492, 1987.

268. **Knochel, J.P., Blachley, J.D., Johnson, J.H., and Carter, N.W.,** Muscle cell electrical hyperpolarization and reduced exercise hyperkalaemia in physically conditioned dogs, *J. Clin. Invest.,* 75, 740, 1985.

269. **Kjeldsen, K., Richter, E.A., Galbo, H., Lortie, G., and Clausen, T.,** Training increases the concentration of [^{3}H] oubain-binding sites in rat skeletal muscle, *Biochem. Biophys. Acta,* 860, 708, 1986.

270. **Klitgaard, H., and Clausen, T.,** Increased total concentration of Na,K pumps in vastus lateralis muscle of old trained human subjects, *J. Appl. Physiol.,* 67, 2491, 1989.

271. **Kjeldsen, K., Nørgaard, A., Gøtsche, C.O., Thomassen, A., and Clausen, T.,** Effect of thyroid function on number of Na-K-pump in human skeletal muscle, *Lancet,* 2, 8, 1984.

272. **Drzevetskaya, I.A., and Limanski, N.N.,** Thyrocalcitonin activity and calcium level in plasma during muscular activity, *Sechenov Physiol. J. USSR,* 64, 1498, 1978 (in Russian).

273. **Aloia, J.F., Rasulo, P., Deftas, L.J., Voswani, A., and Yeh, J.K.,** Exercise-induced hypercalcemia and calciotropic hormones, *J. Lab. Clin. Med.,* 106, 229, 1985.

Chapter 4

POST-EXERCISE RECOVERY PERIOD

OUTLINES OF THE POST-EXERCISE RECOVERY

The end of exercise means the cessation of muscle contractions, but not the cessation of increased functional and metabolic activities. More or less prolonged time is necessary to normalize the functions of various organs. For a comparatively prolonged period the metabolic activities remain far from the resting state. In 1919 it was indicated that during the first 5 to 15 min after exercise, oxygen uptake remains above the basal metabolic rates. This excess oxygen uptake matched the oxygen deficit contracted at the beginning of exercise. After intensive or exhaustive exercise the amount of consumed oxygen is larger than the oxygen deficit.[1] Some years later, the accordance between excess oxygen uptake after exercise (oxygen debt) and lactate accumulation was established.[2] Accordingly, abolishment of oxygen debt was considered the main reason for increased functional activities after exercise.[3] It was also considered that the oxygen debt means a consumption of 'extra oxygen' necessary to supply energy for various restitution processes and particularly for the resynthesis of phosphocreatine and for the oxidative elimination of lactate. However, the problem is more complicated: the oxygen uptake after exercise does not exactly correspond to the amount of energy released during exercise on account of anaerobic processes.[4-6]

In regard to metabolism, the recovery period means not only transition from high to low energy demands, but also restoration of energy reserves, abolishment of the accumulated metabolic intermediants, as well as normalization of water and ionic composition in body compartments. In the course of repletion of energy reserves the phenomenon of supercompensation has been found. This gives a peculiar feature to the delayed stage of the recovery period.[7] Recovery period means also a change in protein metabolism opposite to that happening during exercise. The altered balance between anabolic and catabolic processes has to warrant an effective renewal of exhausted cellular structures and enzyme molecules as well as the opportunity for the increase in active structures and in the number of enzyme molecules. In this meaning as well as in regard to the supercompensation of energy reserves we have to consider the reconstructive function of the recovery period.

Consequently, the main functions of the recovery period are

1. Normalization of functions (their transition from the exercise level to the resting level)
2. Replenishment of energy resources together with temporary supercompensation for them
3. Normalization of homeostatic equilibriums
4. Reconstructive function, particularly in regard to cellular structures and enzyme systems

The first and third functions are actualized within minutes or, in particular cases, within some hours. The corresponding processes constitute the first stage of recovery (Figure 4-1). This stage may be called *the stage of rapid recovery*. The actualization of other tasks consumes far more time. Therefore, they can be considered to constitute the *stage of delayed restitution of bodily resources and working capacity*. However, it would be wrong to think that this stage begins only after the cessation of the first stage. Indeed, it begins with the end of

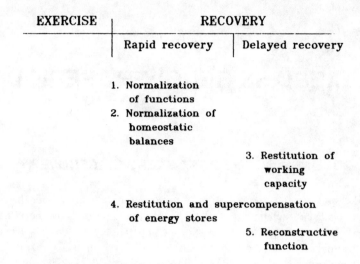

EXERCISE | RECOVERY

Rapid recovery | Delayed recovery

1. Normalization
   of functions
2. Normalization of
   homeostatic
   balances

3. Restitution of
   working
   capacity

4. Restitution and supercompensation
   of energy stores

5. Reconstructive
   function

FIGURE 4-1. A generalized scheme of the post-exercise recovery period.

exercise. In regard to some energy stores, the onset of their replenishment is assumed to be possible already during exercise. Thus the term 'delayed' does not mean a delayed onset but a delayed realization of tasks.

RESTORATION OF NORMAL FUNCTIONAL ACTIVITIES

OXYGEN TRANSPORT SYSTEM

Cessation of muscular contractions at the end of exercise or various kinds of physical work causes a change in regulatory influences. The regulatory actions of central command and proprioceptive impulses drop out. As a result, rapid changes occur in the functions of organs responsible for oxygen transport, despite the persisting high demand for oxygen supply of skeletal muscles having only just acted. These transitory changes are opposite to the initial adjustment at the beginning of exercise in the direction of change, but similar to the general pattern: first there is a rapid and then a gradual decrement of functional activity. While the rapid changes within the first 1 to 2 min express the cessation of the actions of central command and proprioceptive influences, the second gradual and often undulated decrease may be explained by the reduction of influences from metaboreceptors and of hormonal influences. Exercise intensity is a factor that retards the rate of post-exercise changes. After highly intensive exercise during the first 5 to 10 s the heart rate may not change and then the following decrease is not characterized by so steep a slope as after less intensive exercise.[8,9] A possibility of a regulatory inertia seems to exist as well. The duration of exercise may be overridden by the persisting excitement of the cardiac center, stimulating a sino-atrial node through sympathetic discharge. A further increase in the heart rate was noticed during the first 5 to 8 s in 65% of persons after 15 s of cycling at maximal possible rates.[8]

The post-exercise dynamics of heart activity are characterized by enhanced respiratory arrhythmia as well as by pronounced waves in the duration of the cardiac cycle corresponding to the third waves in blood pressure (Figure 4-2). This picture is revealed in association with a steep slope of heart rate decrement and mainly in well-trained persons.[8,9] An increased rate of recovery of heart frequency was found in trained persons also after exercise with increasing intensity up to the individual maximum.[10] It is likely that the steep slope of heart rate expresses not only the decrement of metabolic influences but also the high activity of parasympathetic nerves. Mostly in well-trained persons the heart rate decreases for 20 to 40 s to values below the initial[8] (Figure 4-3). This can be considered an expression of 'hypothalamic tuning' of

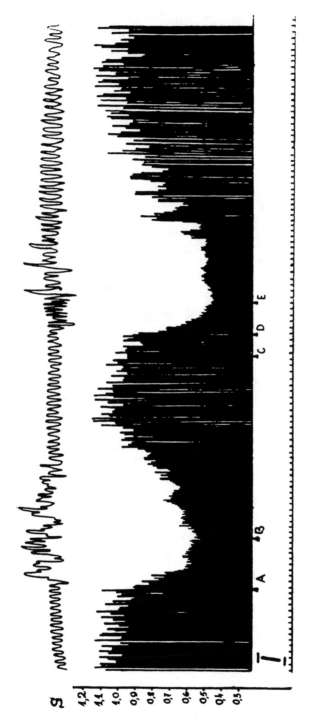

FIGURE 4-2. Dynamics of cardiac cycle duration during exercise of moderate intensity (A-B) and exercise of high intensity (D-E) as well as during post-exercise recovery. From the top: (1) pneumogram, (2) vertical lines corresponding to the duration of the cardiac cycle, (3) time per 2 s. (From Hansson, E., Viru, A., and Sildmäe, H., *4th Estonian Conf. Sports*, Tallinn, 1981, 46. With permission.)

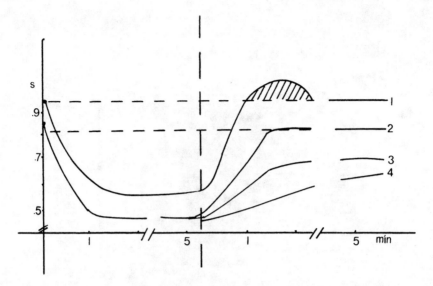

FIGURE 4-3. Dynamics of cardiac cycle duration after exercise: 1—undulated process (a rapid decrease to values of cardiac cycle duration above initial ones), 2 — aperiodic process with restitution of normal heart rate within 1 to 2 min, 3 — aperiodic process with stabilization of cardiac cycle duration on a level below the initial, 4 — torpid process without any stabilization during the first 5 min. Constructed as in the academic dissertation of E. Snoroskaya (Tartu University).

autonomic nervous influences. According to E. Gellhorn,[11] autonomic imbalance due to the prevalence of sympathetic or parasympathetic actions causes the increased sensitivity to change in the opposite direction. The previous prevalence of sympathetic influence during exercise sensitizes the parasympathetic effects. As a result the heart rate decreases below the initial values. However, this change does not appear after very strenuous exercise. Instead of that, after strenuous exercise and in most cases in untrained persons, the heart rate may stabilize to a level of 5 to 20 beats/min higher than the initial.[8]

The significance of the increased vagal tone was emphasized by results indicating that the heart rate decreased exponentially to the initial level during the first post-exercise minute despite the maximal noradrenaline level in the blood at the same time.[12]

By using various methods it was found that a rapid decrease in cardiac output and stroke volume occurs within the first 1 to 2 min post-exercise. Then a less abrupt decrease follows.[13-16]

The transition from exercise to rest is connected with a short-term drop in the intra-arterial pressure, often to values below the initial.[17-19] After only 5 to 10 s a new increase in blood pressure takes place. The latter lasts approximately 20 to 40 s.[19] After that a gradual decrease in arterial pressure follows. The same dynamics were established in the mean arterial pressure using a noninvasive method for its continuous recording.[20] A secondary increase in stroke volume was found during 1 to 2 min post-exercise. During this time period the peripheral resistance remained low and only later did it gradually increase.[16]

By using special equipment, auscultatory recording of blood pressure was obtained after every 8 to 12 s. A comparison of the pattern of auscultatory blood pressure during and after various exercises showed that after exercise the maximal arterial pressure rises to levels higher than those recorded during exercise when the exercise duration was 30 to 60 s and therefore, not enough for blood pressure to increase to the adequate level. After cessation of exercises lasting for 3 to 5 min, maximal arterial pressure decreases without any secondary rise.[21] When the person was in a standing position, the blood pressure drop was common immediately after the end of a 1-min cyclic exercise. The subsequent rise in maximal pressure as well as the decrease in heart rate were less pronounced than in a sitting position. When the blood flow to the legs was prevented by a bandage on the thighs, there was no immediate decrease in blood pressure and the post-exercise increase was the same as in a sitting position.[22] Thus the immediate post-exercise drop in arterial pressure is related to the aggravated venous return due to the cessation of the muscle pump function. As early as the 1930s it was demonstrated that a circulatory collapse called 'gravity shock' is revealed during prolonged standing after intensive exercise. The phenomenon can be avoided by a pressure bandage on the thighs.[23]

Differently from this mechanism, a late mild hypotension may follow within a period from 0.5 to 3 h after the end of exercise.[24-27] An increased sensitivity of vagal baroreflex was found persisting through 24 h of recovery.[25,28] Prostaglandins produced by skeletal muscles and kidney as a result of exercise may contribute to prolonged post-exercise vasodilatation as well.[29]

The transition of lung ventilation and oxygen uptake from exercise level to resting level is usually described by a simple exponent: during the first 1 to 2 min the changes are faster than later on.[30] Immediately after the end of a 5-min cycling at moderate intensity the respiratory frequency and depth decreased in association with reduced bioelectric activity of intercostal muscles.[31] However, the exponential curve may not be found after short-term highly intensive exercises or after static efforts. After a 15-s cycling exercise performed at the highest possible rate, the VO_2 increased during the first 20 to 30 s. Only then did an exponential decline follow. After a 2-min exercise at the highest possible rate the level obtained at the end of exercise persisted for 15 to 20 s before the exponential decline followed. When the exercise duration was enough to obtain the maximal oxygen uptake level (more than 3 min), the recovery period began with a steep decline transferring later to a more gradual decrease.[32,33]

In 1920 Lindhard[34] reported that after static efforts the VO_2 and cardiac output increased to higher levels compared to the values obtained during effort. The lung ventilation remained on the exercise level and respiratory frequency decreased, but tidal volume as well as alveolar ventilation increased. Similarly, after brief tetanic contractions the oxygen consumption by muscle tissue increases and thereafter declines exponentially.[35]

The exponential pattern of post-exercise VO_2 was described with the aid of two straight lines in order to discriminate the fast and slow components of oxygen debt, called alactic and lactic debts, respectively.[36,37] (Figure 4-4) However, there is no direct evidence that the replenishment of ATP and phosphocreatine stores occurs during the time of repayment of the fast component of the oxygen debt. A study of the rat leg muscle by phosphorus nuclear magnetic resonance demonstrated that phosphocreatine concentration rises to the initial level during a rather long-lasting period in accordance with the normalization of VO_2 by muscle tissue.[38] Thus, the restitution of muscle macroergic phosphates lasted not only during the fast component of oxygen debt, but also during the whole period of O_2 debt repayment.

Serious doubts arose also in regard to the exact correspondence between the slow component of O_2 debt and lactate elimination as well as between the total O_2 debt and the amount of energy released in anaerobic processes. The main counterarguments are

1. Elevated body temperature decreases phosphorylative coupling and, consequently, more O_2 is required for a given amount of ATP to be synthesized.[39] The temperature effect is calculated to amount to 1.2 l of O_2 during the first hour of recovery after submaximal and to 0.6 l after supramaximal exercises when the persons exercised in comfortable temperature.[40] The elevated temperature was considered to be the most important factor influencing the mitochondrial O_2 consumption and thereby, excess VO_2 after exercise.[41]

2. Changes in the blood level of adrenaline, thyroxine, and some other hormones may alter the rate of oxygen uptake and the ratio between oxidative phosphorylation and free oxidation, including free radical oxidation. In the canine gastrocnemius-plantaris muscle group the VO_2 increased significantly by noradrenaline infusion during post-contraction recovery.[42] The blockade of adrenoreceptors reduced the VO_2 during post-exercise recovery.[43-45] However, after an exhaustive one-leg exercise, muscle temperature and blood catecholamine concentration returned to the control level within 20 min of recovery, but the VO_2 remained elevated.[46]

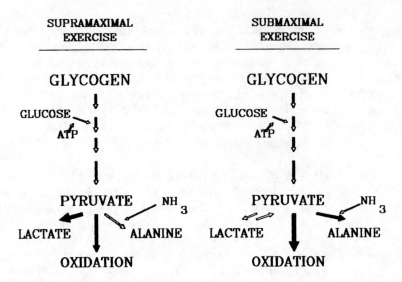

FIGURE 4-4. Dynamics of post-exercise oxygen uptake. The dotted area corresponds to alactic debt and striated area to lactatic debt.

3. Intensive function of the myocardium and respiratory muscles continuing after exercise need additional energy. It was calculated that the O_2 cost of moving an additional blood volume through the circulation for the first hour is about 1.3 l after submaximal and 0.7 l after supramaximal exercises.[40,47] The ventilatory cost constitutes 0.1 l O_2.[48]
4. Altered muscle tone may cause changes in VO_2.

There are reports pointing to a long period of persisting elevated oxygen consumption lasting for up to 12 h or even more after vigorous exercises.[40,48-51] The prolonged component of post-exercise excess oxygen consumption was found both after exhaustive prolonged submaximal and short-term supramaximal exercises. This component is a function of exercise intensity and duration.[40,48,51] Special experiments showed that the thermic effect of the consumed food was not decisive in the prolonged component of post-exercise excess oxygen consumption. It has been suggested that an increase in the rate of substrate cycling, particularly the triglyceride-fatty acid cycle may account for a significant part of the increased energy expenditure after exercise.[50,52-54] Additionally, energy expenditure for the reconstructive function of the recovery period has to be taken into account to explain the prolonged component of excess post-exercise oxygen consumption.

LACTATE DYNAMICS AND PH VALUES IN POST-EXERCISE RECOVERY

Post-exercise lactate values are widely used for evaluation of the participation of anaerobic glycolysis in the attaining of energy during strenuous exercises. However, during exercise lactate accumulates because the increase in the lactate disappearance rate lags behind the increase in the lactate appearance rate.[55] Therefore, the amount of resynthesis of ATP at the expense of anaerobic glycolysis will be underestimated if the calculations are based on the lactate accumulation in the blood or on the post-exercise oxidation of lactate (lactate debt). One must also take into consideration the various pathways of the fate of pyruvate formed during exercise: besides the oxidation of pyruvate and the transformation to lactate, one part is used for alanine synthesis (Figure 4-5). Pyruvate determination does not help because the measured pyruvate gives only its residual amount in a moment of time.

After exercise a part of both the formed pyruvate and lactate is used for glycogen resynthesis in exercised muscles. After supramaximal exercises causing blood lactate levels of

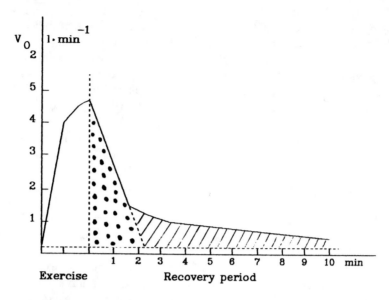

FIGURE 4-5. Fate of pyruvate during supramaximal or submaximal exercises.

10 to 16 mmol·l^{-1} and muscle lactate content of 25 mmol·kg^{-1} the proportion of lactate used for the resynthesis of glycogen has been estimated at 75,[56] 50,[57] and 13 to 27%.[53]

Nevertheless, these sources of errors will not make the use of lactate levels and lactate debt meaningless in evaluating the anaerobic energy production, because in supramaximal exercise the largest part of pyruvate is transferred to lactate and lactate production greatly exceeds its elimination. Only the quantitative estimation of the energy released in anaerobic glycolysis may not be exact.

The rate of lactate removal during recovery is directly related to the lactate concentration at the end of exercise.[58] The three main routes for muscle lactate clearance are (a) release into the capillary bed, (b) conversion to pyruvate, and then (c) either oxidation or further conversion into other compounds.[59] Using a knee-extensor exercise model inducing exhaustion within 2 to 4 min, it was found that at the end of exercise, the femoral vein plasma concentration of lactate is only a half of that accumulated in the muscle (the muscle-blood gradient was 18 mmol·l^{-1}), but 3 min into recovery, the difference was reduced to 5 mmol·l^{-1}, and was zero after 10 min of recovery. During 1 h of recovery as much as 82% of the lactate left the muscle as lactate via the blood stream.[53] These results are in accordance with the other data. After a 4-min exhaustive exercise the lactate release from working muscle gradually decreased. This process continued for at least 8 to 15 min.[60] After a 3-min exhaustive cycling the blood lactate increased during the first 10 min, while a pronounced drop occurred in the muscle lactate concentration. Thereafter, lactate decreased also in the blood. Approximately 0.5 h post-exercise the lactate concentrations in muscles and blood equalized.[61]

In the blood the post-exercise lactate curves could be fitted to a bi-exponential time function, consisting of a rapidly increasing and slowly decreasing component.[62-65] A comparison of lactate pattern after 3- and 60-min exercises showed that with exercise duration the values of velocity constants of lactate increase and decrease were reduced.[66] In exercise intensities over the anaerobic threshold, the blood lactate concentration increased with the prolongation of exercise duration from 3 to 6 min, but the constants of kinetics for both post-exercise increase and decrease of lactate concentration decreased.[65]

During the first 5 min of recovery after cycling with increasing intensity the pyruvate concentration progressively increased in the blood. The lactate/pyruvate ratio decreased.[67] It is yet to be established whether the decreased lactate/pyruvate ratio is a general phenomenon appearing immediately after cessation of muscle contraction, and if it indicates a relative decrease in the pyruvate conversion by corresponding metabolic pathways.

As a result of intensive anaerobic glycogenolysis an accumulation of hydrogen ions appears in the muscles[68-71] and in the blood.[68-72] The changes in pH values after exercise are parallel to the changes in lactate concentrations.[68-72] An intensive 4-min anaerobic exercise resulted in a decrease of the thigh muscle pH from 7.15 ± 0.01 to 6.57 ± 0.04 and that of the blood from 7.39 ± 0.04 to 7.04 ± 0.03. During the first 5 min of recovery the decrease continued and then the pH values began to increase.[73] After another 4-min exhaustive exercise low pH persisted for 4 min in the atrial blood and then began to increase. In the venous blood a gradual increase began from the first post-exercise minute. Both values returned to a level close to the initial within 20 min.[60] Cycling at high intensity (mean heart rate 192) until exhaustion resulted in a pronounced drop of pH values in the m. quadriceps femoris (total muscle pH from 7.08 ± 0.03 to 6.64 ± 0.12), intracellular pH (from 7.00 ± 0.06 to 6.45 ± 0.09), femoral venous blood pH (from 7.08 ± 0.06 to 6.93 ± 0.06), and arterial blood pH (from 7.27 to 7.14). Muscle lactate increased up to 22.0 ± 2.6 mmol/kg (intracellular lactate to 29.1 ± 3.4) and femoral venous blood lactate up to 15 ± 5 mmol/l. At 20 min post-exercise the muscle lactate remained elevated but both total and intracellular pH were normal. The pH values of femoral venous blood normalized within 20 min. At 30 min post-exercise, significantly elevated pH values were found in comparison with the pre-exercise values. At the same time the blood lactate was insignificantly lower than the initial level.[71]

In most cases lactate concentrations normalize within 30 to 60 min after intensive exercise.[56,68,71,72] There is old evidence that activity increases lactate removal from the blood.[74-77] Moderate exercise performed during recovery also causes a faster elimination of lactate from the muscle.[78-81] At first it was supposed to be related to enhanced perfusion.[79] However, stimulation of the oxidation rate against the decline in oxidation intensity may have its significance as well. Mild exercise following a strenuous one enhanced lactate oxidation.[82]

Lactate disappearance after exercise at VO_2max level was intensified by exercise at 40% VO_2max, but not by exercise at 65% VO_2max.[83] However, other studies indicated that the recovery exercise at 65% VO_2max[79] or at 60% VO_2max[78] is optimal for speeding up lactate removal. After a 10-min exercise at 90% VO_2max active rest slightly below the anaerobic threshold improves the lactate removal rate compared to complete rest or active rest above the anaerobic threshold.[84]

ENDOCRINE SYSTEM

A number of studies on blood levels of hormones during the first 10 to 20 min of post-exercise recovery have revealed the continuation of exercise-induced change before the opposite change occurs. Thus, the endocrine response to exercise may be more prolonged than the exercise itself. In other cases opposite changes were found to begin just after the end of exercise. These opposite changes do not mean a fast normalization of hormone levels in the blood. Quite often they reach concentrations significantly differing from the initial value. Thus, the exercise-induced rise or drop may be changed by a decrease or an increase, respectively. The new hormone level may now persist for a long time. There are cases of a secondary rise in the hormone level after a certain time of rest. Of course, there are also cases of gradual normalization of the hormone level to the normal concentration. The hormone changes in the recovery period express, obviously, not only the inertia of regulation in regard to exercise-induced changes, but also the following normalization of the endocrine function. The regulation of metabolic processes during the recovery period may require specific changes in hormone levels.

Catecholamines

During the first minute after the end of 5-min cycling exercises the noradrenaline concentration rose a little. During the following 10 min the hormone concentration decreased rapidly.

Two months of training accelerated, but the following two months of detraining decelerated the restitution rate of the noradrenaline level. Increase in the power output during exercise from 1480 kpm·min⁻¹ to 1920 kpm·min⁻¹ slowed down the disappearance of noradrenaline from the circulation.[85] In a recumbent position the noradrenaline concentration decreased more rapidly than in a sitting position after exercise.[86] A rapid decline in the adrenaline concentration following the highest level has been found after short-term exercise.[87]

After prolonged exercise, high levels of catecholamines may persist for many hours or even for days. Both adrenaline and noradrenaline concentrations remained increased for 2 h after 80-min exercises at 75% VO_2max. After a marathon race adrenaline concentrations above the initial level persisted for at least 24 h.[88] At 24 h after a 24-h endurance run or triathlon competition the blood levels of free and sulfated catecholamines were elevated.[89] During a 6-day cross-country ski hike (daily distance 35 to 50 km) immediately after skiing as well as in the evening, the blood levels of catecholamines were elevated, but catecholamine response to the ergometer test, performed immediately after skiing, was normal. Eleven days after the hike the noradrenaline concentration was above the initial level by 25%.[90]

In rats the noradrenaline levels exceeded the initial one by 229% immediately after 3-h of swimming and by 144 and 238% 1 h and 4 h later, respectively.[91]

According to the results of animal experiments a long time period is necessary for restitution of the catecholamine content in the adrenals. In rats after an 8-h swim the adrenaline content remained low during 7 days due to the disturbed catecholamine synthesis. During the first 5 days of the recovery period the adrenals synthesized mainly noradrenaline. After only a week the adrenaline formation was augmented, but the prevailing adrenaline synthesis, common for the resting state, was not yet observed. The catecholamine content in the heart and the noradrenaline content in the hypothalamus returned to normal levels after 2 days.[92] In the mouse, after a prolonged run (running for 16 and 10 h, interrupted by a 12-h rest period) 6 days was required for the adrenal catecholamine content to return to normal levels.[93]

Glucocorticoids

After short-term exercises the increase in the blood cortisol concentration continues within the first 5 to 30 min.[94-97] This may be due to the inertia of the activation mechanism or of the secondary response of the adrenal cortex. The highest corticotropin level was found immediately after, but the highest cortisol level 15 min after 1 min of cycling at 120% VO_2max.[98] The elevated blood cortisol after exercise has been shown to be related to the decreased rate of hormone elimination from the blood plasma.[99,100] After a 30-min exhaustive exercise the blood cortisol level rose during the first 30 to 60 min, and then declined. The resting level was obtained within 90 to 120 min.[101] After an 80-min exercise at 70% VO_2max a transient increase in the plasma cortisol concentration lasted for 1 h after the exercise.[50] A heavy anaerobic exercise (running 3×300 m) was followed by a high level of cortisol in the blood that persisted for 3 h. Then a drop in the cortisol concentration followed. At 6 h after the end of the exercise it was substantially below the initial level.[96]

At 3 to 6 h after a 13- to 14-km run a low cortisol level was observed.[102] After 2 h of exercise at 60% VO_2max a decreased activity of the pituitary-adrenocortical system was established by levels of both corticotropin and cortisol below the initial ones within 6 to 24 h post-exercise. There were no systematical differences between data obtained from untrained persons and from well-trained sportsmen in endurance events.[103] Low levels of cortisol were found also 24 h after 60-min cycling at 70% VO_2max,[104] marathon race,[88] and 100-km running.[105] At 1,2, and 4 days after running for 34 km, the blood cortisol was insignificantly, and 8 days later significantly, below the initial values.[106]

In rats the corticosterone content in the blood plasma[91,107] and in the adrenals[107] remained augmented for at least 4 h or even 5 days following swimming exercises. The peak values were observed after 2 days in the adrenals and after 5 days in the plasma. One day later, repetition of the same exercise did not elicit any response. After 2 days the response was inverted.

Following 3 to 5 days after the first exercise the response to the new exercise was exaggerated.[107] Is the latter a reflection of supercompensation for biosynthetic activity in the cells of the fascicular zone of the adrenal cortex? Anyway, an elevated content of ascorbic acid in the adrenal tissue was found several days after exercise.[108,109]

Pancreatic Hormones

Exercise is followed by a rapid increase in the blood level of insulin.[104,110-112] This change is so rapid that any measurement of insulin concentration, not carried out while the subject is still exercising, may be misleading in regard to the detection of an insulin drop during exercise.[113] The concomitant increase in the C-peptide level in the blood indicates that insulin secretion increases just after the end of exercise.[114]

After a 100-km run the insulin level in the blood was still increased 24 h later.[105] Running of 34 km was followed by a decreased insulin level 1 day later.[106]

Apart from other results, no significant change in the blood insulin level was observed after an 80-min exercise at 70% VO_2max during the period of post-exercise excess oxygen consumption.[50] In rats, 3 h of swimming was followed by a 4-h period of decreased insulin level.[91]

Using the blockade of the opioid receptor with the aid of naloxone administration, it was shown that in the post-exercise period the glucose-stimulated insulin secretion was enhanced by endogenous opioids. In resting conditions naloxone did not have such effect.[115]

The glucagon level decreases gradually from the highest concentration just after the end of exercise in humans,[110] rats[91] and dogs.[110] In men the glucagon blood levels remained elevated for 90 to 120 min after 30 min of cycling until exhaustion.[101] At 1, 2, 4, and 8 days after running of 34 km the glucagon concentration was close to the initial level.[106]

Somatotropin

In most cases the recovery period is characterized by a rather rapid decrease in the somatotropin concentration in the blood to normal values if the hormone level was augmented during the exercise.[101,103,116,117] The rebinding time is dependent on the fitness level. After the cessation of a 30-min exhaustive exercise the somatotropin concentration returned to the resting level within 30 min in fit persons, but continued to increase for 60 min before declining in unfit ones.[101] A post-exercise increase in the blood somatotropin level was observed mostly after comparatively short-term exercises: after 20-min aerobic exercises or after seven repetitions of a 1-min anaerobic exercise,[118,119] or after intermittent weight-lifting exercises.[120] An anaerobic running exercise (3 × 300 m) induced even in trained persons a persistently high somatotropin level during the first hour of restitution. Subnormal values were found 6, 24, and 72 h later.[96] In athletes the blood level of somatotropin was higher on the night after daytime training exercises than during the control night.[121]

Sex Hormones

Usually, the pituitary-testicular system does not respond until the recovery period. Within the first 6 h of restitution after various endurance exercises, a gradual drop in the blood testosterone[102,103] and androstenedione[102] occurs. Low levels of both components may persist for at least 3 to 4 days.[102,105,106] Prolonged running (15 to 42 km) caused a decrease in the plasma testosterone concentration. The longer the run, the more time it took before the testosterone concentration returned to pre-contest levels.[122]

In rats, short-term swimming with a high additonal load (13% body weight) caused a slight increase in the blood testosterone level but was followed during the first 2 h of restitution by a decrease in the hormone level. At 4 h after the exercise a rise in the hormone concentration was detected, exceeding the resting level by 1.5 to 2.5 times.[123] This exercise bout increased the testosterone, androstenedione, and estradiol contents in the blood, skeletal muscles, and the myocardium. In skeletal muscles the hormone content was close to normal after 2, but increased after 48 h (Figure 4-6). At 72 h after the exercise a decrease was observed in the androstenedione and estradiol content and a further increase in the testosterone content. The number of androgen-binding sites was increased by 20% 2 h and by 80% 72 h after the exercise.[124]

The plasma lutropin level usually returns to the initial values within 1 h and does not change further.[96,102] However, after a 13- to 14-km run the plasma lutropin level decreased within the first 30 min and increased during the next half-hour.[102] After incremental exercise until exhaustion the serum lutropin concentration declined below the basal level reaching nadir values between 60 and 180 min post-exercise. This fall in the serum lutropin concentration appeared to follow a slight but significant elevation of the plasma level of corticoliberin which reached peak values immediately after exercise. The plasma corticotropin paralleled the rise in corticoliberin, but fell to undetectable levels 60 min post-exercise. The plasma cortisol concentration peaked approximately 30 min after the rise in corticotropin, after which they gradually declined to baseline levels. Plasma testosterone concentrations paralleled to concentrations of lutropin. It has been suggested that corticoliberin might suppress the secretion of lutropin after exercise.[125]

Thyroid Hormones

Immediately after a marathon run, increased thyroid activity was evidenced by elevated blood levels of free thyroxine, free triiodothyronine, and thyrotropin. Free thyroxine remained elevated 1 h later as well. At 22 h after the race the thyrotropin concentration was decreased, and thyroxine and triiodothyronine levels were close to pre-race values. Comparison of the changes of free thyroxine or free triiodothyronine to free reverse triiodothyronine indicated that 22 h after the race a favored conversion of active hormones to inactive reverse triiodothyronine still exists.[126] After an 80-min exercise at 75% VO_2max no changes in the free thyroxine levels were found.[50]

In rats, 30 m of running (35 m·min^{-1}) induced increased levels of thyroxine and triiodothyronine in the blood for 48 h, with peak values of thyrotropin 1.5 h after the end of exercise (Figure 4-7). This response was observed even in rats made hypothyroid by repeated injections of mercasolil after 10 min of swimming with additional load of 10% b.w.[127]

Responses to Test Exercises in Men

Substantial changes in the endocrine system during the post-exercise recovery period are evidenced by altered responses to repetition of the same exercise or to test exercise. In swimmers the noradrenaline, adrenaline, corticotropin, cortisol, and somatotropin responses to a 100-m swim, repeated 1 h after the first swim, were suppressed in comparison with response to the first exercise bout. When swimming for 1500 m was repeated, noradrenaline and adrenaline responses were exaggerated, and cortisol and somatotropin responses decreased. In both exercises the insulin response did not change. Increases in lactate, glycerol, and FFA levels were more pronounced after the second repetition of these exercises.[128]

One hour after a 2-h exercise at 53% VO_2max the heart rate response to Stroop conflicting color word test or to a 3-min exercise at 42% VO_2max were elevated, but the blood adrenaline responses to handgrip or the Stroop test were lowered. A reduction in the adrenaline response might reflect either the altered adrenaline removal or changes in the activation of the adrenal medulla. The plasma noradrenaline and blood pressure responses were similar in the control situation and in post-exercise recovery.[129]

When highly qualified weight-lifters performed two strength training sessions in 1 day, an increase in serum cortisol as well as in the total and free testosterone concentrations was observed only after the second training sessions. One hour after the termination of the afternoon session a decrease in the levels of three hormones followed. The studied hormones decreased in response to the morning session. It was suggested that the diurnal variation might mask the exercise-induced changes during the morning session.[130] However, summation of the

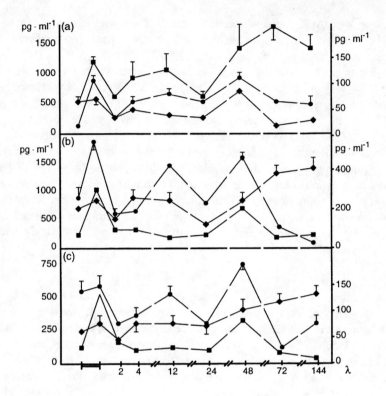

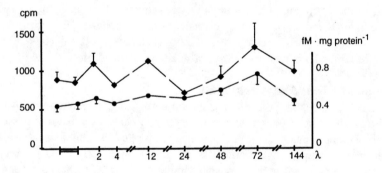

FIGURE 4-6. Testosterone (○–○), androstenedione (●–●) and estradiol (x-x) levels in blood serum (A), cytoplasm of myocardium (B) and skeletal muscle (C) in rats after swimming six to seven times for 1 min with additional load of 12% body weight (rest intervals 90 s). In the lower part of the figure the specific binding of nortestosterone to cytosol proteins (○–○) and number of binding sites (x-x) are indicated. (From Tchaikovsky, V. S., Jevtinova, I. V., and Basharina, O. B., *Acta Comment. Univ. Tartuensis,* 702, 105, 1985. With permission.)

effect of the training session might also have an essential role. This possibility is indicated by a less pronounced increase in the lactate concentration and also by a more pronounced impairment of the maximal isometric force, the maximal rate of force development, and relaxation time after the second rather than after the first training session.[130]

WATER-ELECTROLYTE HOMEOSTASIS

Changes in the water and electrolyte content in the blood plasma and in the muscle and other tissues indicate the rate of restoration of the water-electrolyte balance after exercise. At the same time, changes in the levels of hormones controlling the water-electrolyte balance express the activity of related homeostatic mechanisms.

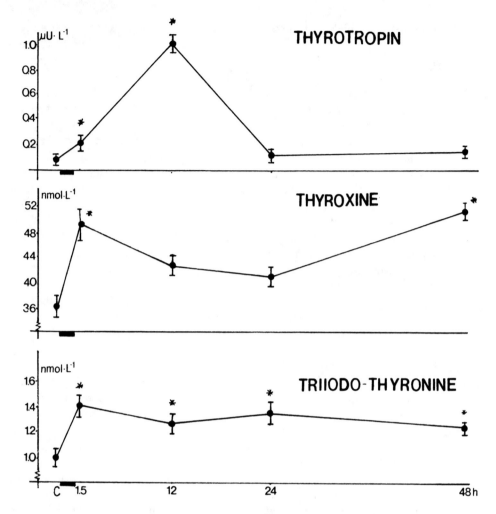

FIGURE 4-7. Dynamics of thyrotropin, thyroxine, and triiodothyronine in the blood after 30 min of running (35 m·min⁻¹) in rats. Asterisks denote statistically significant difference from the control level.

Rapid re-uptake of K^+ by muscles and decrease of plasma K^+ are seen after exercises.[131] The recovery kinetics of K^+ re-uptake by muscles were described by a very fast (<1 min) and a slow component (>1 min). The magnitude of the former was equivalent to what had accumulated in the plasma during exercise.[60] The time of restoration of the normal potassium level in the blood plasma varies from some minutes to 20 to 30 min after various exercises.[112,132,133] During recovery from anaerobic (exhaustion appeared after 4.6 ± 1.3 min of exercise), but not from aerobic exercise (1 h at 65% VO_2max), there was a rapid decrease in the plasma potassium levels while the phosphate values were gradually normalized together with pH.[134]

While concentrations of serum potassium and adrenaline returned to their basal levels immediately after incremental exercise until exhaustion, those of plasma noradrenaline and serum aldosterone remained elevated 30 min later.[112] It was suggested that besides other hormones the increased level of plasma noradrenaline, maintained during the first 30 min post-exercise, might have a function in avoiding excessive hypokalaemia through the stimulation of α-receptors.[112] α-Adrenergic stimulus produces an increase in kalaemia through elevating the hepatic release of potassium. The latter is obviously related to hepatic glycogenolysis. The function of noradrenaline may also be to compensate for the decreased volume of circulating blood by its vasoconstrictor action.

Short-term exercises of high intensity performed until exhaustion caused a decrease in the volume of the circulating blood by 20% in connection with water accumulation in the extra- and intracellular compartments of muscles, and in connection with increased concentrations of sodium and potassium in the blood plasma. At 10 min post-exercise the concentrations of electrolytes decreased despite the fact that the volume of intravascular fluid was still diminished. At 1 h after the end of exercise an increase of 5 to 6% was found in the volume of the circulating blood.[133]

In well-trained swimmers the blood volume that decreased during exercise was restored after a 100- or 800-m swim within 30 min, but plasma sodium within 2.5 min.[132]

After an intensive all-out exercise (duration 10 to 11 min) the increased total muscle water persisted for 20 min. Water accumulation in muscles was associated with an increase in the intracellular water. At 20 min post-exercise the intracellular water was normal, but the amount of extracellular water increased. In muscles both the total and intracellular Na^+ increased, but only the total volume remained beyond the initial level 20 min post-exercise. Total as well as intracellular potassium decreased and did not normalize within 20 min of recovery.[69]

The hormones of renin-angiotensin II-aldosterone, regulating the electrolyte balance, declined slowly after various exercises.[96,103,105]

After short-term exercise the aldosterone and renin normalization rates depend on the body posture. At 15 min after a 20-min exercise bout both the aldosterone and renin levels remained at higher values in a sitting position than in a recumbent position.[135]

Shifts in the water-electrolyte balance, caused by marathon competition, may persist for a prolonged period. Blood volume was increased by 16% on the second post-marathon day. On the third day a tendency to normalization was noticed but the volume remained beyond the initial values. During the first 2 days the sodium concentration was decreased in the plasma, but changes were found neither in the potassium and aldosterone concentration nor in the osmolality of the plasma.[136] At 12 h after a marathon race the increased blood level of atrial natriuretic peptide had changed to a decreased one. At 36 h after the race a secondary rise was observed. The elevated level of the peptide persisted for 7 days.[137]

During the first 1 to 2 h after a 24-h endurance run the plasma volume had decreased by 2%, aldosterone, cortisol, and vasopressin concentrations were increased, and atrial natriuretic peptide was decreased. During 3 days of recovery, plasma volume rose, with a peak on the second day (by 24% over the initial level) and remained elevated on the third day. Cortisol, vasopressin, and atrial natriuretic peptide returned to baseline 24 h later, and aldosterone 72 h later.[138] At 24 h after termination of the 24-h run the plasma Na^+ and K^+ were normal, but the Na^+ level in the urine was very low and the K^+ urinary level was elevated in connection with the increased aldosterone concentration in the blood plasma. Differently, after a 10-h triathlon competition, the high aldosterone level was associated with normal urinary sodium and potassium. High blood cortisol was found 2 days after the triathlon but not after the 24-h run. Increased activities of creatine kinase, lactate dehydrogenase, aspartate aminotransferase, and alanine aminotransferase persisted at least 24 h after the 24-h run.[139]

Erythropoietin concentration in the blood was increased at 3 h and, more impressively, 31 h after a marathon run but not immediately after the race. At 31 h after the race a pronounced increase in the plasma volume was established, which led to a hemodilution together with decreased concentrations of both erythrocytes and hemoglobin.[140] After very prolonged exercise hypocalcemia persisted for 48 h both in rats[141] and in humans.[142] This was associated with a high level of calcitonin in the blood plasma.[141,142]

Highly intensive anaerobic exercise caused an increase in the magnesium concentration in both the blood and urine. These changes correlated with an increase of lactate in the blood. The blood magnesium level normalized within 2 h.[143] During a marathon race serum magnesium increased from 1.44 to 1.68 meq·l^{-1} within the first 2 h. Thereafter the magnesium concentration dropped to 1.07 meq·l^{-1} by the end of the race and returned to its pre-race value by 1 h of recovery. During the first 20 min of recovery a further decrease in the blood magnesium concentration was found.[144] A further decrease in magnesium concentration was also found in cases of its reduction during exercise.[145] Exercise-induced changes in total zinc and zinc derived from carbonic anhydrase type I in erythrocytes as well as in total zinc in the plasma disappeared within 30 min.[146]

CENTRAL NERVOUS SYSTEM

The main features of immediate changes in the status of the central nervous system are a certain inertia of exercise-induced changes in excitability and lability of nervous centers, followed later by undulated changes. The corresponding changes in optical and tactile rheobases[147] and latency of muscle contraction and relaxation[148] are presented in Figure 4-8. Undulated changes were found also in motor chronaxie. For skeletal muscle a relative hypoexcitability for rectangular electrical stimuli has been found in association with low serum Mg level.[149]

The polyphasic nature of changes in the central nervous system after exercise was confirmed by studies of conditioned reflex responses (CRR) on stimuli not related to muscular activity. Immediately after exercise the CRR were more rapid and stronger than before exercise. It was suggested that the first phase of the recovery period expresses the remaining excitation of the central nervous system. This phase was followed by an inhibition phase: the CRR appeared slowly and were less pronounced. When a certain time period elapsed, the third phase appeared, suggesting a normalization of the state of central nervous structures. In a number of cases a further exaltation of reflex responses was later observed. After a hard, fatiguing exercise the first phase was not found and the inhibition phase appeared just after exercise.[150]

H-response of various muscles after all-out exercise (duration less than 10 min) indicated a decreased excitability of spinal motoneurons during the first 3 to 6 min. Then an increased excitability was found. A complete recovery of motoneuron excitability was detected within 8 to 12 min after exercise.[151]

The polyphasic changes appear also in the working capacity during the first minutes or hours after exercise. The recovery of strength is initially rapid with a subsequent two-component pattern.[152] Following rhythmic exercises, the recovery of strength was faster than after a static one.[153] Likewise, the recovery of local muscular endurance is initially fast and then a slow period of normalization follows.[154] After a subject squeezed a hand-grip device for as long as possible at a tension of 50% of his maximum voluntary contraction, the percentage of recovery at various time periods revealed a three-component exponential curve. The percentage of recovery, calculated by dividing the holding time of the first bout by the time of the second, ranged from 20% after 5 s of rest to 87% after 42 min 40 s of rest.[155]

The short-term phases of working capacity and strength are probably associated with changes in the nervous centers, acting through alterations in the recruitment of motor units. The alterations may be related to the various levels of excitability of motoneurons or other nervous cells, participating in the organization of movements. However, besides changes in the central nervous system, one must take into consideration the fact that in the first minutes after exercise there may exist an intracellular electrolytic unbalance due to the lagging behind of the Na,K-pump functions, and the interference of depletion/repletion of intramuscular energy stores and metabolite accumulation of working capacity of muscles. The recovery of force is closely correlated to the decrease in intracellular Na^+. Inhibition of the Na,K-pump favors the net loss of K^+, gain of Na^+, and development of fatigue in the isolated working muscle.[156] In the frog muscle, 15 min after stimulation 30 times per minute (contractile force decreased 36%, lactate content increased from 3.3 to 18.7 $\mu mol \cdot g^{-1}$ of muscle) recovery occurred in two phases. A rapid increase in contractile force (20% of total recovery) took place during the first 15 s concomitantly with an increase in ATP from 3.9 to 4.6 $\mu mol \cdot g^{-1}$. Lactate

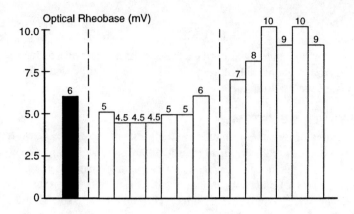

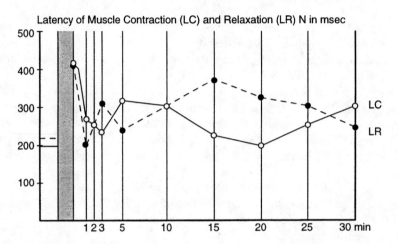

FIGURE 4-8. Post-exercise changes of the optical rheobase (upper part) and latency period of contraction or relaxation (lower part). Upper part: black column — initial level, vertical interrupted lines — 1-min exercise, striated columns — levels determine 20 s, 40 s, 80 s, 100 s, 2 min, 3 min, and 4 min after exercise, respectively. (From Krestovnikov, A. N., *Survey on Physiology of Physical Exercise,* FiS, Moscow, 1951, With permission.)

did not change during this period. The second phase of contractile force recovery was completed in 50 min. The recovery of contractile force lagged behind the decrease in the lactate level. A significant correlation (r = 0.91) was established between the two indices.[157] A direct pH-dependence of force recovery was not observed during the initial phase of recovery but if present, such a relationship might have been masked by other factors like P_i or $H_2PO^-_4$. During the latter phase of recovery a pH-dependent mechanism could come into action directly.[158]

REPLETION OF ENERGY STORES

TIME SEQUENCE OF THE REPLETION OF VARIOUS SUBSTRATES

By a general consensus, more rapid repletion of energy-rich phosphates than that of glycogen is accepted. Within the first 60 s of recovery approximately 70% of the ATP and phosphocreatine were replenished (Figure 4-9). For complete recovery of the ATP store 2 min of recovery was necessary, but for recovery of the phosphocreatine store, more than 3 min was necessary.[159] During highly intensive intermittent exercise 3-min intervals between exercise bouts were not sufficient to avoid a gradual decrease of muscle phosphocreatine content.[160]

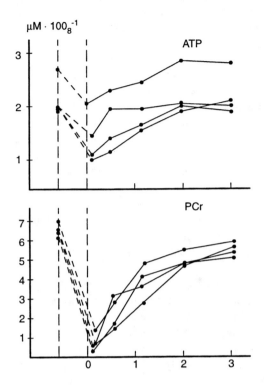

FIGURE 4-9. Restitution of ATP and phosphocreatine contents in skeletal muscles after all-out anaerobic exercise in man. Results of various persons are indicated. (From Hultman, E., Bergström, J., and McLennan-Anderson, N., *Scand. J. Clin. Lab. Invest.*, 19, 56, 1967. With permission.)

After all-out exercise at 100% VO_2max less than 10 min was necessary for the complete recovery of ATP, ADP, and phosphocreatine levels in the quadriceps muscle.[161]

However, there are also results indicating that ATP repletion does not always precede phosphocreatine recovery[162] or even glycogen recovery.[53] After a 3-min one-leg exercise a rapid repletion of ATP and phosphocreatine stores was found in the vastus lateralis muscle during the first 10 min. Later the recovery process slowed down and 1 h after the exercise the levels of energy-rich phosphates as well as glycogen constituted only 90% of the initial.[53] At 9 days after a marathon race decreased levels of ATP, ADP, AMP, and IMP were found in the vastus lateralis muscle, implying that in a late phase of recovery the adenosine deamination was intensified. At the same time, the muscle glycogen level was slightly increased.[163]

At least in rats during the initial 30 min after a short-term running, glycogen synthesis was much slower than during the second 30 min. Between 30 and 60 min after exercising the glycogen synthesis rate was highest in various types of skeletal muscle fibers, heart, and liver. Comparison of glycogen synthesis rates showed that this process is fastest in the fast-twitch oxidative-glycolytic (FOG) fibers and in the myocardium. The rate of slow-twitch oxidative (SO) fibers was 2 times slower. The slowest rate was observed in the fast-twitch glycolytic (FG) fibers (Figure 4-10). The resting level was first reached in the myocardium and FOG fibers, then in SO fibers, and lastly in FG fibers and liver.[164] The same schedule in glycogen repletion was found in rats after other strenuous exercises.[91]

In most cases, the results obtained both in humans[56,165,166] and in rats[167] indicate that the phase of rapid glycogen synthesis occurs within 4 to 6 h after the end of exercise. In this phase the rate of glycogen synthesis is primarily dependent on the amount of glycogen depletion while the subsequent less rapid phase has been reported to be related to the insulin-induced activation of glycogen synthesis.[168]

SUPERCOMPENSATION

The post-exercise supercompensation for muscle glycogen stores was first reported in the late 1940s.[169,170] This phenomenon is dependent on the rate of glycogen depletion during exercise. A little later, supercompensation for the phosphocreatine store was reported (Figure 4-11). When glycogen supercompensation in the rat muscles was found within 1 to 24 h post-exercise, supercompensation for phosphocreatine appeared in the muscle following a shorter time interval, which elapsed after the cessation of exercise.[171,172] After short-term intensive swimming a rapid resynthesis of phosphocreatine occurred, with a pronounced supercompensation, while after long-term swimming the phosphocreatine synthesis was retarded and supercompensation less pronounced. Patterns of glycogen resynthesis were similar in both cases.[173]

Phosphocreatine and glycogen supercompensation appeared in the muscles of slow-twitch fibers earlier than in the muscles of fast-twitch fibers.[174] According to these results, it was later shown that in humans the restitution rate of ATP, ATP/ADP, phosphocreatine, and lactate is in correlation with the oxidative potential of the skeletal muscle, estimated by the activity of citrate synthase.[175]

While immediately after exercise the concentrations of mitochondrial proteins and mitochondrial P/O were decreased, 1 h later both values were significantly higher than in the sedentary control rats. The increase in mitochondrial proteins was associated with an increased concentration of phosphatile inozitol and polyglyceride phosphatide but not of other phospholipids in the mitochondrial fraction of skeletal muscles.[176] The post-exercise increases in the succinate dehydrogenase activity, mitochondrial proteins, and P/O were higher after swimming in water of 22 than of 32°C.[172]

The involvement of mitochondrial function in post-exercise substrate supercompensation has been confirmed in several studies. In rats uncoupling of oxidative phosphorylation by administration of 2.4-dinitrophenole decelerated the recovery process, no supercompensation for glycogen and phosphocreatine was observed, and elimination of lactate was retarded.[177]

The exercise-induced reduction of mitochondrial P/O and respiratory control was followed by an increase in both indices after exercise. Experiments on rats indicated that these changes were accompanied by an elevated ratio of β-hydroxybutyrate/acetoacetate. At that time, increased reductive properties of the mitochondrial pyridine nucleotides and preferably active oxidation of succinate, accumulated in muscles during exercise, were common.[178] At 1 h after 15 min of swimming the ATP content and the ratios of ATP/ADP and ATP/(ADP·P_{inorg}) were elevated.[179] It was concluded that a peculiar 'synthesizing state' of the skeletal muscle mitochondria appeared related to the overproduction of ATP and supercompensation for energy stores. The increased ratios of ATP/ADP and NADH/NAD suppress the catabolic phase of energy metabolism, favoring the substrate supercompensation. However, suppression of the catabolic phase of energy metabolism creates conditions for a decrease in the ATP resynthesis rate, resulting in a reduced ratio of ATP/ADP. Throughout a new intensification of the catabolic phase of energy processes a return to the basal level will be ensured.[180]

The phenomenon of substrate supercompensation has repeatedly been confirmed. Increased levels of glycogen[163,164,181-185] and phosphocreatine[160,162] were found in skeletal muscles after exercises in certain time periods both in humans[160,163,181,183] and rats.[164,184] In the rat soleus muscle glycogen supercompensation appeared to be followed by a secondary decrease.[185] Muscle glycogen supercompensation can be stimulated by carbohydrate feeding.[186-189] Since there is a positive correlation between the pre-exercise muscle glycogen concentration and the ability to perform prolonged severe exercises,[190-192] the glycogen supercompensation enhanced by carbohydrate feeding is correlated to the time of competition in endurance events.

FIGURE 4-10. Post-exercise dynamics of glycogen in the myocardium, FG, FOG, and SO fibers in rats. Arrows indicate the time of return to initial level and the time of onset of supercompensation. Constructed from results of R.L. Terjung et al.[164]

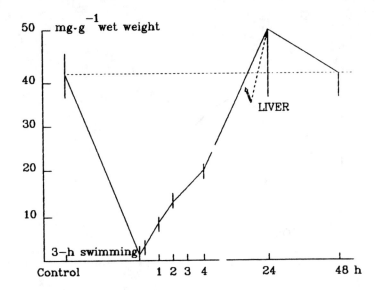

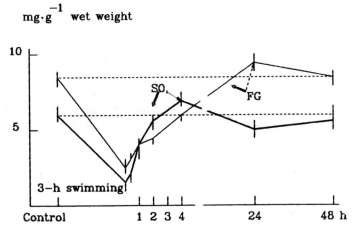

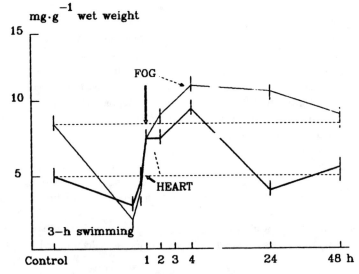

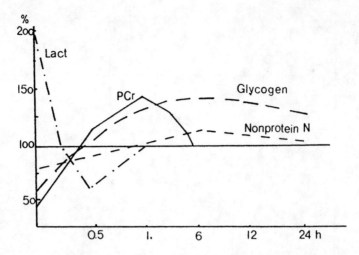

FIGURE 4-11. Substrate supercompensation in rats after exercise. (From Yakovlev, N. N., *Sportbiochemie,* Barta, Leipzig, 1977. With permission.)

In rats supercompensation was demonstrated also in regard to the liver[164,172,193] and myocardial glycogen content.[172,194-196] Glycogen supercompensation was found in a period of 1 to 4 h after exercise in FOG fibers and myocardium, 4 h post-exercise in SO fibers, and 24 h post-exercise in FG fibers and liver.[164]

CONTROL OF GLYCOGEN RESYNTHESIS

Rat experiments demonstrated that after exercise the rate of glycogen synthesis was in good accordance with the activities of glycogen synthase,[164] mainly glycogen synthase I[91] and hexokinase.[164] The activation of glycogen synthase occurs rapidly in a high correlation with an increase in cAMP-phosphodiesterase activity.[193] In humans a significant increase in glycogen synthase fractional activity was found as early as 5 min after cycling at 75% VO$_2$max. At this time the cAMP-dependent protein kinase activity had reverted to the pre-exercise values.[197] Glycogen depletion per se induces an increase in the active form of glycogen synthase[198-200] and stimulates glycogen synthesis.[192,201] Nevertheless, glycogen synthase fractional activity increased markedly during the first 5 min both in conditions of low muscle glycogen (due to previous diet and exercise) and in conditions of high glycogen.[197]

In man the rate of glycogen synthesis was still elevated when the increase in the form I of glycogen synthase had disappeared, indicating that other factors must also contribute to the high rate of glycogen synthesis in the post-exercise period.[200] In rats during an initial phase of post-exercise recovery glucose uptake in skeletal muscles took place despite the lack of endogenous insulin.[202] In this phase a rapid glycogen synthesis occurred despite low insulin and elevated noradrenaline and glycogen levels in the blood plasma.[91] During the second phase, when the glycogen content in the muscles reached the basal level or exceeded it, glucose uptake[202] and glycogen synthesis were insulin-dependent.[168,184]

Insulin has an essential function also in myocardial glycogen resynthesis and supercompensation. Vigorous running for 45 to 75 min caused a decrease in cardiac glycogen in association with increases in glycogen synthase activity and glucose-6-phosphate content. Within 2 to 8 h of recovery the glycogen store was supercompensated, glycogen synthase I activity decreased, and the glucose-6-phosphate content normalized. All these changes were modest in diabetic rats but they became close to normal after treating diabetic rats with insulin.[195]

Post-exercise supercompensation for cardiac glycogen was enhanced with dexamethasone treatment, eliminated by adrenalectomy and restored in adrenalectomized rats that had been given daily doses of dexamethasone.[203] In adrenalectomized rats a slow rate of glycogen post-exercise repletion was found not only in the myocardium, but also in skeletal muscles and liver. Dexamethasone treatment restored the glycogen repletion rate in adrenalectomized rats. The blockade of protein synthesis excluded the dexamethasone effect, suggesting that the glucocorticoid effect was mediated by synthesis of regulatory protein, most likely of glycogen synthase.[204]

SUBSTRATES FOR MUSCLE GLYCOGEN REPLETION

When subjects fasted during the post-exercise recovery, they exhibited a small but significant increase in the muscle glycogen concentration.[205] In fasting rats a preferential resynthesis of muscle glycogen was found.[206] Obviously, the resynthesis of muscle glycogen can proceed by utilizing endogenous substrates. Those substrates may be lactate produced during muscular activity and glucose released from the liver.

Lactate

Lactate has been assumed to serve as a substrate for muscle glycogenesis since the elaboration of the Meyerhof-Hill theory.[2,207] A number of more recent results confirm this old postulation.[56,57,208-213] However, only muscles composed predominantly of FOG or FG fibers have been demonstrated to synthesize glycogen from lactate.[214] In the removal of blood lactate, the main role belongs to SO fibers.[215] The primary fate of absorbed blood lactate is oxidation.[216] For glycogen synthesis in muscles blood glucose is preferred.[53,213,217-219]

Glucose

Intensive refilling of muscle glycogen stores may be associated with a further decrease in liver glycogen during the first post-exercise hours.[206] Obviously, the fast repletion of muscle stores is actualized at the expense of liver glycogen.

The rate of muscle glycogen repletion depends on the blood glucose level,[220] maintained at the expense of liver glucose output or of ingested carbohydrates.[190,191] Fructose ingestion produces a slower rate of glycogen resynthesis than glucose or sucrose ingestion.[189,221] After prolonged exhaustive exercise orally administered glucose was used primarily for muscle rather than hepatic glycogen repletion.[222]

GLUCONEOGENESIS AND LIPID METABOLISM
Hepatic Gluconeogenesis

The rate of liver glycogen restitution is slow until the person or test animal is refed.[211,216,223] In subjects recovering from exercise, glucose infusion raised the blood level of glucose up to 12 mmol·l^{-1}, but the arterio-venous glucose difference across the liver was negligible.[224] The results confirm that the liver defers its glycogen to supply other tissues, such as cardiac and skeletal muscle, by glucose output. After exercise, there is an intensive gluconeogenesis in the liver.[223,225,226] During post-exercise recovery the splanchnic uptake of gluconeogenic substrates is augmented.[223,224,227,228] Convincing evidence is provided for intensive use of blood lactate,[223,229] alanine,[230,231] and glycerol[232] in hepatic gluconeogenesis after exercise. In the post-exercise period the main role in gluconeogenesis belongs to alanine.[230]

While a considerably higher glycogen synthesis has been detected in exercised muscles after glucose than after fructose infusion,[233] fructose infusion gives rise to a four-times-larger increase in liver glycogen synthesis than does glucose infusion in man.[234]

In exercising rats it was found that the increased gluconeogenic flux was the result of the increased activities of gluconeogenic enzymes, pyruvate carboxylase, and fructose-1.6-biphosphatase, with the concomitant inhibition of glycolytic enzymes, 6-phosphofructokinase, and pyruvate kinase. The increased maximal activities of gluconeogenic enzymes were related to changes in the concentrations of several allosteric modulators: increased acetyl-CoA, decreased fructose-2.6-biphosphate, and decreased fructose-1.6-biphosphate.[235]

Lipid Metabolism

Elevated blood levels of glycerol and FFA were found during 24 h after prolonged exercises.[236] By other results, blood glycerol and FFA concentrations returned to the pre-exercise levels within 20 to 60 min, but despite that, a low respiratory exchange ratio persisted.[52,54,237] This was explained by the utilization of intramuscular triglycerides.[52,53,238] It was mentioned earlier that the triglyceride-free fatty acid cycle may proceed intensively during the recovery period.

During 2 h of recovery after moderate cycling for 100 min the insulin effects on carbohydrates and lipid metabolism proved to be altered. While during exercise insulin infusion enhanced carbohydrate oxidation, in the recovery period the insulin effect was negligible. Nonoxidative carbohydrate metabolism increased during the recovery period and became more sensitive to insulin than in resting conditions. However, an exercise-induced increase in fat oxidation did not appear in the first 100 min of the recovery period despite the persisting elevated levels of both glycerol and FFA. Suppression of the FFA level but not of fat oxidation by insulin infusion was enhanced after the exercise.[239] These results suggest that the post-exercise increase in insulin secretion together with the increased sensitivity of lipid metabolism to insulin will limit the amount of fat oxidation, stimulated by the increased level of FFA.

For interpretation of the changes in lipid oxidation one must take into consideration the possible alteration in carnitine metabolism. Exercise-induced increase of esterified carnitine in the muscles persisted for 90 min and was associated with a decrease in free carnitine.[240]

Lipid peroxidation during the post-exercise recovery period has not yet been sufficiently studied. The significance of this problem is indicated by the fact that muscle pain that appeared 24 h after the exercise was preceded by an increase in the serum lipid peroxide concentration.[241]

RECONSTRUCTIVE FUNCTION OF THE RECOVERY PROCESS

PROTEIN SYNTHESIS IN SKELETAL MUSCLES

The renewal of structural and enzymatic proteins in the muscular tissue can be completed only after the end of muscle activity. Accordingly, elevated intensity of protein synthesis is considered to be common for the recovery period after exercise. The exercise-induced decrease of protein nitrogen was found to be reversed after the cessation of contractile activity. Approximately 6 h after swimming it was on a higher level in comparison with the level in sedentary rats.[171,242,243] The studies of whole body metabolism in men point to nitrogen retention in the recovery period.[244-246] The post-exercise intensification of protein synthesis was proved by the elevated rate of amino acid incorporation into various fractions of skeletal muscle proteins[247-259] as well as by enhanced incorporation of labeled precursors into RNA.[256] Accordingly, increases in the ribosomal translational activity[249] and nuclear RNA polymerase activity[257,260] were detected in the recovery period.

However, it would be an oversimplification to regard the post-exercise recovery as a transition from exercise-induced overall catabolism to anabolism. The picture is more complicated.

During the first hours of post-exercise recovery the rate of protein synthesis remains low in the skeletal muscle of man[254] and rat.[252,255,258,259] In rats the duration of this period varied from 6 to 24 h. It is only after this initial period that the rate of protein synthesis increases. There are significant differences in the intensity of protein synthesis between various protein fractions as well as between muscle fibers of various types depending on the character of the performed exercise.[252] The immediate effect of 6 h of swimming was a remarkable decrease in the incorporation of ^{14}C leucine into actin and the myosin heavy chains in the gastrocnemius muscle, but it caused an increase in the incorporation into myosin light chains. An elevation of amino acid incorporation into actin and myosin heavy chain was observed 48 h post-exercise.[255] A post-exercise increase in protein synthesis was also detected in isolated mitochondria.[261]

After endurance exercises the main locus of the increased rate of protein synthesis is the mitochondria of FOG and SO fibers (Figure 4-12). The highest rate was found 24 h post-exercise. Instead of increased synthesis of various proteins, in FG fibers the incorporation of labeled tyrosin into myofibrillar, sarcoplasmic, and mitochondrial proteins was decreased within 24 to 48 h post-exercise.[259] This fact allows us to suggest that during the recovery period the inhibition of protein synthesis in previously less active muscles and fibers makes it possible to concentrate the adaptive protein synthesis for structures that performed the highest load.

The main results of this study were confirmed with the aid of an ultra-autoradiographic study. In this study the comparison of dynamics in label incorporation showed that thyroid hormones may promote post-exercise synthesis of proteins in skeletal muscles. In hypothyroid rats no increase was found in label incorporation during a 48-h recovery period after 30 min of running. In these rats a low level of label was found in the mitochondria as well as in all regions of sarcoplasma and myofibrils during the recovery period.[262] However, after a short-term highly intensive exercise (10 min of swimming with an additional load of 10% b.w.) a post-exercise increase was observed even in rats made hypothyroid by repeated injections of methimazole. The rise in the blood level of triiodothyronine and thyroxine coincided with the increased incorporation of ^{3}H-tyrosine in all types of muscle fibers. The most pronounced increase in label incorporation was found 24 h post-exercise in SO fibers.[262]

These results may be considered to be a justification of the hypothesis about hormonal amplification of adaptive protein synthesis induced by metabolic inductors.[263] Probably, after endurance exercise thyroid hormones ensure hormonal amplifications of this kind. Their function in stimulating the genesis of the mitochondria in skeletal muscles is evidenced by the results of various studies.[264,265] In accordance with the above, mentioned results is also the fact that the thyroxine effect on mitochondrial enzymes is more pronounced in the red muscles than in the white ones.[266] Thyroid hormones may also contribute to the induction of skeletal muscle myosin.[267]

A different situation exists after exercises for improved strength. In these cases the main locus of adaptive protein synthesis is the myofibrillar proteins of fast-twitch glycolytic fibers. In men the action of a resistance training session (4 sets of 6 to 12 repetitions of the biceps curl, preacher curl, and concentration curl with a resistance equal to 80% 1RM) on protein synthesis in the biceps muscle was studied, using the opposite arm as a control. Muscle protein synthesis was significantly elevated 4 h post-exercise. The increased protein synthesis rate persisted for at least 24 h. The increase appeared to be due to changes in post-transcriptional events. The latter conclusion was founded on the unchanged RNA capacity (expressed as total RNA content relative to noncollagenous protein content) and elevated RNA activity (expressed as the amount of protein synthesized per unit time per unit RNA).[268]

In rats a model was employed to imitate the human resistance training: skeletal muscles of anesthetized rats were electrically stimulated to contract against resistance. After a single bout of 'exercise' myofibrillar protein synthesis rate increased 50 to 60% 12 to 17 and 36 to 41 h after the exercise. However, skeletal α-actin mRNA and cytochrome c mRNA were not altered at these times.[269,270] An increase in translation of protein can be inferred from such data.[271]

Stimulation of the synthesis of myofibrillar proteins and RNA polymerase activity[260,272] in skeletal muscles by anabolic steroids makes it possible to assume that in normal conditions the synthesis of myofibrillar proteins is amplified by endogenous androgens. To support this suggestion some evidence is necessary to prove that strength exercises, which cause myofibrillar hypertrophy, specifically stimulate the production of endogenous androgens. There exist variable changes in the blood level of testosterone during and after exercises for improved strength. However, the most essential factor is the dynamics of androgens during the recovery period. It has been indicated (see p. 91) that a general characteristic of testosterone dynamics is its low level during the first hours of the first day after exercises. However, apart

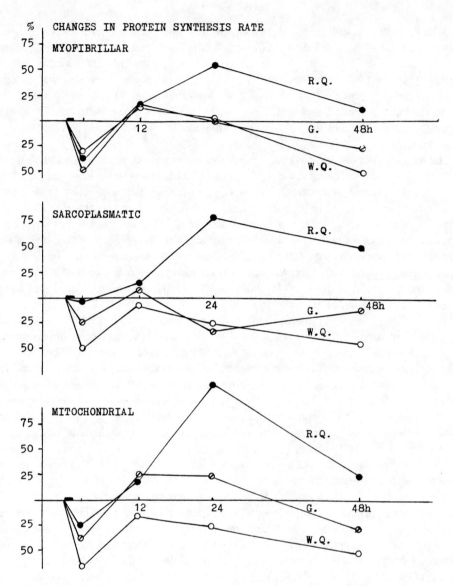

FIGURE 4-12. Synthesis of myofibrillar, sarcoplasmic and mitochondrial proteins in red (R.Q) and white (W.Q) portions of the quadriceps muscle and the gastrocnemius muscle (G) after 30-min running (35 m·min⁻¹) in rats. From Viru, A. and Ööpik, V., in *Paavo Nurmi Congress Book*, Kvist, M., Ed., The Finnish Society of Sports Medicine, Turku, 1989, 55. With permnission.)

from endurance exercises, in case of strength exercises, there follows a tendency to an increased production of testosterone. It is worth repeating that this change is associated with the augmentation of the testosterone and androstenedione content and also with an increase in the number of androgen-binding sites in skeletal muscles.[273] Similarly to the exercise effect, a single injection of testosterone or 10-nortestosterone caused a rapid decrease in the cytoplasmic androgen receptors in skeletal muscles 1 h after treatment, which was followed by its twofold increase 5 to 6 h later. Inhibition of protein synthesis by cyclohexamide 1 h after testosterone treatment led to a less pronounced augmentation of androgen receptors over the control values 5 h later.[274]

Results have been obtained to confirm the role of testosterone and related androgens in the post-exercise synthesis of proteins in skeletal muscles. Repeated 1-min swims with an additional load of 12% b.w. (6 to 7 repetitions over rest intervals of 1.5 min) caused a decrease in the contents of aspartate aminotransferase and myoglobin in the quadriceps muscle during the first 24 h of recovery. At 48 to 56 h post-exercise the content of these proteins was increased by 30%. At the same time testosterone concentrations in the blood and muscle as well as the number of androgens binding sites in the cytoplasm of the muscle were substantially over the control level.[273]

The specific nature of the amplification of protein synthesis in skeletal muscles by testosterone has been confirmed by results obtained by A. Saborido et al.[275] Treatment with anabolic androgens increased succinate dehydrogenase activity in the fast-twitch muscle mitochondria. This effect was not enhanced when anabolic steroids were administered during training. Moreover, the effect of anabolic steroids on the mitochondrial enzyme was not observed in the soleus muscle. Thus, the typical effect of endurance exercises on the mitochondria of oxidative muscles was neither reproduced nor amplified by the administration of steroids.

A stimulatory effect on the protein synthesis (probably on the translational level) is produced by insulin and somatotropin.[276-278] In adults with a somatotropin deficiency, the human growth hormone treatment increased the lean tissue, the total cross-sectional area of the thigh muscle, the strength of the hip flexors, and the limb girdle muscle, but not that of a number of other muscles.[279] Increases were found also in VO_2max, anaerobic ventilatory threshold, and maximal power output.[280] However, one must take into consideration the long period of treatment (6 months) necessary for obtaining the above-mentioned effects as well as the initial hormonal disbalance in the studied patients. In rats, daily injections of somatotropin over 36 days resulted in a significant increase in the diameter of both types of fibers (I and II) in the extensor digitorum longus and soleus muscles. The DNA/protein ratio and the number of satellite cells per muscle fiber cross-sectional area increased as well.[281]

Hind leg perfusion with insulin at 200 $\mu U \cdot ml^{-1}$ but not at 75 $\mu U \cdot ml^{-1}$ stimulated protein synthesis in the white gastrocnemius. After running exercises the insulin effect was not enhanced.[282]

DEGRADATION AND TURNOVER OF PROTEINS

A characteristic feature of post-exercise protein metabolism is the coincidence of an increased rate of protein synthesis with an elevated rate of protein breakdown. While protein synthesis is suppressed immediately after exercise and thereafter enhanced, protein degradation remains elevated for a long period. A high level of urea in the blood and urine persists for many hours after strenuous exercises.[283-287]

After exercises the increased urea level is not necessarily caused by retention of the urea on the level of renal excretion. Contrarily, the post-exercise period was characterized by an increased renal clearance of urea in rats after swims of various duration (Figure 4-13). After only 10 h of swimming a lag period of up to 12 h preceded the increased urea excretion and elevated the renal clearance rate.[288] The post-exercise increase in urea renal elimination is glucocorticoid dependent; it is absent in adrenalectomized rats.[288]

In rats the increased urinary excretion and renal urea clearance persisted for a longer time than was necessary for the normalization of the blood level after swims of various duration.[288] If endogenous production and elimination rates are equal, increased production may lead to an elevated urinary excretion without any increase in the blood level. Therefore, the results obtained in rats point to a persisting elevated urea production for a long period after exercise. Accordingly, the activity of hepatic arginase, an important enzyme in urea biosynthesis, remains elevated for many hours after exercise.[289]

Exercise-induced increase in tyrosine release from muscles may also persist for hours.[290,291] However, alanine output from muscles decreases rapidly after exercise.[292] Since the elevated net uptake of alanine by the splanchnic bed persists,[293] the blood level of alanine decreases.[292]

3-Methylhistidine is released from muscles as a result of myosin and actin degradation. It will be excreted without any conversion or reutilization. Despite the great variability in the

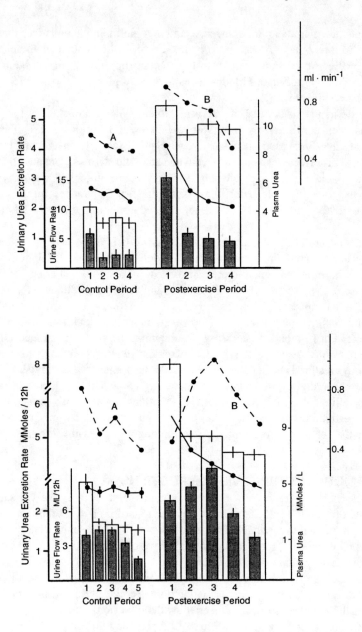

FIGURE 4-13. Urea level of blood plasma (solid line), urinary urea excretion rate (white columns), urine flow rates (striated columns) and renal urea clearance (interrupted line) in rats after swimming for 3 h (upper part) or 10 h (lower part). (From Litvinova, L., Viru, A., and Smirnova, T., *Jpn. J. Physiol.,* 39, 713, 1989. With permission.)

changes that occur in 3-methylhistidine excretion during exercise, the increased excretion is a post-exercise phenomenon[294-298] (Figure 4-14). The excretion dynamics were identical when the persons were on a meat-free ration 3 days prior to the exercise or when from the total 3-methylhistidine excretion the amount of 3-methylhistidine containing the consumed food was substracted.[299] The post-exercise increase in 3-methylhistidine liberation was also revealed in the blood 3-methylhistidine response[294,295] and in the accumulation of the metabolite in muscles.[291]

Increased protein degradation in the recovery period has been confirmed by isotopic methods.[254,255,300] In humans, 5 h after prolonged exercise, the rate of protein synthesis was elevated together with an increased rate of protein degradation.[254] In rats after 10 h of

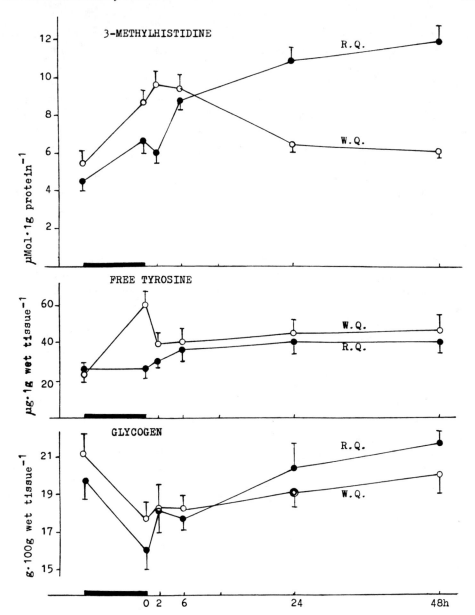

FIGURE 4-14. 3-Methylhistidine, free tyrosin, and glycogen levels in red (R.Q) and white (W.Q) portions of the quadriceps muscle in rats after swimming for 10 h.

swimming a high intensity of protein breakdown persisted for at least 24 h in the soleus muscle. The increased protein degradation was associated with a decrease in the protein content in the muscle during exercise. The increase in the protein synthesis rate followed the period of its suppression and was accompanied by a normalization of the protein content for 24 h after the termination of exercise. A further intensive protein synthesis rate did not lead to an increased protein content due to the persistence of an intensive protein breakdown.[301]

The listed results of various studies justify the conclusion that the increased 3-methylhistidine liberation and excretion after exercise must not be regarded as an index of the prevalent breakdown of contractile proteins, but as a sign of their increased turnover.[298]

G.J. Kasperek and R.D. Snider[300] found a 3-day period of increased 3-methylhistidine excretion after eccentric exercise. They both believe that this reflects protein degradation due to the breakdown of muscle tissue that was damaged during the exercise bout. On the other hand, this process can also be considered part of the general renewal of cellular structures in the muscle after exercise.

The increased protein turnover contributes to the renewal of the molecular content in the actomyosin complex and other muscle proteins in order to eliminate the physiologically exhausted structure elements and to ensure an improvement of the contractile function. However, a question remains of how to interpret the catabolic and antianabolic changes in muscles during and shortly after strenuous exercise. Naturally, it is difficult to assume that the activity causes changes destroying the active organ. Therefore it is reasonable to suggest that the catabolic and antianabolic changes take place mainly in the nonworking or less active muscles. As has been repeatedly demonstrated above, the character, intensity, and duration of the exercise determine the degree of recruitment of muscle fibers of various types. This gives us an opportunity to compare the catabolic changes in muscles containing various types of fibers for evaluating the significance of the degree of muscle activity. The release of 3-methylhistidine and accumulation of free tyrosine occurred in rats during 10 h of swimming mainly in the white portion of the quadriceps muscle. The red portion of the quadriceps muscle, revealing a more pronounced glycogen drop, produced 3-methylhistidine to a little extent during exercises (Figure 4-14).[291] Thus the mobilization of structural proteins is not extended to the contractile apparatus of working muscles. The less active muscles, including their contractile proteins, are used as a reservoir for mobilizing protein resources. Obviously, activity makes muscle tissue less sensitive to catabolic influence. An analogous situation is revealed in the catabolic action of glucocorticoids on muscle tissues: muscle activity decreases their catabolic influence.[302,303]

Compared with the catabolic response during and immediately after exercise, another picture was revealed in protein breakdown in various types of muscle fibers some hours after exercise. In the less active white portion of the quadriceps the 3-methylhistidine content normalized and the increased level of free tyrosine declined after 6 h of post-exercise recovery (Figure 4-14). In the more active red portions of the quadriceps, elevated levels of 3-methylhistidine and free tyrosine were observed after 6 h of recovery. Increased levels were observed 24 and 48 h post-exercise (swimming for 10 h) as well.[291] Thereafter, while during exercise the most active muscle fibers do not contribute to the mobilization of protein resources, in a later stage of post-exercise recovery, catabolic changes take place in most active fibers. These catabolic changes, reasonably, constitute a part of the enhanced protein turnover.

It is tempting to suggest that changes in the testosterone/cortisol ratio are important in the regulation of protein metabolism in skeletal muscles and in the regulation of the protein turnover rate. After endurance exercises the ratio remains low for many hours.[103] An increase in both cortisol and testosterone concentrations was observed during 30 min of strength exercise without change in the testosterone/cortisol ratio. At 1 h post-exercise, cortisol remained on a high level, but the amount of testosterone decreased. At 6 h post-exercise the levels of both hormones were below the initial values. At 24 h post-exercise cortisol remained on a low level; testosterone concentrations returned to the initial levels, causing a significant increase in the testosterone/cortisol ratio.[304] Testosterone has been shown to antagonize the proteolytic effect of exercise through its action on alkaline proteolytic enzymes.[305] Increased urea excretion coincided with a decrease in the blood levels of testosterone and androstenedione in rats after muscular activity.[306] After an intensive anaerobic interval training session the blood urea level was increased from the second to twenty fourth post-exercise hours concomitantly with low levels of testosterone and cortisol.[307]

The increased post-exercise turnover of myofibrillar proteins seems to be ensured by myofibrillar proteinases. Myofibrillar proteinase activity at alkaline pH had already reached its maximum level during the exercise. Moreover, the maximal proteolytic activity at acidic pH was found 6 h, and at neutral pH 24 h post-exercise.[255] After very hard exercises an increased activity of lysosomal enzymes may persist for many days.[308] However, results were reported indicating the post-exercise release of free tyrosine after a blockade of lysosomes. This indicates that the exercise-induced increase in the rate of protein degradation occurs by increasing the flux of proteins through the nonlysosome degradation pathway.[309]

Ca-activated proteinases — calpains — may have contributed to a post-exercise increase in protein turnover. After eight swims of 1 min with an additional load of 12% b.w. (rest intervals between repetitions 90 s) the activity of calpains remained at the control level during the first hours. The following increase in the calpains activity led to the highest level 24 h after the exercise. The high level was maintained for 60 h. A return to the control level was found only 96 h after the exercise.[311]

Glutamine is known to be a direct regulator of muscle protein synthesis[312] and degradation.[313] While alanine and glutamine are synthesized from the same precursor, the relations between alanine and glutamine in muscles may have significance in regulation of protein metabolism. During exercises, the more pronounced production of alanine and, thereby, decreased production of glutamine, promote protein degradation. In the recovery period the increased glutamine production supports the increase in the protein synthesis rate and inhibits protein degradation.

CONCLUSIONS

The recovery period is not only the time for normalizing functional activities and homeostatic equilibriums, but also the time for repletion of energy stores and for constructive alterations. The repletion of energy stores is actualized in a certain sequence and is followed by a transitory phase of supercompensation for energy substrates.

The constructive alterations are founded on increased protein turnover. It is necessary in order to actualize two tasks. First, it speeds up the replacing of physiologically exhausted cellular structure elements with new ones. In this way the enhanced protein turnover warrants the restoration of the functional capacity of cellular structures. The second task is connected with the induction of the adaptive protein synthesis. In order to build something new, one must destroy the old.

The rates of protein synthesis and breakdown may exist in various interrelations during post-exercise recovery. The prevalence of protein synthesis leads to an increase either in the corresponding cellular structures or in the number of enzyme molecules. However, an effective renewal of structural elements may also take place without any changes in the content of the related proteins. After endurance exercises there is a good accordance between the synthesis and degradation of myofibrillar proteins. This might be the reason why endurance exercises do not result in an increase in the size of myofibrils and in muscle hypertrophy. After exercise for improved strength there is another interrelation between the synthesis and degradation of myofibrillar proteins. A more intensive synthesis of these proteins, in compasrison with the degradation rate, warrants an increase in the size of myofibrils and thus also in muscle hypertrophy.

The results presented above demonstrate that the adaptive protein synthesis is specifically related to the previous functional activity. It is natural that after endurance exercises the main locus of adaptive protein synthesis is in the mitochondrial proteins of oxidative or oxidative-glycolytic muscles. After exercises for improved strength, adaptive protein synthesis will take place to the fullest extent in regard to the myofibrillar proteins of glycolytic fibers.

Naturally, exercise-induced adaptive protein synthesis is not limited to skeletal muscle tissue. One of the locuses of the post-exercise adaptive protein synthesis has to be the

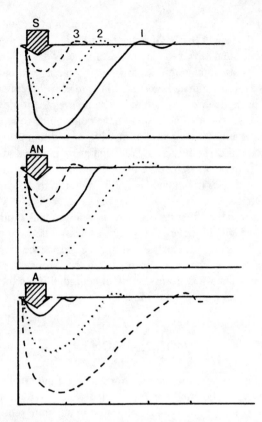

FIGURE 4-15. Restitution of performance capacities in swimmers after training session for improved speed (S), anaerobic endurance (AN) or aerobic endurance (A): 1 — maximal swimming speed, 2 — anaerobic performance capacity, 3 — aerobic performance capacity. Both anaerobic and aerobic capacities were evaluated with special swimming tests. (From Platenov, V. N., Adaptation in Sports, Zdarevya, Kiev, 1988. With permission.)

myocardium. An increased protein synthesis has been found also in the brain tissue during post-exercise recovery.[261]

The reconstructive function is accomplished when the working capacity is completely restored. The restoration of the working capacity is an integral of several processes proceeding in the organism during the post-exercise recovery period. On the one hand, this means the elimination of all fatigue manifestations. On the other hand, it means the refilling of energy stores, the effective renewal of the most exhausted cellular structures, the restoration of the functional capacity of various functional systems and of the central nervous system, and the re-establishment of normal homeostatic balances.

After short-term nonexhausting exercise the restoration of working capacity appears after a couple of minutes or some hours and depends mainly on alterations in the central nervous system. After more strenuous exercises, training sessions, and competitions, much more time is necessary for the restoration of working capacity. After competitions or training sessions three phases of the recovery period were discriminated in athletes: (1) impaired functional state, (2) restitution to the initial level, (3) improved functional state.[314] Due to the heterochronism in the restitution of bodily resources and various functional capacities, working capacity for performance of different exercises is restored after various time intervals. The most delayed is the restitution of working capacity for performance of the same exercise after its previous accomplishment close to exhaustion (Figure 4-15).

REFERENCES

1. **Krogh, J., and Lindhard, J.**, The changes in respiration at the transition from work to rest, *J. Physiol.*, 53, 431, 1919.
2. **Hill, A.V., Long, C.N.H., and Lupton, H.**, Muscular exercise, lactic acid and the supply and utilization of oxygen, *Proc. R. Soc.*, B, 96, 438; 97, 84, 1924.
3. **Hill, A.V.**, *Muscular Movement in Man: The Factors Governing Speed and Recovery from Fatigue*, McGraw-Hill, New York, 1927.
4. **Margaria, R., Edwards, H.T., and Dill, D.B.**, The possible mechanisms of contracting and paying the oxygen debt and the role of lactic acid in muscular contraction, *Am. J. Physiol.*, 106, 689, 1933.
5. **Welch, H.G., and Stainsby, W.N.**, Oxygen debt in contracting dog skeletal muscle in situ, *Respir. Physiol.*, 3, 229, 1967.
6. **Harris, P.**, Lactic acid and the phlogiston debt, *Cardiovasc. Res.*, 3, 381, 1969.
7. **Yakovlev, N.N.**, *Survey of Sports Biochemistry*, FiS, Moscow, 1955 (in Russian).
8. **Hansson, E., Viru, A., and Sildmäe, H.**, Changes of circulation indices in speed and speed-endurance exercises, *4th Estonian Conf. Sports*, Tallinn, 1981, 46.
9. **Sildmäe, H.**, Die Änderung der Herzfrequenz bei Schiläuferinnen auf grund telemetrische Messungen, *Acta Comment. Univ. Tartuensis*, 154, 21, 1964.
10. **Darr, K.C., Bassett. D.R., Morgan, B.J., and Thomas, D.P.**, Effects of age and training status on heart rate recovery after peak exercise, *Am. J. Physiol.*, 254, H340, 1988.
11. **Gellhorn, E.**, *Autonomic Imbalance and the Hypothalamus*, The University of Minnesota Press, Minneapolis, 1957.
12. **Pereni, R., Orizio, C., Comandé, A., Castellano, M., Beschi, M., and Veiesteinas, A.**, Plasma norepinephrine and heart rate dynamics during recovery from submaximal exercise in man, *Eur. J. Appl. Physiol.*, 58, 879, 1989.
13. **Lindhard, J.**, Circulation after cessation of work, with some remarks on the calculation of circulatory rate experiments according to the nitrous oxide method, *J. Physiol.*, 57, 17, 1923.
14. **Cerretelli, P., Piiper, J., Mangio, F., Cuttica, F., and Ricci, R.**, Circulation in exercising dogs, *J. Appl. Physiol.*, 19, 29, 1964.
15. **Cerretelli, P.**, Readjustments in cardiac output during the onset of exercise and recovery, *J. Appl. Physiol.*, 21, 1345, 1966.
16. **DiBello, V., Santoro, G., Cini, G., Pentimore, F., Ginanni, A., Romano, M.F., and Giusti, C.**, Cardiovascular adjustments induced by training evaluated during semisupine isotonic exercise and recovery period: an echocardiographic study, *Int. J. Sports Med.*, 8, 407, 1987.
17. **Peterson, L.H., Schnabel, T.G., Fitzpatrick, H., and Barett, H.C.**, Intra-arterial changes in pressure before, during and after exercise, *Am. J. Physiol.*, 155, 460, 1948.
18. **Eskildsen, P., Götsche, H.E., and Hansen, A.T.**, Measuring intra-arterial blood pressure during exercise, *Acta Med. Scand.*, 138 (Suppl. 239), 245, 1950.
19. **Holmgren, A.**, Circulatory changes during muscular work in man with special reference to arterial and central venous pressures in the systematic circulation, *Scand. J. Clin. Lab. Invest.*, 8 (Suppl. 24), 1956.
20. **Epler, M., Viru, A., and Kurrik, E.**, On dynamics of arterial pressure and heart rhythm in short-term physical exercises, *Conf. Sports Physiol.*, Tiflis, 1960, 224.
21. **Viru, E.**, Dynamics of blood pressure during and after exercise of different intensity, *Acta Comment. Univ. Tartuensis*, 205, 62, 1968.
22. **Viru, E.**, The influence of body position on dynamics of blood pressure and heart rate after work, *Acta Comment. Univ. Tartuensis*, 205, 54, 1968.
23. **Mattef, D.**, Der ortostatische Kreislaufkollaps-Gravitations-shock (gravity shock), *Arbeitsphysiologie*, 8, 595, 1935.
24. **Hannum, S.M., and Kasch, F.W.**, Acute post-exercise blood pressure response of hypertensive and normotensive men, *Scand. J. Sports Med.*, 3, 11, 1989.
25. **Somers, V.K., Conway, J., LeWinter, M., and Sleight, P.**, The role of baroreflex sensitivity in post-exercise hypotension, *J. Hypertens.*, 3 (Suppl.), S129, 1985.
26. **Hagberg, J.M., Montain, S.J., and Mortin, W.H.**, Blood pressure and hemodynamic response after exercise in older hypertensives, *J. Appl. Physiol.*, 63, 270, 1987.
27. **Kaufman, F.L., Hughson, R.L., and Schaman, J.P.**, Effect of exercise on recovery blood pressure in normotensive and hypertensive subjects, *Med. Sci. Sports Exerc.*, 19, 17, 1987.
28. **Convertino, V.A., and Adams, W.C.**, Enhanced vagal baroreflex response during 24 h after acute exercise, *Am. J. Physiol.*, 260, R570, 1991.
29. **Margomroth, M.L., Young, E.W., and Sparks, H.V.**, Prostaglandin and histaminergic mediation of prolonged vasodilatation after exercise, *Am. J. Physiol.*, 233, H27, 1977.

30. **Henry, F.M., and DeMoor, J.**, Metabolic efficiency of exercise in relation to work load at constant speed, *J. Appl. Physiol.*, 2, 481, 1950.

31. **Isaev, G.G.**, Electromyographic analysis of breathing control during muscular exercise, *Fiziol. Chel.*, 12, 219, 1986 (in Russian).

32. **Volkov, N.I.**, Oxygen consumption and lactate acid content of blood during strenuous muscle exercise, *Fed. Proc.*, 22, 118, 1963.

33. **Volkov, N.I.**, *Human Bioenergetics in Strenuous Muscular Activity and Pathways for Improved Performance Capacity in Sportsmen*, Anokhin's Institute of Normal Physiology, Moscow, 1990 (in Russian).

34. **Lindhard, J.**, Untersuchungen über statische Muskularbeit. I, II, *Scand. Arch. Physiol.*, 40, 145, 1920.

35. **Krisanda, J.M., Moreland, T.S., and Kushmerick, M.J.**, ATP supply and demand during exercise, in *Exercise, Nutrition and Energy Metabolism*, Horton, E.S., and Terjung, E.L., Eds., Macmillan, New York, 1988, 27.

36. **Henry, F.M., and DeMoor, J.**, Lactic and alactic oxygen consumption in moderate exercise of graded intensity, *J. Appl. Physiol.*, 8, 608, 1956.

37. **Knuttgen, H.G.**, Oxygen debt after submaximal exercise, *J. Appl. Physiol.*, 29, 651, 1970.

38. **Kushmerick, M.G., and Meyer, R.A.**, Chemical changes in rat leg muscle by phosphorus nuclear magnetic resonance, *Am. J. Physiol.*, 249, C362, 1985.

39. **Brooks, G.A., Hittelman, K.J., Faulkner, J.A., and Beyer, R.E.**, Temperature, skeletal muscle mitochondrial functions, and oxygen debt, *Am. J. Physiol.*, 220, 1053, 1971.

40. **Bahr, R.**, *Excess Postexercise Oxygen Consumption — Magnitude, Mechanisms and Practical Implications*, Academic dissertation, National Institute of Occupational Health, Oslo, 1991.

41. **Gaesser, G.A., and Brooks, G.A.**, Metabolic bases of excess postexercise oxygen consumption: a review, *Med. Sci. Sports Exerc.*, 16, 29, 1984.

42. **Gladden, L.B., Stainby, W.N., and MacIntosh, B.R.**, Norepinephrine increases canine skeletal muscle VO_2max during recovery, *Med. Sci. Sports Exerc.*, 14, 471, 1982.

43. **Barnard, R.J., and Foss, M.L.**, Oxygen debt: effects of beta adrenergic blockade on the lactacid and alactacid components, *J. Appl. Physiol.*, 27, 813, 1969.

44. **Cain, S.M.**, Exercise O_2 debt of dogs at ground level and altitude with and without β-block, *J. Appl. Physiol.*, 30, 838, 1971.

45. **Cain, S.M., and Chapler, C.K.**, Effects of norepinephrine and α-block on O_2 uptake and blood flow in dog hind limb, *J. Appl. Physiol.*, 51, 1245, 1981.

46. **Bangsbo, J., Gollnick, P.D., Graham, T.E., Juel, C., Kiens, B., Mizuno, M., and Saltin, B.**, Anaerobic energy production and O_2 deficit-debt relationship during exhaustive exercise in humans, *J. Physiol.*, 422, 539, 1990.

47. **Åstrand, P.-O., and Rodahl, K.**, *Textbook of Work Physiology. Physiological Bases of Exercise*, McGraw-Hill, New York, 1986, 183.

48. **Bahr, R., Ingnes, I., Vaage, O., Sejersted, O.M., and Newsholme, E.A.**, Effect of duration of exercise on excess postexercise O_2 consumption, *J. Appl. Physiol.*, 62, 485, 1987.

49. **Hermansen, L., Grandmontagne, M., Maehlum, S., and Ingnes, I.**, Post-exercise elevation of resting oxygen uptake: possible mechanisms and physiological significance, in *Physiological Chemistry of Training and Detraining*, Marconnet, P., Poortmans, J., and Hermansen, L., Eds., Karger, Basel, 1984, 119.

50. **Maehlum, S., Grandmontagne, M., Newsholme, E.A., and Sejersted, O.M.**, Magnitude and duration of excess postexercise oxygen consumption in healthy young subjects, *Metabolism*, 35, 425, 1986.

51. **Bahr, R., and Maehlum, S.**, Excess post-exercise oxygen consumption. A short review, *Acta Physiol. Scand.*, 128 (Suppl. 556), 93, 1986.

52. **Bahr, R., Hansson, P., and Sejersted, O.M.**, Triglyceride/fatty acid cycling is increased after exercise, *Metabolism*, 39, 993, 1990.

53. **Bangsbo, J., Gollnick, P.D., Graham, T.E., and Saltin, B.**, Substrates for muscle glycogen synthesis in recovery from intense exercise in man, *J. Physiol.*, 434, 423, 1991.

54. **Bahr, R., Høstmark, A., Newsholme, E.A., Grønnerød, O., and Sejersted, O.M.**, Effect of exercise on recovery changes in plasma levels of FFA, glycerol, glucose, and catecholamines, *Acta Physiol. Scand.*, 143, 105, 1991.

55. **Brooks, G.A.**, Anaerobic threshold: review of the concept and directions for further research, *Med. Sci. Sports Exerc.*, 17, 22, 1985.

56. **Hermansen, L., and Vaage, O.**, Lactate disappearance and glycogen synthesis in human muscle after maximal exercise, *Am. J. Physiol.*, 233, E422, 1977.

57. **Åstrand, P.-O., Hultman, E., Juhlin-Dannfeldt, A., and Reynolds, G.**, Disposal of lactate during and after strenuous exercise, *J. Appl. Physiol.*, 61, 338, 1986.

58. **Jorfeldt, L.**, Metabolism of L(+)-lactate in human skeletal muscle during exercise, *Acta Physiol. Scand. Suppl.*, 138, 1970.

59. **Saltin, B.**, Anaerobic capacity: past, present, and perspective, in *Biochemistry of Exercise VI*, Saltin, B., Ed., Human Kinetics, Champaign, 1986, 387.
60. **Juel, C., Bangsbo, J., Graham, T., and Saltin, B.**, Lactate and potassium fluxes from human skeletal muscle during and after intense, dynamic knee extensor exercise, *Acta Physiol. Scand.*, 140, 147, 1990.
61. **Diamant, B., Karlsson, J., and Saltin, B.**, Muscle tissue lactate after maximal exercise in man, *Acta Physiol. Scand.*, 72, 383, 1968.
62. **Freund, H., and Zouloumian, P.**, Lactate after exercise. I. Evolution kinetics in arterial blood, *Eur. J. Appl. Physiol.*, 46, 121, 1981.
63. **Fujitsuka, N., Yamamoto, T., Ohkuva, T., Saito, M., and Miyamura, M.**, Peak blood lactate after short periods of maximal treadmill running, *Eur. J. Appl. Physiol.*, 48, 289, 1982.
64. **Freund, H., Oyono-Enguelle, S., Heitz, A., Marbach, J., Ott, C., Zouloumian, P., and Lampert, E.**, Work rate dependent lactate kinetics after exercise in humans, *J. Appl. Physiol.*, 61, 932, 1986.
65. **Freund, H., Oyono-Enguelle, S., Heitz, A., Ott, S., Marbach, J., Gartier, M., and Pape, A.**, Comparative lactate kinetics after short and prolonged submaximal exercise, *Int. J. Sports Med.*, 11, 284, 1990.
66. **Freund, H., Oyono-Enguelle, S., Heitz, A., Marbach, J., Ott, S., and Gartner, M.**, Effect of exercise duration on lactate kinetics after short muscular exercise, *Eur. J. Appl. Physiol.*, 58, 534, 1989.
67. **Wasserman, K., Beaver, W.L., Davis, J.A., Pu Jum-Zong, Heber, D., and Whipp, B.J.**, Lactate, pyruvate and lactate-to-pyruvate ratio during exercise and recovery, *J. Appl. Physiol.*, 59, 935, 1985.
68. **Hermansen, L., and Osnes, J.-B.**, Blood and muscle pH after maximal exercise in man, *J. Appl. Physiol.*, 32, 304, 1972.
69. **Sahlin, K., Harris, R.C., Nylind, B., and Hultman, E.**, Lactate content and pH in muscle obtained after dynamic exercises, *Pflügers Arch. ges. Physiol.*, 367, 143, 1976.
70. **Sahlin, K.**, Intracellular pH and energy metabolism in skeletal muscles of man, with special references to exercise, *Acta Physiol. Scand. Suppl.*, 455, 1978.
71. **Sahlin, K., Alverstrand, A., Brandt, R., and Hultman, E.**, Intracellular pH and bicarbonate concentration in human muscle during recovery from exercise, *J. Appl. Physiol.*, 45, 474, 1978.
72. **Kindermann, W., and Keul, J.**, *Anaerobic Energiebereitstellung im Hochleistungssport*, Hoffman, Schorndorf, 1977.
73. **Allsop, P., Chetham, M., Brooks, S., Hall, G.M., and Williams, C.**, Continuous intramuscular pH measurement during the recovery from brief maximal exercise in man, *Eur. J. Appl. Physiol.*, 60, 465, 1990.
74. **Jervell, O.**, Investigation of the concentration of lactic acid in blood and urine, *Acta Med. Scand. Suppl.*, 24, 1928.
75. **Barry, O.**, The lactate content of the blood during and after muscular exercise in man, *Scand. Arch. Physiol.*, 74, 51, 1936.
76. **Johnson, R.E., and Edwards, H.T.**, Lactate and pyruvate in blood and urine after exercise, *J. Biol. Chem.*, 118, 427, 1937.
77. **Newman, E.V., Dill, D.B., Edwards, H.T., and Webster, F.A.**, The rate of lactic acid removal in exercise, *Am. J. Physiol.*, 118, 457, 1937.
78. **Gollnick, P.D., Bayly, W.M., and Hodgson, D.R.**, Exercise intensity, training, diet, and lactate concentration in muscle and blood, *Med. Sci. Sports Exerc.*, 18, 334, 1986.
79. **Hermansen, L., and Stensvold, I.**, Production and removal of lactate during exercise in man, *Acta Physiol. Scand.*, 86, 191, 1972.
80. **Belcastro, A.N., and Bonen, A.**, Lactic acid removal rates during controlled and uncontrolled recovery exercise, *J. Appl. Physiol.*, 39, 932, 1975.
81. **Bonen, A., and Belcastro, A.N.**, Comparison of self-selected recovery methods on lactic acid removal rates, *Med. Sci. Sports*, 8, 176, 1976.
82. **Hatta, H., Atomi, Y., Yamamoto, Y., Shinohara, S., and Yamada, S.**, Oxidation of lactate in rats after short-term strenuous exercise, *Int. J. Sports Med.*, 9, 403, 1988.
83. **Weltman, A., Stamford, B.A., and Fulco, C.**, Recovery from maximal effort exercise: lactate disappearance and subsequent performance, *J. Appl. Physiol.*, 47, 677, 1979.
84. **McLellan, T.M., and Skinner, J.S.**, Blood lactate removal during active recovery related to the aerobic threshold, *Int. J. Sports Med.*, 3, 224, 1982.
85. **Hagberg, J.B., Hickson, R.C., McLane, J.A., Ehsani, A.A., and Winder, W.W.**, Disappearance of norepinephrine from the circulation following strenuous exercise, *J. Appl. Physiol.*, 47, 1311, 1979.
86. **Moorman, E.J., Bogart, M.G., and De Schrepdryver, A.F.**, Estimation of plasma catecholamines in man, *Clin. Chim. Acta*, 72, 89, 1976.
87. **Jezova, D., Vigas, M., Tatár, P., Kvetsansky, R., Nazar, K., Kaciuba-Uscilko, H., and Kozlowski, S.**, Plasma testosterone and catecholamine responses to physical exercise of different intensities in men, *Eur. J. Appl. Physiol.*, 54, 62, 1985.
88. **Maron, M.B., Horwath, S.M., and Wilkerson, J.E.**, Blood biochemical alteration during recovery from competitive marathon running, *Eur. J. Appl. Physiol.*, 36, 231, 1977.

89. **Sagnol, M., Claustre, J., Cottet-Emard, J.M., Pequignot, J.M., Fellmann, N., Coudert, J., and Pevyin, L.,** Plasma free and sulphated catecholamines after ultra-long exercise and recovery, *Eur. J. Appl. Physiol.,* 60, 91, 1990.

90. **Vuori, J., Marniemi, J., Rahkila, P., and Vainikka, M.,** The effect of a six-day ski-hike on plasma catecholamine concentrations and on their response to submaximal exercise, *Med. Biol.,* 57, 362, 1979.

91. **Conlee, R.V., Hickson, R.G., Winder, W.W., Hagberg, J.M., and Holloszy, J.O.,** Regulation of glycogen resynthesis in muscle of rats following exercise, *Am. J. Physiol.,* 235, R145, 1978.

92. **Matlina, E.S., Vaisman, S.M., Bôkhovskaya, K.N., and Vassilyev, V.N.,** About the mechanisms of disturbed synthesis of catecholamines in adrenals in physical fatigue and during recovery in trained rats, *Byull. Exp. Biol. Med.,* 5, 34, 1975 (in Russian).

93. **Eränko, O., and Härkönen, M.,** Long-term effects of muscular work on the adrenal medulla of the mouse, *Endocrinology,* 69, 186, 1961.

94. **Follenius, M., and Brandenberger, G.,** Influence de l'exercise musculaire sur l'evolution de la cortisolémie et de la glycémie chez l'homme, *Eur. J. Appl. Physiol.,* 33, 23, 1974.

95. **Mullin, J.P., and Howley, E.T.,** Dynamics of serum cortisol in response to high intensity exercise in man, *Med. Sci. Sports,* 6, 72, 1974.

96. **Adlercreutz, H., Härkönen, M., Kuoppasalmi, K., Kosunen, K., Näveri, H., and Rehumen, S.,** Physical activity and hormones, *Adv. Cardiol.,* 18, 144, 1976.

97. **Bullén, B.A., Skirinar, G.S., Beitins, I.Z., Carr, D.B., Reppert, S.M., Dotson, C.O., Fencl, M. de M., Gervino, E.V., and McArthur, J.W.,** Endurance training effects on plasma hormonal responsiveness and sex hormone excretion, *J. Appl. Physiol.,* 56, 1453, 1984.

98. **Buono, M.J., Yeager, J.E., and Hodgdon, J.A.,** Plasma adrenocorticotropin and cortisol responses to brief high-intensity exercise in humans, *J. Appl. Physiol.,* 61, 1337, 1986.

99. **Davies, C.T.M., and Few, J.D.,** Effect of exercise on adrenocortical function, *J. Appl. Physiol.,* 35, 887, 1973.

100. **Few, J.D.,** Effect of exercise on the secretion and metabolism of cortisol in man, *J. Endocrinol.,* 62, 341, 1974.

101. **Sutton, J.R., Young, J.D., Lazarus, L., Hickie, J.B., and Maksvytis, J.,** The hormone response to physical exercise, *Aust. Ann. Med.,* 18, 84, 1969.

102. **Kuoppasalmi, K., Näveri, H., Härkönen, M., and Adlercreutz, H.,** Plasma cortisol, androstenedione, testosterone and luteinizing hormone in running exercise of different intensities, *Scand. J. Clin. Lab. Invest.,* 40, 403, 1980.

103. **Viru, A., Karelson, K., and Smirnova, T.,** Stability and variability in hormonal responses to prolonged exercise, *Int. J. Sports Med.,* 13, 230, 1992.

104. **Holm, G., Björntrop, B., and Jagenburg, R.,** Carbohydrate, lipid, and amino acid metabolism following physical exercise in man, *J. Appl. Physiol.,* 45, 128, 1978.

105. **Keul, J., Kohler, B., von Glutz, G., Luthi, U., Berg, A., and Howald, A.,** Biochemical change in a 100-km run: carbohydrates, lipids, and hormones in serum, *Eur. J. Appl. Physiol.,* 47, 181, 1981.

106. **Dufaux, B., Assman, G., Order, U., Holderath, A., and Hollmann, W.,** Plasma lipoproteins, hormones, and energy substrates during the first day after prolonged exercise, *Int. J. Sports Med.,* 2, 256, 1981.

107. **Viru, A., and Kôrge, P.,** Study of adrenocortical functions in training process, in *Metabolism and Biochemical Assessment of the Fitness of Sportsmen,* Yakovlev, N., Ed., Leningrad, 1974, 160 (in Russian).

108. **Ratsimamanga, R.,** Variations de la teneur en acide ascorbique dans la surrénale au cours du travail, *C.S. Soc. Biol.,* 131, 863, 1939.

109. **Karaulova, L.K., and Golovina, L.V.,** Hypothalamic regulations of the pituitary-adrenocortical system during recovery period after physical exercise, *Sechenov Physiol. J. USSR,* 61, 55, 1975 (in Russian).

110. **Böttinger, J., Sehlein, E.M., Faloona, G.R., Knochel, J.R., and Myer, R.H.,** The effect of exercise on glucagon secretion, *J. Clin. Endocrin.,* 35, 117, 1972.

111. **Rennie, M.J., and Johnson, R.H.,** Alteration of metabolic and hormonal responses to exercise by physical training, *Eur. J. Appl. Physiol.,* 33, 215, 1974.

112. **Laso, F.J., Conzález-Buitrago, J.M., Ruiz, C.M., and Castro, de S.,** Hormonal regulation of potassium shifts during graded exhaustive exercise, *Eur. J. Appl. Physiol.,* 62, 292, 1991.

113. **Pruett, E.D.R.,** Insulin and exercise in non-diabetic and diabetic man, in *Exercise Endocrinology,* Fotherby, K., and Pal, S.B., Eds., Gruyter, Berlin, New York, 1985, 1.

114. **Wirth, A., Diehm, C., Mayer, H., Mörl, H., Vogel, I., Björntrop, P., and Schlierf, G.,** Plasma C-peptide and insulin in trained and untrained subjects, *J. Appl. Physiol.,* 50, 71, 1981.

115. **Farrell, P.A., Sonne, B., Mikines, K., and Galbo, H.,** Stimulatory role for endogenous opioid peptides on postexercise insulin secretion in rats, *J. Appl. Physiol.,* 65, 744, 1988.

116. **Sutton, J., and Lazarus, L.,** Effect of adrenergic blocking agents on growth hormone response to physical exercise, *Horm. Metab. Res.,* 6, 428, 1974.

117. **Viru, A., Smirnova, T., Tomson, K., and Matsin, T.,** Dynamics of blood levels of pituitary trophic hormones during prolonged exercise, in *Biochemistry of Exercise IV-B,* Poortmans, J., and Niset, G., Eds., University Park Press, Baltimore, 1981, 100.

118. **Vanhelder, W.P., Goode, R.C., and Radomski, R.C.**, Effect of anaerobic and aerobic exercise of equal duration and work expenditure on plasma growth hormone levels, *Eur. J. Appl. Physiol.*, 52, 255, 1984.

119. **Vanhelder, W.P., Goode, R.C., Radomski, R.C., and Casey, K.**, Hormonal and metabolic response to three types of exercise of equal duration and external work output, *Eur. J. Appl. Physiol.*, 54, 337, 1985.

120. **Vanhelder, W.P., Radomski, M.W., and Goode R.C.**, Growth hormone responses during intermittent weight lifting exercises in men, *Eur. J. Appl. Physiol.*, 53, 31, 1984.

121. **Adamson, L., Hunter, W.M., Ogurremi, O.O., Oswald, I., and Percy-Robb, I.W.**, Growth hormone increase during sleep after daytime exercise, *J. Endocrinol.*, 62, 473, 1974.

122. **Keizer, H., Janssen, G.M.E., Menheere, P., and Kranenburg, G.**, Changes in basal plasma testosterone, cortisol, and dehydroepiandrosterone sulfate in previously untrained males and females preparing for a marathon, *Int. J. Sports Med.*, 10 (Suppl. 3), S139, 1989.

123. **Kocegub, T.P., and Feldkoren, B.I.**, Effect of exercise on the level of testosterone in blood of trained albino rats, *Acta Comment. Univ. Tartuensis*, 543, 138, 1980.

124. **Tchaikovsky, V.S., Jevtinova, I.V., and Basharina, O.B.**, Action of physical exercise on steroid content and reception of androgens in skeletal muscles, *Acta Comment. Univ. Tartuensis*, 702, 105, 1985.

125. **Elias, A.N., Wilson, A.F., Pandian, M.R., Chune, G., Utsumi, A., Kayaleh, R., and Stone, S.C.**, Corticotropin releasing hormone and gonadotropin secretion in physically active males after acute exercise, *Eur. J. Appl. Physiol.*, 62, 171, 1991.

126. **Sander, M., and Röckar, L.**, Influence of marathon running on thyroid hormone, *Int. J. Sports Med.*, 9, 123, 1988.

127. **Konovalova, G.M., Viru, A.A., Masso, R.A., and Riuhhina, O.F.**, Changes of the concentration of thyroid hormones in the blood of rats after a single bout of intensive exercise of short duration, in *Hormonal Regulation of Adaptation to Muscular Activity*, Tartu University, Tartu, 1991, 40.

128. **Weiss, M., Jockers, M., Barwich, D., and Weicker, H.**, Das Stoffwechselverhalten, seine hormonelle Regulation auf der kurzen and langen Wettkampfstracke im Schwimmen, *Schweiz. Z. Sportmed.*, 33, 5, 1985.

129. **Pèronnet, F., Massicotte, D., Paquet, J.E., Brisson, G., and de Champlain, J.**, Blood pressure and plasma catecholamine responses to various challenges during exercise-recovery in man, *Eur. J. Appl. Physiol.*, 58, 551, 1989.

130. **Häkkinen, K., Pakarinen, A., Alen, M., Kauhanen, H., and Komi, P.V.**, Neuromuscular and hormonal responses in elite athletes to two successive strength training sessions in one day, *Eur. J. Appl. Physiol.*, 57, 133, 1988.

131. **Lindiger, M.J., and Sjøgaard, G.**, Potassium regulation during exercise and recovery, *Sports Med.*, 11, 382, 1991.

132. **Goodman, C., Rogers, G.G., Vermaak, H., and Goodman, M.R.**, Biochemical response during recovery from maximal and submaximal swimming exercise, *Eur. J. Appl. Physiol.*, 54, 346, 1985.

133. **Sejersted, O.M., Vøllestad, N.K., and Medbø, J.I.**, Muscle fluid and electrolyte balance during and following exercise, *Acta Physiol. Scand.*, 128 (Suppl. 556), 119, 1986.

134. **Ljunghall, S., Joborn, H., Rastad, J., and Akerström, G.**, Plasma potassium and phosphate concentration — influence by adrenaline infusion, β-blockade and physical exercise, *Acta Med. Scand.*, 221, 83, 1987.

135. **Wolf, J.P., Nguyen, N.U., Dumoulin, G., and Berthelay, S.**, Plasma renin and aldosterone changes during twenty minutes moderate exercise. Influence of posture, *Eur. J. Appl. Physiol.*, 54, 602, 1986.

136. **Schmidt, W., Maassen, N., Tegtbur, U., and Brauman, K.M.**, Changes in plasma volume and red cell formation after a marathon competition, *Eur. J. Appl. Physiol.*, 58, 453, 1989.

137. **Lijnen, P., Hospel, P., M'Buyamba-Kabangu, J.R., Goris, M.L.R., Van der Ende, E., Fagard, R., and Amery, A.**, Plasma atrial natriuretic peptide and cyclic nucleotide levels before and after a marathon, *J. Appl. Physiol.*, 63, 1180, 1987.

138. **Fellmann, N., Bedu, M., Giry, Pharmakis-Amadieu, M., Bezou, M.-J., Barlet, J.-P., and Coudert, J.**, Hormonal, fluid, and electrolyte changes during a 72-h recovery from a 24-h endurance run, *Int. J. Sports Med.*, 10, 406, 1989.

139. **Fellmann, N., Sagnol, M., Bedu, M., Falgarrette, G., Van Praagh, E., Goullard, G., Jougnel, P., and Coudert, J.**, Enzymatic and hormonal responses following a 24-h endurance run and a 10-h triathlon race, *Eur. J. Appl. Physiol.*, 57, 545, 1988.

140. **Schwandt, H.-J., Heyduck, B., Gungh, H.-C., and Röcker, L.**, Influence of prolonged physical exercise on the erythropoietin concentration in blood, *Eur. J. Appl. Physiol.*, 63, 463, 1991.

141. **Drzevetskaya, I.A., and Beljayev, N.G.**, Comparison of changes in calcium and glucose homeostasis in recovery period after muscular exercises of various duration in rats, *Acta Comment. Univ. Tartuensis*, 702, 164, 1985 (in Russian).

142. **Beljayev, N.G.**, Endocrine regulation of calcium homeostasis in recovery period, *Teor. Prakt. Fiz. Kult.*, 4, 18, 1985 (in Russian).

143. **Dekster, P.A., Dolev, E., Kyle, S.B., Anderson, R.A., and Schoemaker, E.B.**, Magnesium homeostasis during high-intensive anaerobic exercise in men, *J. Appl. Physiol.*, 62, 545, 1987.

144. **Franz, K.B., Rüddel, H., Todd, G.L., Dorheim, T.A., Buell, J.C., and Eliot, R.S.**, Physiologic changes during a marathon with special reference to magnesium, *J. Am. Coll. Nutr.*, 4, 187, 1985.

145. **Haralambie, G.**, Changes in electrolytes and trace elements during long-lasting exercise, in *Metabolic Adaptation to Prolonged Exercise*, Howald, H., and Poortmans, J.R., Eds., Birkhäuser Verlag, Basel, 1975, 340.

146. **Ohno, H., Yamashita, K., Doi, R., Yamamura, K., Kondo, T., and Taniguci, N.**, Exercise-induced changes in blood zinc and related proteins in humans, *J. Appl. Physiol.*, 58, 1453, 1985.

147. **Krestovnikov, A.N.**, *Survey on Physiology of Physical Exercise*, FiS, Moscow, 1951 (in Russian).

148. **Fedorov, V.L.**, Dynamics of recovery process after training sessions in sportsmen of high qualification, in *Problems of Sports Physiology*, Hippenreiter, B., Ed., FiS, Moscow, 1963, 131 (in Russian).

149. **Haralambie, G., and Keul, J.**, Der Einfluss von Muskelarbeit auf den Magnesiumspiegel and die neuromuskuläre Erregbarkeit beim Menschen, *Med. Klin.*, 65, 1445, 1970.

150. **Danko, J.I.**, *Survey of Physiology of Physical Exercises*, Medizina, Moscow, 1974 (in Russian).

151. **Zaitsev, A.A.**, Recovery processes in spinal motor centres, in *Physiological Foundation of Training*, Zimkin, N.V., Korobkov, A.V., and Farfel, V.S., Eds., FiS, Moscow, 1965, 161 (in Russian).

152. **Stull, G.A., and Clarke D.H.**, Patterns of recovery following isometric and isotomic strength decrement, *Med. Sci. Sports*, 3, 135, 1971.

153. **Kearney, J.T.**, Strength recovery following rhythmic or sustained exercise, *Am. Correct. Ther. J.*, 27, 163, 1973.

154. **Lind, A.R.**, Muscle fatigue and recovery from fatigue induced by sustained contractions, *J. Physiol.* (London), 147, 162, 1959.

155. **Stull, G.A., and Kearney, J.T.**, Recovery of muscular endurance following submaximal, isometric exercise, *Med. Sci. Sports*, 10, 109, 1978.

156. **Clausen, T.**, Na^+,Ka^+-exchange in working skeletal muscle and its significance for contractility, in *Abst. 32nd Congr. Int. Union Physiol. Sci.*, Sunday, Glasgow, 1993, 60.

157. **Fitts, R.H., and Holloszy, J.O.**, Lactate and contractile force in frog muscle during development of fatigue and recovery, *Am. J. Physiol.*, 231, 430, 1976.

158. **Belivau, L., Van Hoecke, J., Helal, J.-N., Gaillard, E., Garapon-Bas, C., Herry, J.-P., Atlan, G., Dubray, C., and Boissou, P.**, Recovery of fatigued muscle: possible relationship between mechanical, electrical and metabolic changes, *8th Int. Biochem. Exerc. Conf.*, Nagoya, 1991, 92.

159. **Hultman, E., Bergström, J., and McLennan-Anderson, N.**, Breakdown and resynthesis of phosphocreatine and adenosine triphosphate in connection with muscular work in man, *Scand. J. Clin. Lab. Invest.*, 19, 56, 1967.

160. **Saltin, B., and Essen, B.**, Muscle glycogen, lactate, ATP and CP in intermittent exercise, in *Muscle Metabolism During Exercise*, Pernow, B., and Saltin, B., Eds., Plenum Press, New York, 1971, 419.

161. **Katz, A., Broberg, S., Sahlin, K., and Wahren, J.**, Muscle ammonia and amino acid metabolism during dynamic exercise in man, *Clin. Physiol.*, 6, 365, 1986.

162. **Söderlund, K., and Hultman, E.**, ATP content in single fibres from human skeletal muscle after electrical stimulation and during recovery, *Acta Physiol. Scand.*, 139, 459, 1990.

163. **Vusse van der, G.J., Janssen, G.M.E., Coumans, W.A., Kuipers, H., Does, R.J.M.M., and Hoorten, T.**, Effect of training and 15-, 25- and 42-km contests on the skeletal muscle content of adenine and guanide nucleotides, creatine phosphate, and glycogen, *Int. J. Sports Med.*, 10 (Suppl. 3), S146, 1989.

164. **Terjung, R.L., Baldwin, K.M., Winder, W.W., and Holloszy, J.D.**, Glycogen repletion in different types of muscle and in liver after exhausting exercise, *Am. J. Physiol.*, 226, 1387, 1974.

165. **Piehl, K.**, Time course of refilling of glycogen-induced glycogen depletion, *Acta Physiol. Scand.*, 90, 297, 1974.

166. **Keizer, H.A., Kuipers, H., Kranenburg van, G., and Geurten, P.**, Influence of liquid and solid meals on muscle glycogen resynthesis, plasma fuel, hormone response and maximal physical working capacity, *Int. J. Sports Med.*, 8, 99, 1987.

167. **Fell, R.D., Terblanche, S.E., Ivy, J.L., Young, J.C., and Holloszy, J.O.**, Effect of muscle glycogen content on glucose uptake following exercise, *J. Appl. Physiol.*, 52, 434, 1982.

168. **LeMarchard-Brustel, Y., and Freychet, P.**, Relation of glycogen synthase activity in the isolated mouse soleus muscle. Effect of insulin, epinephrine, glucose and anti-insulin receptor antibodies, *Biochim. Biophys. Acta*, 677, 13, 1981.

169. **Jampolskaya, L.I.**, Muscle glycogen supercompensation in restitution period after exercises of various character and duration, *Byull. Eksp. Biol. Med.* (Moscow), 11, 358, 1948.

170. **Yakovlev, N.N.**, Biochemical foundations of the training of muscles, *Usp. Sovrem. Biol.* (Moscow), 27, 257, 1949.

171. **Chagovets, N.R.**, Biochemical changes in muscles in restitution period after physical work, *Ukr. Biokhim. Zh.* (Kiev), 29, 450, 1957.

172. **Yakovlev, N.N.**, *Sportbiochemie*, Barta, Leipzig, 1977.

173. **Batuner, L.S.**, Restitution of energy potential of muscles after exercises close to maximal, *Sechenov Physiol. J. USSR*, 63, 406, 1977.

174. **Yakovlev, N.N.**, The expenditure and resynthesis of energy sources in muscles of various functional profile in regard to the character of load, *Sechenov Physiol. J. USSR*, 65, 1796, 1979.

175. **Jansson, E., Dudley, G.A., Norman, B., and Tesch, P.A.**, Relationship of recovery from intense exercise to the oxidative potential of skeletal muscle, *Acta Physiol. Scand.*, 139, 147, 1990.

176. **Yakovlev, N.N., Krasnova, A.F., Lenkova, R.I., Leshkevitch, L.G., Samodanova, G.I., and Chagovetz, N.R.**, Effect of the adaptation to intensive muscle activity on the functional state of skeletal muscle mitochondria, *Cytologia* (Moscow), 14, 197, 1978.

177. **Chagovets, N.R.**, Action of 2,4-dinitrophenole on resynthesis of phosphocreatine and glycogen in muscle during rest period after work, *Sechenov Physiol. J. USSR*, 48, 1260, 1962.

178. **Kondrashova, M.N., and Chagovets, N.R.**, Succinate in skeletal muscles during intensive work and rest period, *Proc. Acad. Sci. USSR*, 198, 249, 1971.

179. **Chagovets, N.R.**, Adenonucleotides NAD^+ and NAD·H in skeletal muscles during intensive work and rest, *Proc. Acad. Sci. USSR*, 207, 739, 1972.

180. **Chagovets, N.R.**, The after physical work "synthesizing state" of skeletal muscle mitochondria as a basis for the energy expenses supercompensation, in *Metabolism and Biochemical Evaluation of Fitness of Sportsmen*, Yakovlev, N.N., Ed., Leningrad Research Institute of Physical Culture, Leningrad, 1974, 32.

181. **Hermansen, L., Hultman, E., and Saltin, B.**, Muscle glycogen during prolonged severe exercise, *Acta Physiol. Scand.*, 71, 129, 1967.

182. **Gollnick, P.D., Armstrong, R.E., Saubert, C.W., Semberowich, W.L., Shephard, R.L., and Saltin, B.**, Glycogen depletion patterns in human skeletal muscle fibres during prolonged work, *Pflügers Arch. ges. Physiol.*, 344, 1, 1973.

183. **MacDowall, J.D., Ward, G.R., Sale, D.G., and Sutton, J.R.**, Muscle glycogen repletion after high-intensity intermittent exercise, *J. Appl. Physiol.*, 42, 129, 1977.

184. **Garetto, L., Richard, E.A., Goodman, M.N., and Ruderman, N.B.**, Enhanced muscle glucose metabolism after exercise in rat: the two phases, *Am. J. Physiol.*, 246, E471, 1984.

185. **Henrikson, E.J., Kirby, C.R., and Tischler, M.E.**, Glycogen supercompensation in rat soleus muscle during recovery from nonweight bearing, *J. Appl. Physiol.*, 66, 2782, 1989.

186. **Hultman, E.**, Physiological role of muscle glycogen in man, with special reference to exercise, *Circ. Res.*, 20 (Suppl. 1), 99, 1967.

187. **Roch-Norlund, A.E., Bergström, J., and Hultman, E.**, Muscle glycogen and glycogen synthase in normal subjects and in patients with diabetes mellitus. Effect of intravenous glucose and insulin administration, *Scand. J. Clin. Lab. Invest.*, 30, 77, 1972.

188. **Maehlum, S., Hostmark, A.T., and Hermansen, L.**, Synthesis of muscle glycogen during recovery after prolonged severe exercise by diabetic and non-diabetic subjects, *Scand. J. Clin. Lab. Invest.*, 37, 309, 1977.

189. **Costill, D.L., Sherman, W.M., Fink, W.J., Maresh, C., Witten, M., and Miller, J.M.**, The role of dietary carbohydrates in muscle glycogen resynthesis after strenous running, *Am. J. Clin. Nutr.*, 34, 1831, 1981.

190. **Ahlborg, B., Bergström, J., Brohult, J., Ekelund, L.G., Hultman, E., and Machio, G.**, Human muscle glycogen content and capacity for prolonged exercise after different diets, *Forsvarsmedicin*, 3, 85, 1967.

191. **Bergström, J., Hermansen, L., Hultman, E., and Saltin, B.**, Diet, muscle glycogen and physical performance, *Acta Physiol. Scand.*, 71, 140, 1967.

192. **Hultman, E.**, Muscle glycogen stores and prolonged exercise, in *Frontiers of Fitness*, Shephard, R.J., Ed., Thomas, Springfield, 1971, 37.

193. **Yakovlev, N.N., Aleksandrova, G.V., Batuner, L.S., Krasnova, A.F., Lenkova, R.I., Usik, S.V., and Chagovets, N.R.**, Metabolic structure of the restitution process after physical exercises of various character, *Sechenov Physiol. J. USSR*, 64, 1160, 1978.

194. **Poland, J.L., and Trauner, D.A.**, Effects of prior exercise on myocardial glycogenesis during a fast, *Proc. Soc. Exp. Biol. Med.*, 131, 1100, 1971.

195. **Conlee, P., and Tipton, C.M.**, Cardiac glycogen repletion after exercise: influence of synthase and glucose-6-phosphate, *J. Appl. Physiol.*, 42, 240, 1977.

196. **Poland, J.L., Throwbridge, C., and Poland, J.W.**, Substrate repletion in rat myocardium, liver and skeletal muscle after exercise, *Can. J. Physiol. Pharmacol.*, 58, 1229, 1980.

197. **Yan, Z., Spencer, M.K., and Katz, A.**, Effect of low glycogen on glycogen synthase in human muscle during and after exercise, *Acta Physiol. Scand.*, 145, 345, 1992.

198. **Danforth, W.H.**, Glycogen synthase in skeletal muscle, *J. Biol. Chem.*, 240, 588, 1965.

199. **Bergström, J., Hultman, E., and Roch-Norlund, A.E.**, Muscle glycogen synthase in normal subjects. Basal values, effect of glycogen depletion by exercise and of a carbohydrate-rich diet following exercise, *Scand. J. Clin. Lab. Invest.*, 29, 231, 1972.

200. **Zachuraja, J.J., Costill, D.L., Pascoe, D.D., Robergs, R.A., and Fink, W.J.**, Influence of muscle glycogen depletion on the rate of resynthesis, *Med. Sci. Sports Exerc.*, 23, 44, 1991.

201. **Bergström, J., and Hultman, E.**, Muscle glycogen synthesis after exercise: an enhancing factor localized to the muscle cell in man, *Nature*, 210, 309, 1966.

202. **Zorzano, A., Balon, T., Goodman, M.N., and Ruderman, N.B.**, Additive effects of prior exercise and insulin on glucose and AIB uptake by rat muscle, *Am. J. Physiol.*, 254, E21, 1986.

203. **Poland, J.L., and Trauner, D.A.**, Adrenal influence on the supercompensation of cardiac glycogen following exercise, *Am. J. Physiol.*, 224, 540, 1973.

204. **Kôrge, P., Eller, A., Timpmann, S., and Seppet, E.**, The role of glucocorticoids in the regulation of postexercise glycogen repletion and the mechanism of their action, *Sechenov Physiol. J. USSR*, 68, 1431, 1982.

205. **Maehlum, S., and Hermansen, L.**, Muscle glycogen concentration during recovery after prolonged severe exercise in fasting subjects, *Scand. J. Clin. Lab. Invest.*, 38, 557, 1978.

206. **Fell, R.D., McLane, J.A., Winder, W.W., and Holloszy, J.O.**, Preferential resynthesis of muscle glycogen in fasting rats after exhaustive exercise, *Am. J. Physiol.*, 238, R328, 1980.

207. **Meyerhof, O.**, Über die Energieumwandlungen in Muskel. II. Das Schicksal der Erholungsperiode des Muskels, *Pflügers Arch. ges. Physiol.*, 182, 284, 1920.

208. **Sacks, J., and Sacks, W.C.**, Carbohydrate changes during recovery from muscular contraction, *Am. J. Physiol.*, 112, 565, 1935.

209. **Bendell, J.R., and Taylor, A.A.**, The Meyerhof quotient and the synthesis of glycogen from lactate in frog and rabbit muscle. A reinvestigation, *Biochem. J.*, 118, 887, 1970.

210. **McGrail, J.C., Bonen, A., and Belcastro, A.N.**, Dependence of lactate removal on muscle metabolism in men, *Eur. J. Appl. Physiol.*, 39, 89, 1978.

211. **Brooks, G.A., and Gaesser, G.A.**, End points of lactate and glucose metabolism after exhausting exercise, *J. Appl. Physiol.*, 49, 1057, 1980.

212. **Shiota, M., Golden, S., and Katz, J.**, Lactate metabolism in the perfused rat hindlimb, *Biochem. J.*, 222, 281, 1984.

213. **Stevensson, R.W., Mitchell, D.R., Hendrick, D.K., Rainey, R., Cherrington, A.D., and Frizzel, R.T.**, Lactate as substrate for glycogen resynthesis after exercise, *J. Appl. Physiol.*, 62, 2237, 1987.

214. **McLane, J.A., and Holloszy, J.O.**, Glycogen synthesis from lactate in three types of skeletal muscle, *J. Biol. Chem.*, 254, 6548, 1979.

215. **Bonen, A., Campbell, C.J., Kirby, R.L., and Belcastro, A.N.**, Relationship between slow-twitch muscle fibers and lactic acid removal, *Can. J. Sports Sci.*, 3, 160, 1978.

216. **Brooks, G.A., Brauner, K.E., and Caesser, R.G.**, Glycogen synthesis and metabolism of lactic acid after exercise, *Am. J. Physiol.*, 224, 1162, 1973.

217. **Hatta, H., Atomi, Y., Yamamoto, Y., Shinohara, S., and Yamada, S.**, Incorporation of blood lactate and glucose into tissues in rats after short-term strenuous exercise, *Int. J. Sports Med.*, 10, 275, 1989.

218. **Gaesser, A.G., and Brooks, G.A.**, Glycogen repletion following continuous and intermittent exercise to exhaustion, *J. Appl. Physiol.*, 79, 722, 1980.

219. **Bonen, A., McDermott, J.C., and Tan, M.H.**, Glycogenesis and gluconeogenesis in skeletal muscle: effects of pH and hormones, *Am. J. Physiol.*, 21, E693, 1990.

220. **Blom, P., Vollestad, N.K., and Costill, D.L.**, Factors affecting changes in muscle glycogen concentration during and after prolonged exercise, *Acta Physiol. Scand.*, 125 (Suppl. 556), 67, 1986.

221. **Blom, P.C.S., Høstmark, A.T., Vaage, O., Kardel, K.R., and Maehlum, S.**, Effect of different post-exercise sugar diets on the rate of muscle glycogen synthesis, *Med. Sci. Sports Exerc.*, 19, 491, 1987.

222. **Wahren, J., Maehlum, S., and Felig, P.**, Glucose metabolism during recovery after exercise: primary of muscle rather than hepatic glycogen repletion, *Am. J. Clin. Nutr.*, 30, 623, 1977.

223. **Brooks, G.**, The lactate shuttle during exercise and recovery, *Med. Sci. Sports Exerc.*, 18, 360, 1986.

224. **Maehlum, S., Felig, P., and Wahren, J.**, Splanchnic glucose and muscle glycogen metabolism after glucose feeding during postexercise recovery, *Am. J. Physiol.*, 235, E255, 1978.

225. **Hultman, E.**, Carbohydrate metabolism during hard exercise and in the recovery period after exercise, *Acta Physiol. Scand.*, 128 (Suppl. 556), 75, 1986.

226. **Johnson, J.L., and Bagdy, G.J.**, Gluconeogenic pathway in liver and muscle glycogen synthesis after exercise, *J. Appl. Physiol.*, 64, 1591, 1988.

227. **Wahren, J., Felig, P., Hendler, R., and Ahlborg, G.**, Glucose and amino acid metabolism during recovery after exercise, *J. Appl. Physiol.*, 34, 838, 1973.

228. **Ahlborg, G., Wahren, J., and Felig, P.**, Splanchnic and peripheral glucose and lactate metabolism during and after arm exercise, *J. Clin. Invest.*, 77, 690, 1986.

229. **Wasserman, D.H., Brooks, L.D., Green, D.R., Wilbams, P.E., and Cherrington, A.D.**, Dynamics of hepatic lactate and glucose balances during prolonged exercise and recovery in the dog, *J. Appl. Physiol.*, 63, 2411, 1987.

230. **Favier, R.J., Kouh, H.E., Mayet, M.H., Semore, B., Sumi, B., and Flandrois, R.**, Effects of gluconeogenic precursors flux alteration on glycogen resynthesis after prolonged exercise, *J. Appl. Physiol.*, 63, 1733, 1987.

231. **Wasserman, D.H., Williams, P.E., Brooks, L.D., Green, D.R., and Cherrington, A.D.**, Importance of intrahepatic mechanisms to gluconeogenesis from alanine during exercise and recovery, *Am. J. Physiol.*, 254, E518, 1988.

232. **Terblanche, S.E., Fell, R.D., Juhlin-Dannfeldt, A.C., Craig, B.W., and Holloszy, J.O.**, Effect of glycerol feeding before and after exercise, *J. Appl. Physiol.*, 50, 94, 1981.

233. **Bergström, J., and Hultman, E.**, Synthesis of muscle glycogen in man after glucose and fructose infusion, *Acta Med. Scand.*, 182, 93, 1967.

234. **Nilsson, L.H., and Hultman, E.**, Liver and muscle glycogen in man after glucose and fructose infusion, *Scand. Clin. Lab. Invest.*, 33, 5, 1974.

235. **Dohm, G.L., and Newsholme, E.A.**, Metabolic control of hepatic gluconeogenesis during exercise, *Biochem. J.*, 212, 633, 1983.

236. **Annuzzi, G., Jansson, E., Kaijser, L., Holmquist, L., and Carlson, L.A.**, Increased removal rate of exogenous triglycerides after prolonged exercise in man: time course and effect of exercise duration, *Metabolism*, 36, 438, 1987.

237. **Krzentowski, G., Pirnay, F., Luyckx, S., Pallikaris, N., Lacroix, M., Morora, E., and Lefebvre, P.J.**, Metabolic adaptations to postexercise recovery, *Clin. Physiol.*, 27, 277, 1982.

238. **Newsholme, E.A.**, A possible metabolic basis for the control of body weight, *N. Engl. J. Med.*, 302, 400, 1980.

239. **Wasserman, D.H., Geer, R.J., Rice, D.E., Bracy, D., Flakoll, P.J., Brown, L.L., Hill, J.O., and Adumard, N.N.**, Interaction of exercise and isulin action in humans, *Am. J. Physiol.*, 260, E37, 1991.

240. **Carlin, J.I., Reddan, W.G., Sanjak, M., and Hodach, R.**, Carnitine metabolism during prolonged exercise and recovery in humans, *J. Appl. Physiol.*, 61, 1275, 1986.

241. **Donnelly, A.E., Gleesor, M., Maughan, R.J., Walker, K.A., and Whiting, R.H.**, Delayed-onset rise in serum lipid peroxidase concentration following eccentric exercise in man, *J. Physiol.*, 392, 51P, 1987.

242. **Rogozkin, V.A., and Yakovlev, N.N.**, Nitrogen metabolism during muscular activity of various character, *Ukr. Biokhim. Zh.*, 32, 899, 1960 (in Russian).

243. **Chagovets, N.R.**, Sarcoplasmic proteins of muscles during exercise and recovery, *Vopr. Med. Khim.*, 8, 599, 1962 (in Russian).

244. **Chailley-Bert, P., Plas, F., Henry, M.A., and Bugard, P.**, Les modifications métaboliques au cours d'effort prolonges chez le sportif, *Rev. Pathol. Gen.*, 61, 143, 1961.

245. **Conzolazio, C.F., Johnson, H.L., and Nelson, R.A.**, Protein metabolism during intensive physical training in the young adult, *Am. J. Clin. Nutr.*, 28, 29, 1975.

246. **Narable, N.L., Hickson, J.F., Korslund, M.K., Herbert, W.G., and Desjardins, R.F.**, Urinary nitrogen excretion as influenced by a muscle building exercise program and protein intake variation, *Nutr. Rep. Int.*, 19, 795, 1979.

247. **Litvinova, V.N., and Rogozkin, V.A.**, Action of muscular activity on the rate of leucine-C^{14} and alanine-C^{14} incorporation into muscle proteins, *Ukr. Biokhim. Zh.*, 42, 450, 1970.

248. **McManus, B.M., Lamb, D.R., Jundis, J.J., and Scala, J.**, Skeletal muscle leucine incorporation and testosterone uptake in exercised guinea pigs, *Eur. J. Appl. Physiol.*, 34, 149, 1975.

249. **Rogers, P.A., Jones, G.H., and Faulkner, J.A.**, Protein synthesis in skeletal muscle following acute exhaustive exercise, *Muscle Nerv.*, 2, 250, 1979.

250. **Dohm, G.L., Kasperek, G.J., Tapscott, E.B., and Beacher, G.R.**, Effect of exercise on synthesis and degradation of muscle protein, *Biochem. J.*, 188, 255, 1980.

251. **Rennie, M.J., Edwards, R.H.T., Davies, C.T.M., Krywawych, S., Halliday, D., Waterlow, J.C., and Millward, D.J.**, Protein and amino acid turnover during and after exercise, *Biochem. Soc. Trans.*, 8, 499, 1980.

252. **Wenger, H.A., Wilkinson, J.G., and Dallaire, J.**, Uptake of ^{3}H-leucine into different fractions of rat skeletal muscle following acute endurance and sprint exercise, *Eur. J. Appl. Physiol.*, 47, 83, 1981.

253. **Booth, F.W., Nicholsen, W.F., and Watson, P.A.**, Influence of muscle use on protein synthesis and degradation, *Exerc. Sports Sci. Rev.*, 10, 27, 1982.

254. **Millward, D.J., Davies, C.T.M., Halliday, D., Wolman, S.L., Matthews, D.M., and Rennie, M.**, Effect of exercise on protein metabolism in humans as explored with stable isotopes, *Fed. Proc.*, 41, 2686, 1982.

255. **Seene, T., Alev, K., and Pehme, A.**, Effect of muscular activity on the different types of skeletal muscle, *Int. J. Sports Med.*, 7, 287, 1986.

256. **Silber, M.L., Pliskin, A.V., and Rogozkin, V.A.**, Action of physical exercise on synthesis of nuclear RNA in skeletal muscles, *Vopr. Med. Khim.*, 17, 280, 1972 (in Russian).

257. **Silber, M.L., and Rogozkin, V.A.**, Action of physical exercise on the activity of nuclear RNA-polymerase of skeletal muscles and liver, *Ukr. Biokhim. Zh.*, 431, 588, 1971.

258. **Bates, P.C., DeCoster, T., Grimble, G.K., Holloszy, J.O., Millward, D.J., and Rennie, M.**, Exercise and muscle protein turnover in the rat, *J. Physiol.*, 303, 41P, 1980.

259. **Viru, A., and Ööpik, V.**, Anabolic and catabolic responses to training, in *Paavo Nurmi Congress Book,* Kvist, M., Ed., The Finnish Society of Sports Medicine, Turku, 1989, 55.

260. **Rogozkin, V., and Feldkoren, R.I.**, The effect of retabolil and training on activity of RNA polymerase in skeletal muscle, *Med. Sci. Sports*, 11, 345, 1979.

261. **Hamberger, A., Gregson, N., and Lehninger, A.L.**, The effect of acute exercise on amino acid incorporation into mitochondria of rabbit tissue, *Biochim. Biophys. Acta*, 186, 373, 1969.

262. **Viru, A., Konovalova, G., Ööpik, V., and Masso, R.**, Thyroid hormones in protein synthesis during postexercise recovery, in *8th Int. Biochem. Exerc. Conf. Progr. Abstr.*, Nagoya, 1991, 107.

263. **Viru, A.**, The mechanism of training effects: a hypothesis, *Int. J. Sports Med.*, 5, 219, 1984.

264. **Gustafson, R., Tata, J.R., Lindberg, O., and Ernester, L.**, The relationship between the structure and activity of rat skeletal muscle mitochondria after thyroidectomy and thyroid hormone treatment, *J. Cell. Biol.*, 26, 555, 1965.

265. **Winder, W.W., Baldwin, K.M., Terjung, R.L., and Holloszy, J.O.**, Effects of thyroid hormone administration on skeletal muscle mitochondria, *Am. J. Physiol.*, 228, 1341, 1975.

266. **Winder, W.W., and Holloszy, J.O.**, Response of mitochondria of different types of skeletal muscle to thyrotoxicosis, *Am. J. Physiol.*, 232, C180, 1977.

267. **Ianuzzo, C.D., Petel, G., Chen, V., O'Brien, P., and Williams, C.**, Thyroid trophic influence on skeletal muscle myosin, *Nature*, 270, 74, 1977.

268. **Chesley, A., MacDougall, J.D., Tarnopolsky, M.A., Atkinson, S.A., and Smith, K.**, Changes in human muscle protein synthesis after resistance exercise, *J. Appl. Physiol.*, 73, 1383, 1992.

269. **Wong, T.S., and Booth, E.W.**, Protein metabolism in rat gastrocnemius muscle after stimulated chronic concentric exercise, *J. Appl. Physiol.*, 69, 1718, 1990.

270. **Wong, T.S., and Booth, E.W.**, Protein metabolism in rat tibialis anterior muscle after stimulated chronic eccentric exercise, *J. Appl. Physiol.* 69, 1709, 1990.

271. **Booth, F.W., and Thomason, D.B.**, Molecular and cellular adaptation of muscle in response to exercise: perspectives of various models, *Physiol. Rev.*, 71, 541, 1991.

272. **Rogozkin, V.**, Metabolic effects of anabolic steroids on skeletal muscle, *Med. Sci. Sports*, 11, 160, 1979.

273. **Tchaikovsky, V.S., Astratenkova, I.V., and Basharina, O.B.**, The effect of exercise on the content and receptor of the streoid hormones in rat skeletal muscle, *J. Steroid Biochem.*, 24, 251, 1986.

274. **Feldkoren, R., and Osipova, H.**, Exercise, testosterone blood levels and androgen receptor in skeletal muscle, in *Hormonal Regulation of Adaptation to Muscular Activity*, Tartu University, Tartu, 1991, 25.

275. **Saborido, A., Vila, J., Molano, F., and Megias, A.**, Effect of anabolic steroids on mitochondria and sarcotubular system of skeletal muscle, *J. Appl. Physiol.*, 70, 1088, 1991.

276. **Wool, I.G., and Cavicchi, P.**, Insulin regulation of protein synthesis by muscle ribosomes, *Proc. Natl. Acad. Sci. USA*, 56, 991, 1966.

277. **Check, D.B., and Hill, D.E.**, Effect of growth hormone on cell and somatic growth, in *Handbook of Physiology*, Knobil, E. and Sawyer, W.H., Eds., American Physiological Society, Washington, D.C., 1974, 159.

278. **Fryburg, D.A., Gelfand, R.A., and Barrett, E.J.**, Growth hormone acutely stimulates forearm muscle protein synthesis in normal humans, *Am. J. Physiol.*, 260, E499, 1991.

279. **Cuneo, R.C., Salomon, F., Wills, C.M., and Sönksen, P.H.**, Growth hormone treatment in growth hormone-deficient adults. I. Effects on muscle mass and strength, *J. Appl. Physiol.*, 70, 688, 1991.

280. **Cuneo, R.S., Salomon, P., Wills, C.M., Hesp, R., and Sönksen, P.H.**, Growth hormone treatment in growth hormone-deficient adults. II. Effects on exercise performance, *J. Appl. Physiol.*, 70, 695, 1991.

281. **Ullman, M., and Oldfors, A.**, Effects of growth hormone on skeletal muscle. I. Studies on normal adult rats, *Acta Physiol. Scand.*, 135, 531, 1986.

282. **Balon, T.W., Zorzano, A., Treadway, J.L., Goodman, M.N., and Ruderman, N.B.**, Effect of insulin on protein synthesis and degradation in skeletal muscle after exercise, *Am. J. Physiol.*, 258, E92, 1990.

283. **Refsum, H.E., and Strömme, S.E.**, Urea and creatine production and excretion in urine during and after prolonged heavy exercise, *Scand. J. Clin. Lab. Invest.*, 33, 247, 1974.

284. **Gorokhov, A.L.**, A study of acid-base balance and urea in blood of sportsmen, *Teor. Prakt. Fiz. Kult.*, 1, 22, 1976 (in Russian).

285. **Buhl, H., Newmann, G., Gerber, G., and Gottschalk, K.**, Der extreme Dauerleistung. Fall-stude eines 24-Stunden bzw 100-km Laufes, *Med. Sport*, 18, 354, 1978.

286. **Janssen, G.M.E., Degenaur, C.P., Mensheere, P.P.C.A., Habets, H.M.L., and Gervesten, P.**, Plasma urea, creatinine, uric and albumin and total protein concentrations before and after 15-, 25- and 42-km contests, *Int. J. Sports Med.*, 10 (Suppl. 3), S132, 1989.

287. **Lenkova, R.I., Usik, S.K., and Yakovlev, N.N.**, Changes in urea content in blood and tissues during muscular activity in dependence on the adaptation of organism, *Sechenov Physiol. J. USSR*, 59, 1097, 1973 (in Russian).

288. **Litvinova, L., Viru, A., and Smirnova, T.**, Renal urea clearance in normal and adrenalectomized rats after exercise, *Jpn. J. Physiol.*, 39, 713, 1989.

289. **Yakovlev, N.N.**, Ornithine metabolism and adaptation to augmented muscular activity, *Sechenov Physiol. J. USSR*, 65, 979, 1979 (in Russian).

290. **Kasperek, G.J., and Snider, R.D.**, The effect of exercise on protein turnover in isolated soleus and extensor digitorum longus muscle, *Experimentia*, 41, 1399, 1985.

291. **Varrik, E., Viru, A., Ööpik, V., and Viru, M.**, Exercise-induced catabolic responses in various muscle fibers, *Can. J. Sports Sci.*, 17, 125, 1992.

292. **Wahren, J., Felig, P., Hendler, R., and Ahlborg, G.**, Glucose and amino acid metabolism during recovery after exercise, *J. Appl. Physiol.*, 34, 838, 1973.

293. **Brooks, G.A.**, Amino acid and protein metabolism during exercise and recovery, *Med. Sci. Sports Exerc.*, 19, S150, 1987.

294. **Dohm, G.L., Williams, R.T., Kasperek, G.J., and van Rij, A.M.**, Increased excretion of urea and N¹-methylhistidine by rats and humans after a bout of exercise, *J. Appl. Physiol.*, 52, 27, 1982.

295. **Dohm, G.L., Israel, R.G., Breedlove, R.L., Williams, B.L., and Askew, E.W.**, Biphasic changes in 3-methylhistidine excretion in humans after exercise, *Am. J. Physiol.*, 248, 588, 1985.

296. **Varrik, E., and Viru, A.**, Excretion of 3-methylhistidine in exercising rats, *Biol. Sport*, 5, 195, 1988.

297. **Dohm, G.L., Tapscott, E.B., and Kasperek, G.J.**, Protein degradation during endurance exercise and recovery, *Med. Sci. Sports Exerc.*, 19, S166, 1987.

298. **Viru, A.**, Mobilization of structural proteins during exercise, *Sports Med.*, 4, 95, 1987.

299. **Seli, N. and Viru, A.**, 3-Methylhistidine excretion in training for improved power and strength, *Sports Med. Training Med. Rehab.*, 3, 183, 1992.

300. **Kasperek, G.J., and Snider, R.D.**, Increased protein degradation after eccentric exercise, *Eur. J. Appl. Physiol.*, 54, 30, 1985.

301. **Varrik, E., Ööpik, V., and Viru, A.**, Protein metabolism in muscles after their activity, *Med. Sport*, 46, 27, 1993.

302. **Hickson, R.C., and Davis, J.R.**, Partial prevention of glucocorticoid-induced muscle atrophy by endurance training, *Am. J. Physiol.*, 241, E226, 1981.

303. **Seene, T., and Viru, A.**, The catabolic effect of glucocorticoids on different types of skeletal muscle fibers and its dependence upon muscle activity and interaction with anabolic steroids, *J. Steroid Biochem.*, 16, 349, 1982.

304. **Jürimäe, T., Karelson, K., Smirnova, T., and Viru, A.**, The effect of a single-circuit weight-training session on the blood biochemistry of untrained university students, *Eur. J. Appl. Physiol.*, 61, 344, 1990.

305. **Dahlman, B., Widjaja, A., and Reinauer, H.**, Antagonistic effects of endurance training and testosterone on alkaline proteolytic activity in rat skeletal muscles, *Eur. J. Physiol.*, 46, 229, 1981.

306. **Dohm, G.L., and Louis, T.M.**, Changes in androstenedione, testosterone and protein metabolism as a result of exercise, *Proc. Soc. Exp. Biol. Med.*, 158, 622, 1978.

307. **Fry, R.W., Morton, A.P., Garcia-Webb, P., and Keast, D.**, Monitoring exercise stress by changes in metabolic and hormonal responses over a 24 h period, *Eur. J. Appl. Physiol.*, 63, 228, 1991.

308. **Vihko, V., Salminen, A., and Rantamäki, J.**, Acid hydrolase activity in red and white skeletal muscle of mice during a two-week period following exhausting exercise, *Pflügers Arch. ges. Physiol.*, 378, 99, 1978.

309. **Salminen, A., and Vihko, V.**, Acid hydrolase activities in mouse cardiac and skeletal muscle following exhaustive exercise, *Eur. J. Appl. Physiol.*, 47, 57, 1981.

310. **Kasperek, G.J., and Snider, R.D.**, Effect of exercise on total and myofibrillar protein degradation in isolated soleus muscle, *Can. J. Sports Sci.*, 13, 20P, 1988.

311. **Nazarov, I.B., Baboshina, O.V., Rogozkin, V.A., and Tsyplenkov, N.V.**, Influence of physical exercises on the activity of calpains and the content of myeloperoxidase in skeletal muscles of rats, *Ukr. Biokhim. Zh.*, 62, 101, 1990 (in Russian).

312. **MacLennan, P.A., Brown, R.A., and Rennie, M.J.**, A positive relationship between protein synthetic rate and intracellular glutamine concentration in perfused rat skeletal muscle, *FEBS Lett.*, 215, 187, 1987.

313. **MacLennan, P.A., Smith, K., Weryk, B., and Rennie, M.J.**, Inhibition of protein breakdown by glutamine in perfused rat skeletal muscle, *FEBS Lett.*, 237, 133, 1988.

314. **Platonov, V.N.**, *Adaptation in Sports*, Zdarovya, Kiev, 1988.

Chapter 5

SPECIFIC NATURE OF TRAINING
ON SKELETAL MUSCLES

The principle of specific adaptation to various kinds of muscular activity was first formulated and argued by N.N. Yakovlev.[1-5] Later, striking evidence of the specific nature of training effects was obtained from a great number of studies carried out in several laboratories.

Each exercise determines the degree of activity of various organs, different type of muscles, and motor units. Within each active cell the main metabolic pathways that permit the accomplishment of necessary functional tasks also depend on the nature of training exercises. The activity of the metabolic control system at various levels as well as the activity of the system directly regulating bodily functions is also dependent on the nature of training exercise. Correspondingly, the organism's adaptation bears the imprint of the type of exercise systematically used in training (Figure 5-1).

HYPERTROPHY OF MYOFIBRILS

The most prominent result of training for improved strength is hypertrophy of skeletal muscles.[6-9] A very pronounced muscle hypertrophy is displayed by athletes exposed to long-term vigorous strength training.[10-13] Muscular hypertrophy is primarily the result of an increased size of the individual fibers.[14-20] In its turn, the latter is based on the enlargement of myofibrils,[21,22] obviously due to the augmentation of myofibrillar proteins.[3,4,5,23,24] Also, an increased number of myofibrils has been found, indicating some hyperplasia.[4,21,25-27] It is assumed that the myogenic response to strength training involves mainly the synthesis of new contractile proteins.[4,5,28-31]

In rats a model of strength training, consisting of a repeated series of fast climbing up a slope with an attached load (100 to 400 g), induced an increased rate of synthesis of actinomyosin proteins in fast-twitch glycolytic (FG) and fast-twitch oxidative-glycolytic (FOG) fibers.[32] Accordingly, a period of strength training resulted in an increase in the cross-sectional area mainly in the fast-twitch fibers of the rat.[16,18, 20,33-36] Olympic weight-lifters may possess fast-twitch fibers that are two times larger in diameter than slow-twitch fibers of the same muscle.[14,37] The great growth potential of fast-twitch fibers allows the area of muscle occupied by fast-twitch fibers to increase by 90% with strength training, despite retaining a fiber-type composition within the normal range.[37,38] However, a moderate enlargement of slow-twitch fibers cannot be excluded from having contributed to this hypertrophy.[19,36]

The effect of training for improved strength differs from that of aerobic endurance training, which does not cause a substantial increase in the cross-sectional area of muscle fibers.[31,39] The cross-sectional area of thigh muscles remained essentially unchanged during about 6 months of strenuous bicycling.[40] In one study even a decrease in the volume fraction of myofibrils occurred after endurance training of 2 months duration.[41] However, a selective and moderate enlargement of slow-twitch oxidative (SO) fibers and in some cases also FOG fibers is possible in endurance training.[42-44] In endurance training no enlargement of myofibrils was found. The increase in the fiber diameter is mainly due to the elevated volume of sarcoplasma.[27,31] The increase in the sarcoplasmic space is thought to be due to the glycogen content increase.[31] The elevated glycogen content also explains the increase in the volume density of cytoplasm as a result of strength training.[45]

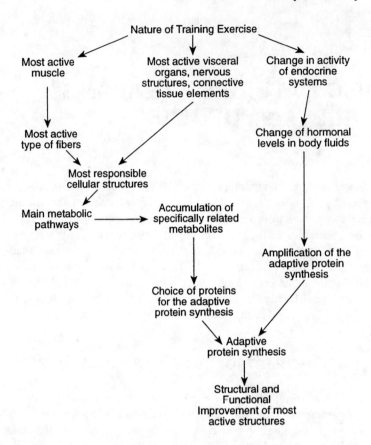

FIGURE 5-1. Factors determining the specificity of the influence of training exercises.

Endurance training induces an elevated rate of myosin heavy chain and actin turnover in all fiber types. In sprint-trained rats a more rapid turnover of the myosin heavy chain was found only in FG and FOG fibers in comparison with sedentary rats.[46]

No increase in the content of myosin or actin has been found after endurance training.[3,4]

Sprint training increases the cross-sectional area of both slow- and fast-twitch fibers.[47] This effect is greatest for the fast-twitch fibers. The end result is that they occupy a slightly greater area in the sprint trained athletes.[48] The effect of sprint training on fiber size is less pronounced than that of strength training.

The area of slow-twitch fibers constituted 51 to 76% of muscle in distance runners, the percentage of slow-twitch fibers was 63 to 74%, and in sprinters the respective values were 15 to 32 and 21 to 27%, with no significant difference in individual fiber area between the two groups of athletes. In middle-distance runners, long and high jumpers, shot-putters, and javelin and discus throwers, the corresponding values were somewhere between those in sprinters and distance runners. The area of individual fibers was largest in shot-putters and discus throwers, particularly in regard to fast-twitch fibers.[49] In comparison with elite long-distance runners, middle-distance runners have a smaller percentage of slow-twitch fibers (62 ± 2.9 vs. $70 \pm 3.5\%$), slow-twitch fiber area (6378 ± 400 vs. 8342 ± 724 μM^2), and percentage of slow-twitch fiber area (62 ± 2.6 vs. $83 \pm 3.1\%$). There were no differences in the fast-twitch fiber area.[50]

A significant increase in the numerical density of myonuclei was observed in both rats[26,27] and dogs[51] with endurance training. According to other data, in rats the quantity of nuclei in a cross section of 100 muscle fibers increased as a result of models of power training but not of models of endurance and sprint training.[3,4,21] However, training in swimming resulted in an increase in nuclei dimensions.[21]

Running training induced greater areas of nerve terminals in the extensor digitorum longus muscle and the soleus muscle.[26, 27,51,52] The quantity of terminal branches[4,26,27,53] as well as the cross-sectional area of motor nerve fibers[4,51] increased as a result of speed or power training but not as a result of endurance training. In case of endurance training even a decrease of 15% in the cross-sectional area of motor nerve fibers was observed.[4,53]

HYPERTROPHY VS. HYPERPLASIA

Results of a number of studies indicate the possibility of a longitudinal division of muscle fibers in training.[26,27,54-58] Data have been obtained suggesting that motor nerve endings on newly formed muscular fibers develop from collateral branch endings springing from preterminal departments of motor axons.[59]

Calculations of total numbers of fibers were performed in the human biceps from measurements of the total cross-sectional area of the muscle determined by computerized tomography. The area of the individual fibers was determined from biopsy samples. The obtained data demonstrate the existence of considerable variations between the fiber numbers of subjects. However, there was no evidence of a systematic difference between sedentary and trained persons. The greater total cross-sectional area in athletes was attributable to the larger cross-sectional area of individual fibers.[60,61] In rats the number of fibers per muscle was determined by direct counts of individual fibers dissected from HNO_3-treated muscles. Ablation of a synergist produced enlargements of about 25, 45, and 29% in the soleus, plantaris, and extensor digitorum longus muscles respectively. Treadmill running after synergist ablation produced increases in wet weight of about 44 and 88% in the soleus and plantaris muscles, whereas no further increases were observed in the extensor digitorum longus muscle. Intraanimal comparisons revealed that no differences existed in the total fiber number or the incidence of fibers with bifurcations between enlarged and contralateral muscles.[62] Against the background of these results it has been affirmed that the increased muscle mass is produced by further increases in the total cross-sectional area of individual fibers and not by addition of more muscle fibers.[63]

In some studies an increase in the DNA content was found in association with work-induced hypertrophy.[28,64] However, the DNA was augmented without any increase in the number of fibers per muscle cross-sectional area.[65] It is reasonable to assume that the augmented DNA was not due to the extra muscle fibers content. The bulk of the increase in DNA arises from the additions of connective tissue to support the enlarged fibers.[66] Part of the increase in DNA is associated with a proliferation of the satellite muscle cells.[67,68] Blocking of DNA synthesis did not stop hypertrophy of muscle fibers in the rat soleus muscle after tenotomy of the synergists.[69]

In conclusion, the stimulus for muscular hypertrophy depends on the resistance to muscle contraction as well as the total number of contractions performed against high resistance. Therefore, the main tool for muscle hypertrophy is high-resistance exercise (Figure 5-2). The effect of power and sprint exercises is less pronounced. Endurance exercise is ineffective. Muscle hypertrophy appears most of all in FG fibers, to a lesser degree in FOG fibers, and inconsistently in SO fibers.

CONTRACTILE MECHANISM

In regard to the contractile mechanism there are three main conditions that determine the effectiveness of muscular contraction in sports performance:

1. Total number of cross-bridges formed between myosin and actin protofibrils during contraction — determines the force of contraction
2. The rate of formation of cross-bridges (number of cross-bridges formed per unit time) — determines the velocity of contraction and power output
3. Energy liberation for the contraction

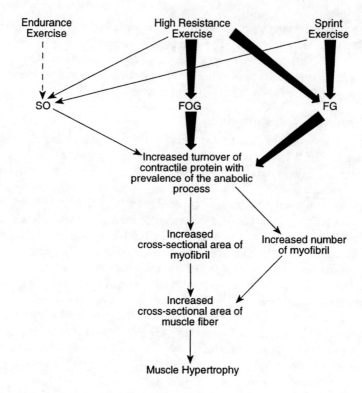

FIGURE 5-2.   Stimulation of the hypertrophy of muscle fibers by various exercises. The width of arrows shows the degree of influence.

It is logical to assume that the maximal number of cross-bridges formed depends on the amount of myofibrillar contractile proteins. At the same time mechanisms of excitation and excitation/coupling are also highly significant. Both mechanisms are closely related to ionic shifts through the plasma membrane as well as within cells through the membranes of the sarcoplasmic reticulum. While the total amount of calcium ions released from the sarcoplasmic reticulum may limit the number of the formed cross-bridges and then the generated force, the power output has to be dependent on the rate of calcium ions release and thereby on the rate of formation of cross-bridges. The rate of calcium release also determines the myosin ATPase activity and thus the energy liberation for contraction.

SARCOLEMMA

No data are available for evaluating the specific training effect on the excitation mechanism. It may only be speculated that there exist individual differences in acetylcholine synthesis and release, cholinesterase activity, and maybe even in ionic gradients. If this is the case, these differences may limit the transfer of high frequencies of nerve discharges to events initiating the contraction and determining the force or power output. Anyway, highly effective ionic pumps are necessary for avoiding decreases in the ionic gradient and thereby ensuring optimal conditions for excitation and excitation/coupling events. The plasma membrane of skeletal muscles has been frequently implicated in the process of fatigue.[70] It was suggested that low-intensity fatigue may be the result of alterations in membrane structure in response to the activation of phospholipases and/or the production of free radicals. The latter can induce lipid peroxidation as well as direct modification of the transport systems.[70] Training-induced adaptive response involves lipid peroxidation and alterations in scavenger enzyme activity.[71] The action on cellular membranes is obviously accentuated by a concomitant increase in the activity of proteases.[72]

Highly effective ionic pumps are necessary for good performance in athletes. In rats a very long exercise (swimming for up to 24 h) caused a decreased activity of Na,K-ATPase in association with the accumulation of sodium and water in the skeletal muscle and myocardial cells.[73,74] Endurance training did not alter the activity of myocardial Na,K-ATPase but excluded the changes induced by prolonged exercise.[73] An 11-week training program decreased the K_m of the Na^+-Ca^{2+} exchanges in sarcolemmal vesicles of the myocardium with no alterations of Vmax.[75]

In humans a biopsy study showed that persons who for many years systematically exercised had increased concentrations of Na,K-pumps in the vastus lateralis muscle. In comparison with age-matched untrained subjects, the swimming-, running-, and strength-trained subjects demonstrated increased concentrations of ^{3}H-ouabain binding sites by 30, 32, and 40% respectively.[76] An intensive cycle-sprint training of 7 weeks resulted in an increase in ^{3}H-ouabain binding sites in the vastus lateralis muscle.[77] In rats intensive swimming training of 3 weeks produced 25 to 64% increases in the concentration of Na,K-pumps.[78] In dogs subjected to a moderate training program, the activity of Na,K-ATPase in the sarcolemma was found to be 2.6-fold higher than in controls.[79]

It was suggested that up-regulation of the Na,K-pump concentration might contribute to the reduction in exercise-induced hyperkalemia observed in trained subjects.[77,80]

SARCOPLASMIC RETICULUM (SR)

The protein content of the SR increased in rat muscles as a result of swimming training when the exercise intensity was gradually elevated by increasing additional loads, but not when the exercise intensity remained modest even if its duration was gradually prolonged.[5] In this study the capacity of the SR to absorb Ca^{2+} remained unchanged when calculated per milligram of protein. If calculated per unit of muscle weight, the capacity increased in training with elevated intensity of swimming. In another study the calcium transport capacity was found to have decreased as a result of analogous training programs.[81]

During endurance training Ca^{2+} uptake by the SR decreased in FG fibers, but did not change in FOG or SO fibers.[82]

A comparison of effects of various training regimes in rats demonstrated increased rates of Ca^{2+} accumulation by the SR (calculated per milligram of protein) in the soleus muscle after training in continuous aerobic running, sprint training, interval training, and strength training in fast clambering (Figure 5-3). In the white portion of the quadriceps muscle significantly increased rates were obtained after sprint, interval, or strength training, but not after continuous running. In both muscles the highest changes were caused by sprint and strength training. Training in continuous swimming decreased the Ca^{2+} accumulation in both muscles.[83] Consequently, the training effect on the SR depends on the types of exercises used. As could be expected, adaptation to systematic use of highly intensive exercises stimulated an improvement in the function of the SR.

Electron microscope studies gave controversial results. In one study, dilation of the terminals of the SR and of the T-tubes were found with training.[84] In another study, endurance training of moderate intensity did not cause any changes in the volume density of the tubular system of the SR.[85]

After 10 weeks of endurance running changes in tropomyosin isoforms subunit structure and functions were found in the rat hind leg muscles.[86]

ACTOMYOSIN ATPASE ACTIVITY

In rats the activity of muscle ATPase was increased[87] or remained without any changes after endurance training.[88,89] No changes were found after running training in nonhuman primates.[90] Strenuous running training (continuous running with periodic sprints) decreased the enzyme activity by 20% in FOG fibers and increased it approximately to the same extent

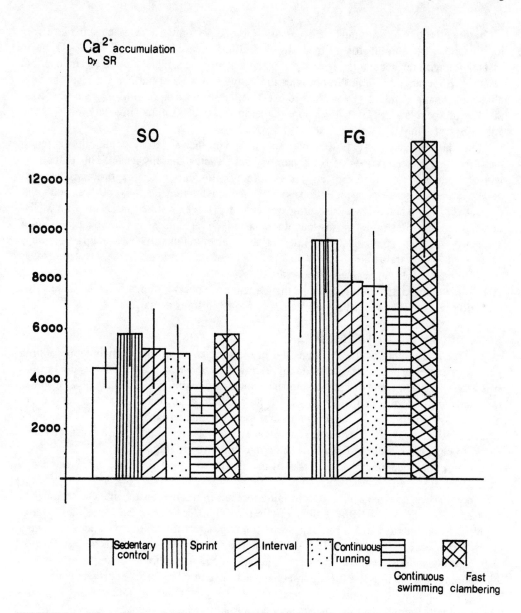

FIGURE 5-3. Effect of various training programs on Ca^{2+} accumulation by SR. Ca^{2+} accumulation was evaluated by cpm per milligram of protein (mean ± SEM). (From Viru, M., *J. Sports Med. Phys. Fitness,* 34, 1994. With permission.)

in SO muscles. No changes have been found in FG fibers.[91] Training with intensive exercises increased the activity of myofibrillar ATPase in humans[92] but not in rats.[89] When training exercise consisted of repeated jumps, the myofibrillar ATPase activity increased in rats.[33]

Myofibrillar Ca^{2+}-ATPase activity was increased in the soleus muscle after sprint, interval, or strength training. In the white quadriceps the same changes have also been found after continuous running in addition to the effect obtained after sprint, interval, and strength training (Figure 5-4). The greatest increase has been caused by strength training in glycolytic muscle. The effect of repeated short-term intensive running (sprint and interval training) was more pronounced than that of continuous running. Continuous swimming caused a decrease in the enzyme activity.[83] Electrostimulation of muscles, simulating endurance training, also caused a reduction in the enzyme activity.[93]

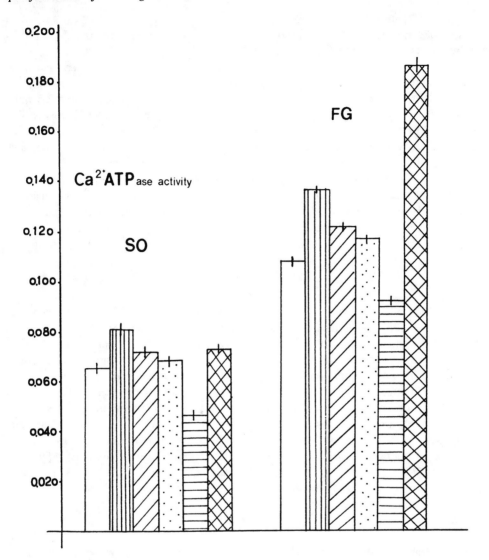

FIGURE 5-4. Effect of various training programs (see Figure 5-4) on myofibrillar Ca^{2+}-ATPase activity (micromoles of released phosphate per milligram of protein in 1 min; mean ± SEM).

In humans the effect of strength training on the activity of myofibrillar ATPase is variable, showing both an increase[35] and a decrease.[94] P.A. Tesch et al.[95] showed that neither concentric nor combined eccentric and concentric resistance training regimes caused any changes in the Mg^{2+}-ATPase activity.

Thus, training may induce two different adaptations at the level of myofibrillar ATPase. One of them consists of an elevation of the enzyme activity, making possible a rapid liberation of energy for muscular contractions at a level of high-power output. This adaptation seems to be common for sprint and interval training as well as for strength training, if we do not consider the opposite results of a study mentioned above. The second adaptation takes place in adaptation to continuous exercises of moderate intensity. The decreased myofibrillar ATPase may be considered essential for a more economical utilization of ATP stores.

CHARACTERISTICS OF CONTRACTION

Strength training induces changes in force-velocity curves of muscles.[96] After heavy resistance training the increase in the maximal voluntary force was most pronounced at slow velocities of contraction.[97-99] After explosive type of strength (power) exercises the improvement was greater in the high velocity portion of the curve.[99,100]

The time for producing a 30, 60, or 90% force level was shorter for wrestlers and body-builders than for power-lifters.[101] These differences were explained by various training exercises used. The training of body-builders and especially that of wrestlers involves more submaximal lifting at a higher speed, whereas the training of power-lifters involves high resistance, slow contraction velocity exercises.

In cats a weight-lifting program increased the time to peak tension in fast-twitch muscles.[102]

A program of sprint training shortened the time to peak tension of the rat soleus muscle, but did not alter the contractile properties of the fast-twitch rectus femoris muscle.[103] Treadmill endurance training resulted in a 14% decrease in the time to peak tension of the rat soleus muscle[104] and increased the ability to maintain tetanic tension during a series of fatiguing contractions.[104,105] Various other contractile properties remained without change during endurance training.[105]

MITOCHONDRIA AND OXIDATIVE ENZYMES

Typical for endurance training is an augmented number and volume of mitochondria observed[4,40,43,85,106-109] and an increased activity of oxidative enzymes.[2-5,40,42,48-50,107,110-119] One may add that a training-induced increase in oxidation rate was first reported as early as in 1935.[120] These changes are in association with increased working capacity and endurance.[63,115,116,121] A preferential proliferation of subsarcolemmal mitochondria in comparison with interfibrillar mitochondria was found.[40,41,85,122] The results of endurance training are an increased rate of oxidative phosphorylation evidenced by P/O value of isolated muscle mitochondria[4,108] as well as an increased ATP production rate in skeletal muscles calculated per milligram of mitochondrial proteins or per gram of muscle weight.[4]

Endurance training enhanced the intensity of muscle cell respiration by 53%, pyruvate oxidation by 200%, succinate oxidation by 40%, palmitate oxidation by 120%, ATP production per 1 mg of mitochondrial protein by 30% and per 1 g of muscle weight by 85%.[4] Similar results about training effects on oxidation rate were obtained by K.M. Baldwin et al.[112] In this study the increased rate of pyruvate and palmitate oxidation was recorded in all types of muscle fibers.

Increased activity of enzymes of β-oxidation[85,107,112,114,117,123-125] as well as a general enhancement of oxidative potential of muscle fibers[63,112,115,121,126,127] makes possible an elevated use of lipids during prolonged exercise despite the high level of muscle lactate.[4,114,119] A greater use of fat as a fuel after endurance training seems to be related to a more rapid translocation of the ATP generated during contractions into the mitochondria. The consequence of this is a tighter control over the glycolytic process, thereby creating more favorable conditions for the entry of acetyl units derived from β-oxidation of fatty acids into the citric acid cycle.[127]

Bearing in mind the function of phosphocreatine in energy transport from mitochondria through the mitochondrial membrane into the sarcoplasma,[128,129] it is interesting that endurance training does not enhance the activity of mitochondrial creatine kinase.[130] However, in another study an increase in mitochondrial creatine kinase activity was found as a result of swimming training under an additional weight of 4% b.w. in rats.[131]

When the endurance exercises are sufficiently intense, the increases in mitochondrial enzymes occur somewhat parallel in all fiber types in the muscle.[132] Consequently, glycolytic fibers become 'more oxidative'.[125] This fact is related to the peculiarity in motor units recruitment during prolonged exercise. Endurance exercises at approximately 60% VO_2max are initially performed through involvement of the activity of slow-twitch motor units. As the exercise continues, there is a progressive recruitment of fast-twitch motor units. If exercise is carried out until exhaustion, all of the motor units in the muscle can be utilized.[133,134] However, if the training exercise is moderate in intensity and duration, a difference may be found in the enzyme profile between various types of muscle fibers; for example, the β-hydroxybutyrate dehydrogenase activity increased 2.6-fold in SO and 6-fold in FOG fibers, whereas no changes could be detected in FG fibers.[135] An endurance-training effect on carnitine palmityltransferase activity has been found in slow-twitch but not in fast-twitch fibers of the gastrocnemius muscle.[136]

Training for improved strength usually does not cause a significant change in mitochondria number.[31,35,101,113,137,138] After an intensive weight-training program a significant reduction has been found in mitochondrial volume density and mitochondrial to myofibrillar volume.[20,22,101,137] Due to the increase in total muscle volume, the calculated absolute volume of mitochondria remained constant.[137] Mitochondrial density is reduced also in the muscles of body-builders and power-lifters.[139] In some reports an increased activity of enzymes catalyzing oxidative processes has been reported.[140] However, these findings are not consistent.[14,18,141] Decreased activity of citrate synthase has been found in the vastus lateralis muscle after 6 months of strength training.[94] In a more recent study from the same laboratory, citrate synthase activity changed neither with concentric nor combined eccentric and concentric resistance training regimes.[95] In rats training by high-power exercises caused a small increase in succinate dehydrogenase and cytochrome oxidase activities but not in citrate synthase activity. This kind of training elevated pyruvate but not succinate oxidation in the muscle tissue.[3,4] In endurance trained athletes the O_2 diffusion distance was shorter in the vastus lateralis muscle in comparison with strength trained athletes.[142]

A comprehensive study performed by G. A. Dudley and co-workers[143] on rats used the concentration of cytochrome c as an index of mitochondrial adaptation. Nineteen groups of animals were trained by different programs of treadmill running. In rats running at a speed of 10 to 20 m·min^{-1} (final duration of exercise 30 to 90 min of running) no change in cytochrome c concentration of FG fibers was observed. When the running velocity was 30, 40, 50, or 60 m·min^{-1}, the training effect appeared despite the decrease in final exercise duration to 5 to 25 min (Figure 5-5). In FOG fibers an increased cytochrome c concentration was found at all exercise intensities. The training effect increased with running velocity up to 30 m·min^{-1} and then the effect leveled off at a steady-state level. In SO fibers the training effect was negligible when the running velocity was 10 m·min^{-1}. The effect was highest at a running velocity of 30 or 40 m·min^{-1}. A lower running velocity (20 m·min^{-1}) as well as a higher velocity (50 or 60 m·min^{-1}) gave a less pronounced effect. Likewise, the variable effect found in different types of fibers was related to motor unit recruitment depending on exercise intensity.[143] An important point for rats is the running velocity of 30 m·min^{-1}. By the results of E.R. Shephard and P.D. Gollnick[144] rats use 83% of their maximal oxygen uptake at this running intensity. This percent value seems to be close to their anaerobic threshold. If it is the case, then from the anaerobic threshold onward:

1. Training becomes effective in increasing oxidative potential in FG fibers.
2. The training effect levels off in regard to FOG fibers.
3. A further increase in exercise intensity reduces the training effect in SO fibers.

A linear increase was found in oxidative potential as the duration of training exercise increases.[115] The results presented in Figure 5-6 reveal that an increase in the duration of exercise brings about a greater adaptive response. However, when the running duration was 60 min, a further prolongation of exercise did not enhance the increase in cytochrome c concentration any more.[143] Thus a 'saturation' response was found. An analogous saturation response was detected in the training effect on the activity of succinate dehydrogenase (Figure 5-7). In case of more intensive interval training, 'saturation' was observed at less durable training bouts than in continuous running at moderate velocity.[145]

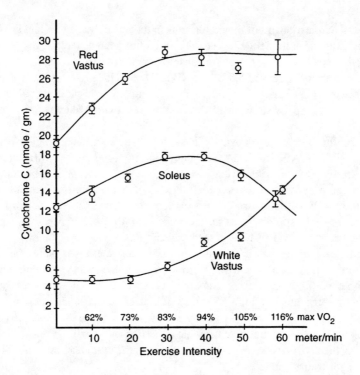

FIGURE 5-5. Influence of exercise intensity on adaptive increase in oxidative capacity in working muscles of rat. On the abscissa the intensity of training exercises is shown as the running velocity (in $m \cdot min^{-1}$) and as the percentage of VO_2max. (From Dudley, G. A., Abram, W. M., and Terjung, R. L., *J. Appl. Physiol.*, 53, 844, 1982. With permission.)

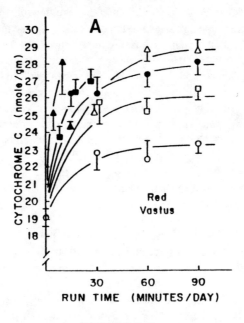

FIGURE 5-6A

FIGURE 5-6. Increase in cytochrome c concentration in FOG (panel A), FG (panel B), and SO (panel C) fibers as a function of duration of training exercises. The exercise intensity is indicated in the following manner: (○) 10 $m \cdot min^{-1}$, (□) 20 $m \cdot min^{-1}$, 30 $m \cdot min^{-1}$, 40 $m \cdot min^{-1}$, 50 $m \cdot min^{-1}$, 60 $m \cdot min^{-1}$ (From Dudley, G. A. Abram, W. M., and Terjung, R. L., *J. Appl. Physiol.*, 53, 844, 1982. With permission.)

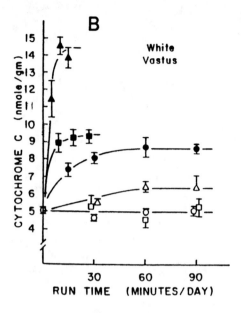

FIGURE 5-6B

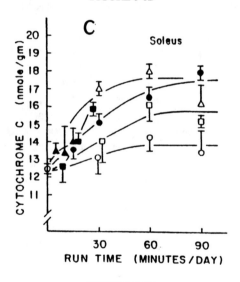

FIGURE 5-6C

It was also found that it is important to employ a training program utilizing an exercise frequency approaching one per day, if a maximal adaptation is sought.[146]

The abbreviated running times in rats obligated when exercise intensity is inordinately high (approximately 100 m·min⁻¹), yield minimal or no mitochondrial changes.[147] Accordingly in man, sprint exercise does not improve the oxidative capacity of muscles. In boys aged 16 to 17 years, a 3-month endurance training resulted in significant increases in VO_2max, SO and FOG fibers area, and succinate dehydrogenase activity in the vastus lateralis muscle. However, none of these changes were found after a 3-month period of sprint training.[148] In previously untrained male persons during 8 weeks of sprint training (30-s spurts repeated over 4-min rest intervals) the succinate dehydrogenase activity remained unchanged.[149]

In the activities of citrate synthase and hydroxyacyl CoA dehydrogenase, significant differences were not found between elite sprint cyclists and nonathletes.[47]

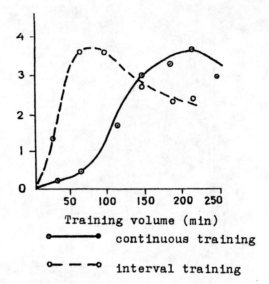

FIGURE 5-7. Changes in succinate dehydrogenase activity in quadriceps muscle of rats in function of the total volume of performed aerobic training (solid line) or interval training (interrupted line). (From Volkov, N. I., *Metabolism and Biochemical Evaluation of Sportsmen's Fitness*, Yakovlev, N. N., Ed., Leningrad Research Institute of Physical Culture, Leningrad, 1974, 213. With permission.)

However, some studies indicate that a modest adaptation of mitochondrial enzymes is not excluded following sprint training.[48,147,150] The possibility of a positive effect of sprint training seems to be related to the intermittent character of sprint exercises when a short period of activity with great power output is followed by a more prolonged recovery period for restoration of the levels of the muscle concentration of high-energy phosphate, furnished from oxidation energy. When performed intermittently, isometric strength training also induces a modest increase in mitochondrial enzymes.[92] However, the effect of sprint training on mitochondrial enzymes is far from the effect of endurance training.

A study of muscle enzymes in track and field athletes showed that the succinate dehydrogenase activity was highest in long- and middle-distance runners. Slightly increased activity was also observed in sprinters but not in field athletes compared to untrained persons.[49]

In rats sprint training produced only modest augmentation of the oxidative pathways. Eleven weeks of such training did not alter the succinate dehydrogenase activity in any of the fiber types.[151] A 16-week period of sprint training increased the fumarase activity in the soleus, the white portion of gastrocnemius, and the plantaris muscles. However, the effect of endurance training was more pronounced.[147]

After 12 weeks of training the succinate dehydrogenase activity was increased in the group continuously running (32 m·min^{-1}, 85% VO$_2$max, 120 min) in the soleus and vastus lateralis profundus, containing SO and FOG fibers, respectively. A less pronounced change occurred in the vastus lateralis superficialis (FOG fibers). In a group undergoing sprint training (10-s dashes at 82 m·min^{-1}, 160% VO$_2$max) the enzyme activity increased only in the vastus lateralis superficialis.[152]

Training by short-term intensive swimming increased the activities of citrate synthetase, succinate dehydrogenase, and cytochrome oxidase, as well as the rate of oxidation of pyruvate, succinate, and palmitate. Comparison with results of training by prolonged continuous swimming revealed that the effect of intensive swimming on oxidative enzymes was two to three times lower than the effect of continuous swimming.[4]

While as a result of aerobic endurance training the activity of oxidative enzymes increases in combination with reduced activities of enzymes for anaerobic processes,[119,153] anaerobic interval training increases the activities of enzymes catalyzing both processes.[153] Greater

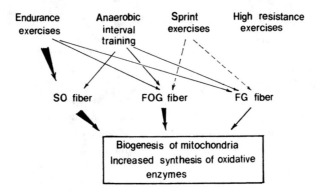

FIGURE 5-8. Exercise-dependent specificity of effect on mitochondrial proliferation and activity of oxidative enzymes.

mitochondrial changes were found following low power compared with high-power interval training programs.[147]

In conclusion, the adjustments on the mitochondrial level are rather common for training connected with a long exercise period of continuous or interrupted muscular activity (Figure 5-8). The most effective seem to be continuous aerobic exercises close to the anaerobic threshold. Interrupted muscular activity becomes an effective tool for mitochondrial improvement when a high intensity of oxidation is necessary during the rest periods between the activity periods. This is the case with interval training. In sprint or strength training, prolonged rest periods are needed to warrant optimal conditions for high force or power output during the next repetition of exercise. Usually, only a part of these prolonged rest periods are necessary for recovery processes requiring a high oxidation rate. It is reasonable to suggest that the mitochondrial adjustments depend (1) on the total time of the persisting high level of oxidation in skeletal muscles, including the time for contractile activity, as well as the time for restitution based on high oxidation rate, and (2) on the oxidation rate during these periods (the closer to the maximum of oxidation rate, the more effective the training).

As a result of endurance training, active muscle starts to produce less lactate despite the same rate of glycogenolysis.[116,125] Partly, at least, it is related to the increased oxidation capacity. Additionally, one must take into consideration that endurance training influences lactate elimination from the blood rather than lactate production.[154]

ENZYMES OF ANAEROBIC PATHWAYS OF ATP RESYNTHESIS

The effect of training on the amount of sarcoplasmic enzymes may be expected because of the essential role of anaerobic pathways of ATP resynthesis in energetics of sports performance in most events. Data were obtained indicating that various kinds of training increase the concentration of sarcoplasmic proteins in skeletal muscles.[3-5]

CREATINE KINASE AND MYOKINASE

The most rapid pathway of ATP resynthesis, the phosphocreatine mechanism, is related to the activity of creatine kinase. It should be expected that sprint training increases the activity of this enzyme. This possibility is supported by the fact that animals adapted to rapid dashes possess a high percent of fast-twitch fibers and very high activities of creatine kinase, myokinase, and glycolytic enzymes in FG fibers.[155] In the studies of N.N. Yakovlev[4,5] an increased activity of creatine kinase was found in rat skeletal muscles both after training with prolonged exercises of moderate intensity and after training with short-term intensive exercises. These results have been partly confirmed. In rats 11 weeks of sprint training resulted in an increased activity of creatine kinase in the soleus but not in the rectus femoris muscle.[103]

Thus, the enzyme activity was stimulated only in SO fibers, which possess a lower activity of the enzyme than other fiber types.[130] However, in another study no changes were found in SO, FOG, and FG fibers as a result of sprint training.[152] No changes were found as a result of daily prolonged exercises of moderate intensity either.[130,152] Both creatine kinase and myokinase activities remained constant after daily exercise of high intensity.[89]

In humans sprint training did not change the activity of muscle creatine kinase.[150] When fast maximal contractions were repeated 5 to 8 times with brief rest intervals, creatine kinase and myokinase activities in muscle increased.[92] Another program of strength training either did not cause these changes[156] or a small increase in myokinase was observed.[157]

Changes were found in creatine kinase isozymes in humans. The results of a study showed that a program of endurance training did not affect the total activity of the enzyme in the soleus and extensor digitorum longus muscles, but resulted in an increased creatine kinase MB isozyme content of muscle.[158] In SO fibers of endurance-trained athletes an increased creatine kinase MB isozyme content was detected.[159,160]

GLYCOLYTIC ENZYMES

In exercises of submaximal power output lasting more than 30 s and less than 5 min, anaerobic glycogenolysis becomes critical for ATP resynthesis. Correspondingly, adaptive changes in enzymes of glycogenolysis are expected in the first order in training for improvement of sports performance in corresponding competitive exercises.

In the practice of sports training the main tool for improvement of anaerobic working capacity is interval training (highly intensive exercises are repeated over rest intervals too short for elimination of accumulated lactate and for prevention of summation from bout to bout of the consequences of anaerobic energy processes in the internal environment of the organism). The influence of systematical use of interval training involves both aerobic and anaerobic enzymes. The effect of interval training on enzymes of aerobic processes was discussed earlier. It was pointed out that in case of interval training the effect on aerobic and anaerobic enzymes is unidirectional. In a number of studies the enzymatic adaptation of glycogenolysis by interval training has been documented.[119,153,161,162]

After a 5-week period of interval training (8 × 200-m runs at 90% of maximal speed, 2-min rest intervals) significant increases were found in the activities of phosphorylase, phosphofructokinase, glyceraldehyde phosphate dehydrogenase, lactate dehydrogenase, and malate dehydrogenase.[162] During 9 weeks of interval training the phosphofructokinase activity increased in the soleus muscle, first decreased and then normalized in the red part of the vastus lateralis muscle, and did not change in the white part of the vastus lateralis muscle.[163]

Interval training models used in rats gave various results. When only two 45-s running bouts (final running speed 80 m·min^{-1}) were performed twice daily during 3 weeks, 24 h after the last exercise session the activity of triosephosphate dehydrogenase was increased in the soleus but not in the rectus femoris muscle. Activities of physphorylase and lactate dehydrogenase changed in neither muscle.[103] When training consisted of 18 alternate periods of 30 s of running (the running speed attained during the 11th week was 80 m·min^{-1}) and 30 s of rest, the activities of phosphorylase, phosphofructokinase, and pyruvate kinase remained unchanged in FOG and FG fibers. In SO fibers the phosphorylase and pyruvate activities increased.[151] In a study, systematical repetition of short-term intensive exercises caused elevated phosphofructokinase activity in both FG and FOG but not in SO fibers.[152]

Training with the aid of repeated 4-min swims with additonal load increased phosphorylase activity by 40% (continuous swimming by 28%), hexokinase by 25% (continuous swimming by 35%), pyruvate kinase by 20% (continuous swimming by 10%), phosphofructokinase by 30%, and aldolase by 27% (continuous swimming was ineffective in regard to both these enzymes).[3,4]

Less variable was the effect of sprint training, which differs from interval training by (1) less durable exercises (10 to 20 s dashes), (2) almost the highest exercise intensity, and (3) more prolonged rest intervals between repetitions. In humans 6 to 12 weeks of sprint training resulted in an increase in phosphofructokinase activity,[148-150] and the increase in phosphorylase activity was insignificant.[149] In rats sprint training increased the phosphofructokinase activity in FOG and FG but not in SO fibers. The activity of lactate dehydrogenase did not alter,[152] and the hexokinase activity increased.[151] Continuous running with periodic sprints increased the activities of phosphofructokinase, pyruvate kinase, and α-glycerophosphate in the soleus muscle and decreased the activities of these enzymes as well as phosphorylase in the red portion of the quadriceps muscle. The activities of these enzymes remained unchanged in the white portion of the quadriceps. Hexokinase activity increased in all muscles. Lactate dehydrogenase activity did not change in the soleus but was lowered in both parts of the quadriceps muscle.[164]

Endurance training with continuous exercises did not change the phosphofructokinase activity in slow-twitch fibers, but decreased the activity in fast-twitch fibers.[136] In another study the phosphofructokinase activity did not change and lactate dehydrogenase activity decreased in all types of muscle fibers.[152] Small but significant reductions in lactate dehydrogenase activities of the soleus and white portion of the gastrocnemius muscle were reported after both sprint and endurance training.[147] An increase in the hexokinase activity with endurance and sprint training was confirmed in rats[3,4,103] and guinea pigs.[165]

As a result of sprint training the activity of lactate dehydrogenase increased in association with augmentation of the M_4 isozyme content in horses.[166] In humans an augmentation[167] or a lack of alteration in the total activity of lactate dehydrogenase was found after sprint training.[63] However, sprinters and jumpers usually have elevated activity of the enzyme.[49] Their muscles contain a relatively high percent of LDH_{4-5} whereas muscles from endurance athletes are high in LDH_{1-2}.[168] A marathon training induced increased activity of LDH_{1-2} and decreased activity of LDH_{3-5}.[169]

No significant changes were found in phosphorylase, phosphofructokinase, aldolase, or pyruvate kinase in the quadriceps muscle after one-leg endurance training.[170] In contrast, a more strenuous program of training resulted in a greater than twofold increase in phosphofructokinase activity of the same muscle.[42] Also, in swimmers of 11 to 13 years an intensive training increased the enzyme activity.[171]

Strength training usually does not produce alterations in the activity of phosphorylase, phosphofructokinase, or lactate dehydrogenase.[35] However, when the resistance was lowered and the exercise extended to 30 s, there was an elevation in phosphorylase and phosphofructokinase activities but lactate dehydrogenase was unchanged. Shot-putters, weight-lifters, and discus throwers have phosphorylase, phosphofructokinase, and lactate dehydrogenase activities well within the range of sedentary subjects,[49] whereas sprinters, jumpers, and runners of 400 to 800 m usually have elevated levels of these enzymes.[49] However, the enzyme activity was not higher in qualified competitive cyclists, distance runners, and swimmers than in sedentary persons.[113]

The variability of results of training effects on glycogenolytic enzymes is likely related to the strain in the glycolytic process during the training exercise used. However, a pronounced variability was also present in the results of anaerobic interval training. Consequently, there must be other sources of variability. Nevertheless, even in case of interval training the exercises used might not be severe enough to stress the glycolytic pathway. This seems to be rather likely in case of experiments on rats.[63] On the other hand, the results are influenced by the time at which the tissue samples were obtained after the final training session, since the turnover rate of the glycolytic enzymes lies between about 1.5 h and a few days.[172] Therefore, a principal question arises: does the adaptation of glycolytic enzymes signify an increased number of enzyme molecules or an enhanced sensitivity of rapidly renewing enzymes to regulatory influences? The latter possibility is underlined by the following results.

In rats phosphofructokinase activity decreased as a result of a 10-week period of interval or continuous aerobic training both in SO and FG fibers. Sprint training also caused this

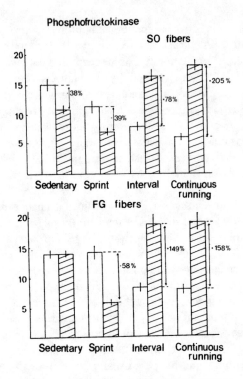

FIGURE 5-9. Effects of sprint, interval, or continuous running (see Figure 5-4) on phosphofructokinase activity in the resting state and after a 4-min test running at 60 m·min^{-1} in rats.[83] Phosphofructokinase activity is evaluated by the change in optical density during 30 s periods per 1 g protein (mean ± SEM).

change in SO but not in FG fibers. Since 48 h passed after the final training session before muscle samples were obtained, the time elapsed was enough to suggest that a rapid enzyme turnover eliminated the increased enzyme activity. However, an important result of this study was the fact that 4 min of intensive running (at 60 m·min^{-1}) changed the muscle phosphofructokinase activity differently, depending on the training regimen used. In untrained control rats the test exercise induced a decrease in the enzyme activity in the oxidative muscle. In glycolytic muscle the activity did not change. Instead a two- or threefold increase was found in muscles of rats trained by either interval or continuous running (Figure 5-9). After test exercise the enzyme activity was not only over the resting levels in these trained rats but also over the resting levels in sedentary control rats. The effect of sprint training was different. The effect of the test exercise was to decrease muscle enzyme activities in both types of fibers, but in SO fibers the change was greater than in the control group.[83]

Phosphofructokinase activity is controlled by AMP, ADP, ATP, citrate, ammonium, and fructose biphosphate.[173] The enzyme is also sensitive to decrease in pH.[174] The enzyme concentration itself may also modulate the activity: a cell with a high concentration of the enzyme will exhibit a higher activity than could be expected from the simple linear relationship between enzyme concentration and activity.[175] It may be speculated that training-induced increase in the enzyme concentration sensitizes the enzyme activity to stimulatory factors. This explanation implies that the enzyme sensitivity to inhibitory factors is also increased. Thus, despite the elevated number of enzyme molecules, the activity was reduced in resting conditions. Final conclusion of the obtained results points to an enhanced effectiveness of the regulation of phosphofructokinase activity in the organism trained by interval or continuous exercises.

E.A. Newsholme[176] assumes that one important factor in improving the sensitivity of the control of enzymes that catalyze nonequilibrium reaction (phosphorylase, 6-phosphofructokinase, pyruvate kinase) is the operation of substrate cycles between glycogen and glucose-phosphate, phosphoenolpyruvate and pyruvate, and fructose-6-phosphate and fructose biphosphate. The role of the cycle between 6-phosphate and fructose biphosphate is considered to be in the increase of the sensitivity of metabolic control at the level of fructose-6-phosphate phosphorylation to changes in the concentrations of the regulators of 6-phosphofructokinase. Evidence has been obtained that the rate of this cycle can be increased by catecholamines.[177] Further, the increase in ATP hydrolysis rate will lead to decreases in the concentrations of creatine phosphate, ATP, and citrate, and to increases in the concentrations of AMP, phosphate, and NH^{+4}. This in turn will increase the activity of phosphofructokinase towards its maximum. E.A. Newsholme[176] believes that one reason for the remarkable performance of elite sportsmen is the fact that their metabolic control mechanisms are so well developed that they provide maximum sensitivity when required in the control of energy-producing pathways in muscle.

The increased sensitivity of the metabolic control mechanism may be related to (1) increased catecholamine response to supramaximal exercise (see p. 32), (2) increased sensitivity of muscle tissue to catecholamine action connected with the exaggerated increase in the activity of adenylate cyclase after adrenaline administration,[178] and (3) a possible increase of the number of enzyme molecules.

The specific adaptation to anaerobic exercises may concern the formation of isozymes less sensitive to a lowered pH value. However, this question has only been investigated in regard to hexokinase in one study.[179] An interval training program (training sessions caused an increase in the blood lactate concentration up to 18 to 22 mmol·l⁻¹ and a decrease in the blood pH to 6.98 to 6.90) resulted in an increase in hexokinase activity in the medium pH range of 8.0 to 6.5. This change was found in both SO and FG fibers as well as in the brain tissue. In FG fibers the enzyme activity increased most of all at pH 6.5. After training with continuous aerobic exercises the increase in the enzyme activity was also found at various medium pH, but at pH 6.5 predominanting increase was not observed. In association with these events, an augmentation of muscle type II hexokinase occurred in muscles and the brain tissue.[179]

BUFFER CAPACITY

Since the possibilities of anaerobic glycolysis will be utilized during supramaximal exercises, training should increase the buffer capacity of skeletal muscles and the blood. Actually, this is a typical result of anaerobic interval training as well as sprint training.[180] The buffer capacity is a contributing factor of enhanced anaerobic performance capacity.[181]

Assessing the buffer capacities of the blood by Van Slyke's method it was found that a 2-month period of interval training or repeated uphill runs resulted in a pronounced increase in 'reserve alkali'. Two months of continuous aerobic running were ineffective, but 2 months of sprint training was effective in this respect.[182] In previously untrained male persons 8 weeks of sprint training (30-s sprints repeated over 4-min rest intervals) increased muscle buffer capacity calculated from the changes in lactate concentrations and pH of the vastus lateralis during incremental exercise. The same period of endurance training by continuous aerobic cycling did not change the buffer capacity.[149] Accordingly, runners of 800 m had significantly higher muscle buffer capacity than untrained persons or marathon runners. No difference was found in buffer capacity between marathon runners and untrained persons.[183] A difference was found in the ability of blood to buffer lactate during exercise in endurance-trained and untrained subjects.[184]

In accordance with the above-presented results, increased muscle buffer capacity was detected in sprinters and rowers but not in marathon runners. The buffer capacity was significantly related to carnosine concentration in the vastus lateralis muscle. Both indices were also related to the results of the anaerobic speed test as well as with the percent of fast-twitch fibers.[185] These results indicate that within the human skeletal muscle, carnosine levels may be related to the glycolytic capacity of the muscle, substantially contributing to buffer capacity.

A comparison of buffer capacity in vertebrates' muscles confirms a correlation with the potential for ATP resynthesis by anaerobic glycolysis.[186] It is assumed that in the muscle tissue of vertebrates the main role of intracellular buffer belongs to indisol groups of histidine.[155] The proteins-bound histidyl residues, histidine-containing dipeptides, and free histidine are considered the most important buffers within the skeletal muscle.[187] In mammal muscles approximately half of the total histidine is in proteins, and the remainder is bound by dipeptides as carnosine, anserine, or optidine.[155] In this connection the adaptive synthesis of histidine-rich proteins as well as the metabolism of carnosine and other related dipeptides may contribute to specific adaptation to anaerobic exercises.

ANAEROBIC WORKING CAPACITY

Anaerobic working capacity is the ability to perform highly intensive exercises using anaerobic processes for ATP resynthesis. Anaerobic working capacity implies (1) the highest possible power output during a certain time, and (2) the prevalence of anaerobic production of energy (resynthesis of ATP). The time factor discriminates the application of the anaerobic working capacity into three purposes: (1) energy attaining of the maximal power output during exercises lasting up to 10 to 20 s, (2) energy attaining of the submaximal power output during exercises lasting more than 20 to 30 s and less than 5 min, (3) energy attaining of great power output during exercises lasting from 5 to 30 min.

Accordingly, the first purpose of anaerobic working capacity concerns sprint exercises. In this case, anaerobic working capacity may be understood as the sprinting or sprinters' capacity. ATP resynthesis has to be at the highest rate. This is provided by degradation of phosphocreatine. Due to the limited amount of phosphocreatine in muscles, the phosphocreatine mechanism of ATP resynthesis has to be complemented by anaerobic glycogenolysis. Therefore, the biochemical foundation for sprint performance consists in the phosphocreatine store and the activity of creatine kinase. It was mentioned earlier that animals adapted to rapid dashes possess a high activity of creatine kinase. However, a training experiment did not provide unanimous evidence of the increase of the creatine kinase activity as a result of sprint training. Obviously, more important is the utilization of the highest rate of ATP resynthesis for actualization of contractions ensuring a high level of power output. Accordingly, highly significant are the excitation-contraction mechanism, membrane functions including the possibilities of the Na,K-pump, function of the SR, the rate of cross-bridge formation, and the rate of ATP hydrolysis. Of course, the essential precondition for all of these is a high percent of FG fibers.

The second purpose of anaerobic working capacity needs anaerobic glycogenolysis and glycolysis. Frequently, the term 'anaerobic working capacity' is used in the sense of realization of the anaerobic working capacity for performance of exercises using anaerobic glycogenolysis as prevalent. The difference between the second and third purposes consists mainly in the ratio between contributions of anaerobic glycogenolysis and oxidative phosphorylation in ATP resynthesis. In exercises lasting from 30 s to 5 min, prevalence belongs to anaerobic glycolysis, and in exercises of 5 to 30 min it belongs to oxidative phosphorylation.

In both groups of exercises the contribution of anaerobic glycogenolysis is quantitatively related to the accumulation of lactate in the working muscles and blood. As was discussed on p. 87, lactate accumulation is not a precise quantitative estimate of the contribution of anaerobic glycogenolysis in energy attaining of exercising muscles, but at least semiquantitatively it sufficiently characterizes anaerobic working capacity. Therefore, the specific nature of training actions on anaerobic working capacity may be studied using lactate accumulation during short-term anaerobic (supramaximal) exercise.

In humans, 8 weeks of sprint training increased the accumulation of lactate in muscles and noradrenaline in the blood plasma during test exercise at 110% VO_2max.[188] Sprint training in running increased the blood lactate response in the Wingate test.[150] Enhanced lactate response was also observed after sprint training in swimming.[189] In top athletes, lactate concentrations

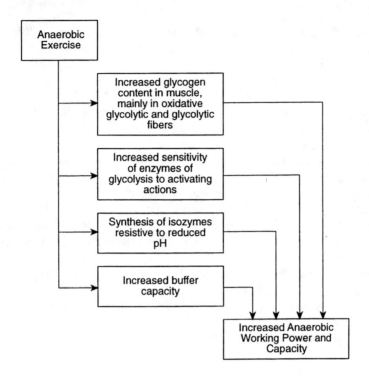

FIGURE 5-10. Adaptation to anaerobic exercise.

of up to 25 mmol·l⁻¹ in the blood and 30 to 35 mmol·kg⁻¹ in the muscle tissue were recorded at the finish of 400- and 800-m races. At the same time, pH was 6.9 (in some cases 6.8) in the blood and 6.4 in the muscle tissue.[190]

Training experiments on rats have shown that a 4-min intensive run (60 m·min⁻¹) caused in interval trained rats a less pronounced lactate acccumulation in FG fibers, and in rats trained with short-term dashes or continuous running, a more pronounced one than in control rats. In SO fibers an elevated lactate accumulation was revealed only in sprint-trained rats.[83] These results obviously emphasize the significance of improved lactate elimination in lactate response to exercise.

The increase in anaerobic working capacity as a result of using concerned exercises is summarized in Figure 5-10.

INTRAMUSCULAR ENERGY STORES AND MYOGLOBIN

ATP

There is no convincing evidence that training increases the ATP store in muscles. No changes were detected in rat muscles with either endurance or strength training.[3,4] A mild increase in ATP concentration has been reported in the limb muscles of adolescent[171] and adult[191-193] males after a program of endurance training. However, these reports seem to describe the initial effect of training.

PHOSPHOCREATINE

There are old evidences that training elevates the phosphocreatine content in skeletal muscles.[194,195] Rats trained by repeated short-term intensive exercise increased the phosphocreatine content in skeletal muscles, but the effect of continuous exercise was only modest.[3,4] Some of the human biopsy studies confirm the increase in muscle phosphocreatine.[171,191-193] However, an increased phosphocreatine store is not considered a common result of training.[63]

It was suggested that in humans an increased amount of phosphocreatine will be achieved by a moderate hypertrophy without any change in the substrate concentrations. It was considered a second way for the increased total amount of energy for fast contractile activity.[155]

GLYCOGEN

The training effect on muscle glycogen store has been known since 1927.[196] In rats no difference was found between training with continuous exercises and interval training, but the effect of high-power exercises was less pronounced.[3,4] In one study no effect of sprint training on the glycogen content of any of the fiber types was found.[151] A comparison of various kinds of training effects confirmed that sprint training does not alter the glycogen store of either SO or FG fibers. Aerobic training with continuous running or swimming was highly effective. In SO fibers these effects were more pronounced than the response to interval or strength training. In FG fibers all the training variants produced approximately the same changes. Also, in this study glycogen compartmentalized to the SR was detected. It increased as a result of all the training variants used, including sprint training, which was otherwise ineffective in regard to inducing a total glycogen increase. The largest increase in glycogen compartmentalized to the SR resulted from interval training in both SO abd FG fibers.[83]

In humans a higher value of muscle glycogen stores in trained than in sedentary individuals has been demonstrated repeatedly since the first biopsy studies.[197,198] Both longitudinal and cross-sectional studies indicate that subjects undergoing strength-, sprint-, or endurance-training programs possess a larger store of muscle glycogen than untrained persons or the same person before training.[42,192,193] The augmentation of glycogen stores may be related to the increase in glycogen synthase activity in trained muscles.[199-200]

TRIGLYCERIDES

In humans an increase in the triglyceride content of the quadriceps muscle was detected after endurance training.[203] This change was not confirmed in a one-leg training experiment.[204] In rats a reduced triglyceride content was observed in both the white and red parts of the gastrocnemius muscle after training.[205]

MYOGLOBIN

This protein increases the rate of O_2 diffusion in muscles through the cytoplasma to the mitochondria.[116] Endurance training increased the concentration of myoglobin in skeletal muscles of rats.[3,4,146,206,107] Analogous results were obtained with speed and power training.[3,4] In contrast, biopsy studies did not demonstrate an increased myoglobin content in endurance-trained humans.[208,209] Six weeks of sprint training decreased the intramuscular myoglobin content in human muscles.[150]

MUSCLE CAPILLARIZATION

An endurance training-induced increase in capillary densities was detected in animal muscles during 1934 to 1936.[210,211] Later it was shown that the human skeletal muscle also adapts to increased use by increasing the number of capillaries.[61,210-216] This effect of endurance training becomes apparent in regard to increases of capillaries per fiber, capillaries per square millimeter, or number of capillaries found around a fiber.[63] Soccer players, as compared with untrained persons, also possess a significantly greater mean number of capillaries surrounding each fiber.[217] The number of capillaries per fiber in trained muscle is closely linked to the whole body maximal oxygen uptake of a subject.[63,218] If during exercise all fiber types are involved, both the number of capillaries around the various fiber types and the size of the fibers are increased.[216,219] The increase in capillaries is larger than the increase in the fiber area each capillary has to supply.[63]

Endurance training induces an increased number of capillaries in animal skeletal muscles,[220,221] mainly around slow, not fast, fibers.[222] In experiments of chronic stimulation of muscles it was found that capillaries begin to proliferate before changes can be noted in the oxidative enzymes.[223,224] A close coupling is assumed between the number of capillaries and the capacity for oxidative metabolism of the fibers they supply.[223,224]

Heavy resistance training does not change capillarity.[22] Olympic weight-lifters and power-lifters display lower capillary density than untrained subjects, whereas the number of capillaries per fiber of m. vastus lateralis was equal in these athletes and nonathletes.[225] The increased muscle capillarity seems to be a specific phenomenon characteristic of endurance training.[226]

There is undoubtedly a true proliferation of capillaries associated with prolonged muscular activity. The adaptation occurs in the exercised muscle and only around fibers that are recruited in the training schedule.[220]

Hypoxia is known to increase the growth rate of cultured vascular cells. Therefore it was suggested that hypoxia may play a role in blood vessel growth *in vivo*.[227] However, in motorically highly active Japanese waltzing mice, a 2-week period in lowered atmospheric pressure (approximately 3000 m altitude) gave no evidence of the development of new capillaries. The capillaries became tortuous and many capillary cross-bridges were developed, hence enlarging the endothelial surface.[228] On the basis of these results it was suggested that higher capillary counts on cross sections are mostly derived from the altered capillary pattern but not actually from new capillaries.[228] This situation will not occur in endurance training, at least in rats. After 4 weeks of endurance training the number of capillaries per muscle fiber increased by 30% in association with an increased citrate synthase activity in the soleus muscle. Capillary tortuosity was not affected by endurance training.[229]

Against the significance of hypoxia in increased capillarization of active muscles speak the results of an investigation of permanent high-altitude residents (3700 m). When the high-altitude residents were divided into physically active and inactive groups, the first group had a higher number of capillaries per fiber, similar to the results found in sea-level residents.[230]

In rats a 13- to 17-week period of endurance training increased the total blood flow in hind limb vessels by 50%. The highest was the increase in the blood flow of the red part of the gastrocnemius muscle (up to 200%). Maximal capillary infusion was in trained rats 70% higher than in untrained ones. Thus, endurance training warrants a total increase in vascular transport capacity and mainly in muscles of high oxidative potential.[231]

FIBER TYPE TRANSFORMATION PROBLEM

Fast- and slow-twitch fibers can be distinguished by their specific myosin light chain patterns.[232] Both 'fast' and 'slow' myosin were found in fast- as well as in slow-twitch fibers, but in different ratios.[233] Changes of these ratios are not excluded in training. However, there are limited possibilities for this.[155]

In guinea pigs 30 days of treadmill running influenced the specific myosin light chain pattern and probably also the myosin isoenzymes content. While running at 0.7 m·s⁻¹ on a 5° slope decreased the DTNB light chains and increased the A2 light chains both in m. psöas major and m. vastus lateralis, running at 0.4 m·s⁻¹ on a 45° slope caused an increase in the DTNB light chains and a decrease in the A2 light chains.[234]

Under appropriate conditions muscle fibers are mutable indeed.[63] Perhaps the first of these situations occurs during maturation after birth. Data obtained indicate the change of slow- to fast-twitch fibers during the early postnatal period.[235] Fiber type transformation is possible with cross-innervation[236] and specific electrical stimulation.[237,238]

Chronically increased contractile activity by low-frequency stimulation induces a transformation of fast- into slow-twitch muscle fibers in the rabbit. Early changes in enzyme activities and isozymes of energy metabolism result in a 'white-to-red' metabolic transformation. Simultaneously, cytosolic Ca^{2+} binding and Ca^{2+} sequestering are reduced by a decrease in paralbumin and a transformation of the sarcoplasmic reticulum membranes. The fast-to-slow transformation is completed by an exchange of fast- with slow-type myosin isoforms. Changes in total RNA and qualitative and quantitative alterations in translatable mRNA indicate that the various transitions result from altered translational and transcriptional activities.[238] The phenotype of a muscle fiber thus appears to be dynamic and is modified according to the actual functional demands.[238-240] More recent studies have confirmed that endurance training can change the isomyosin pattern in fast- and slow-twitch muscles[241] and in the diaphragm[242] and thereby alter the myosin phenotype of muscle fiber.

Results were obtained indicating that training may also produce changes similar to fiber type transformation. In prolonged endurance training a transformation of type IIc fibers into type I fibers[243] and type IIb fibers into type IIa fibers [244] was suggested. A 50-day program of skiing induced a reduction of the total population of IIa and IIb fibers that was partly compensated for by an increase in the IIc fiber population.[124] When the intensity of endurance exercises was over the anaerobic threshold, the training result was a decrease in type I fibers accommodated by an increase in type IIc fibers.[243] A study of skiers demonstrated the coexistence of slow and fast isoforms of myosin and troposin in various types of muscle fibers.[245] According to the obtained results, it was suggested that in endurance training the following fiber type transformations may exist: IIa $\rightarrow$ IIc$\rightarrow$ I. Anaerobic interval training during a 15-week period also increased the percent of type I fibers (from 41 to 47%). The percent of type IIb decreased from 17 to 12%, and the percent of type IIa did not change in the vastus lateralis muscle.[246] The endurance training-induced increase in myofibrillar ATPase intermediate fibers was confirmed in another paper.[247]

With sprint or strength training, changes in different fiber types are mainly restricted to alterations in the myofibrillar to mitochondrial volume ratio.[138] Nevertheless, data were obtained about an increase in fast-twitch fibers,[248] mainly type IIa fibers,[150] as a result of sprint training. After 16 weeks of isokinetic training the percent of fast-twitch fibers decreased when one training session consisted in 5 sets of 5 repetitions, while in the case of 15 sets of 10 repetitions no changes were revealed.[249]

In contrast, 6 months of bicycle exercises did not alter the percent of fast- and slow-twitch fiber despite the doubling of the oxidative potential of the studied vastus lateralis muscle.[42] Differences in the percent of fast- or slow-twitch fibers were not found after endurance or sprint training practice with one leg either.[48] In the distribution of type I, IIa, and IIb fibers, no change was found in the same muscle after endurance training of 6 months.[250]

In rats no changes were detected in a population of various types of fibers in the gastrocnemius muscle after either an endurance or sprint training program.[251] This result was not confirmed in another study. After 18 weeks of endurance training the percent of type I and type IIa fibers increased and the percent of type IIb fibers decreased in the plantaris and extensor digitorum longus muscle. In the deep portion of the vastus lateralis a pronounced increase from 10 to 27% in type I fibers occurred. A rise in slow type myosin light chains accompanied the histochemically observed fiber type transition in the deep vastus lateralis muscle. Changes in peptide pattern of the SR occurred both in the deep and superficial portion of the vastus lateralis muscle, suggesting a complete transition from type IIb to IIa in the superficial portion and from type IIa to I in the deep portion. A complete type IIa transition to type I in the deep vastus lateralis muscle was also suggested by the failure to detect parvalbumin in this muscle after 15 weeks of training. Changes in the parvalbumin content and in the SR tended to precede the transition in myosin light chains. It was concluded that high-intensity endurance training is capable of transforming specific characteristics of muscle fibers beyond the commonly observed changes in the enzyme activity pattern of energy metabolism.[252] The fiber type-specific transition in the enzyme activity pattern by this kind of training was previously established in a study of this group.[253]

In 3-week-old rats during 8 weeks following heavy resistance training, the type I fiber population decreased significantly and fiber IIb population insignificantly in the deep vastus lateralis muscle. In the superficial portion of the muscle the ratio between type IIa and IIb fibers did not change.[254]

Presently, it seems correct to assume that under certain appropriate conditions, an influence on the muscle cell genetic apparatus might be born by training, resulting in switching of muscle fibers from one subgroup to another.

CONCLUSION

In skeletal muscles, the main manifestations of various forms and regimens of training are

- Myofibrillar hypertrophy
- Adaptation of myofibrillar ATPase
- Increased possibilities of the SR
- Improved function of Na,K-pumps
- Increased activity of glycolytic enzymes or alterations of their susceptibility to activators and inhibitors
- Increased volume density of mitochondria and activity of oxidative enzymes
- Augmented capillarization
- Increased energy stores

Resistance to muscle conraction is the main factor stimulating myofibrillar hypertrophy. Repeated strong contractions (heavy resistance exercises) are necessary for actualization of this change.

Continuous exercises of moderate intensity stimulate increases in the volume density of mitochondria, activity of oxidative enzymes, and capillarization. However, these alterations also appear in interrupted exercises of rather high intensity. Therefore, the most essential condition is a prolonged period of a high rate of oxidation. It may be warranted by a prolonged continuous exercise, but also by interrupted exercises if a high rate of oxidation persists during rest periods between exercise bouts. However, a question remains whether there exists a limit for exercise intensity, bearing in mind the possibility that exaggerated accumulation of lactate and proteins may suppress oxidation.

Adaptation of myofibrillar ATPase means, first of all, an increased activity of the enzyme. It is a typical result of strength or speed training. This change is less pronounced in endurance training. In this case a possibility for decreased enzyme activity arises. While the increased myofibrillar ATPase activity is necessary for rapid and augmented transfer of chemical energy to mechanical energy, the decreased activity of myofibrillar ATPase enables economizing the utilization of the produced energy. Further studies are necessary in regard to this aspect.

Possibilities for both rapid sequestering and rapid reaccumulation of calcium ions are essential conditions in performance of sprint or power exercises. The velocity of muscle contraction as well as the necessity to form a high number of cross-bridges in a short time have to be the factors stimulating the improvement of the function of the SR. Less effective are heavy resistance exercises. Endurance exercises may even exhibit an opposite effect. Again a question arises whether the latter is related to the sparing effect of endurance training.

Evidence has been obtained on the improved functions of Na,K-pumps in trained muscles. However, further detailed studies are necessary to specify the dependence of the improved Na,K-pump functions on the exercises used.

The stimulus for adaptation at the level of glycolytic enzymes is provided by exercises founded on a high rate of anaerobic glycogenolysis. However, the life span of glycolytic enzymes is rather short. Therefore, the increased activity of these enzymes, resulting from corresponding exercise, may persist only for some days. Recently, a possibility was indicated that anaerobic exercises may elevate the susceptibility of glycolytic enzymes to their activators and inhibitors, or induce a synthesis of isozymes resistive to low pH. This possibility needs further confirmation and specification.

The training effect on intramuscular energy stores is the most pronounced in regard to glycogen content. Endurance exercises seem to be more effective than sprint or strength exercises. However, the differences are not always convincing. Results are not unanimous in regard to increased phosphocreatine content. One may suggest that sprint exercises have to be the most effective in regard to augmentation of the phosphocreatine store. Up to now, this has not been convincingly evidenced. The increase of the ATP store is doubtful. Besides the function of energy donor, ATP possesses an essential role in control of intracellular metabolism. The increased ATP content would mean decreased possibilities for mobilization of cellular resources during exercise performance.

All these training manifestations are dependent on the type of muscle fibers. Some of them are favorable in FG and others in SO fibers. This dependence is founded on the differences in recruiting various motor units and, thereby, fibers of various types. The increase in force application or intensity of performance makes it necessary to recruit more motor units. In heavy resistance as well as highly intensive exercises, the recruiting of motor units is close to maximal. Thereby, the training effects of these exercises are less specific in regard to the influence on muscle fibers of various types.

REFERENCES

1. **Yakovlev, N.N.**, Biochemical foundations of muscle training, *Usp. Sovrem. Biol.*(Moscow), 27, 257, 1949 (in Russian).
2. **Yakovlev, N.N.**, Problem of biochemical adaptation of muscles in dependence on the character of their activity, *Zh. Obshch. Biol.*, 19, 417, 1958 (in Russian).
3. **Yakovlev, N.N.**, Biochemical mechanisms of adaptation of skeletal muscles to muscular activity, *Ukr. Biokhim. Zh.*, 48, 388, 1976 (in Russian).
4. **Yakovlev, N.N.**, *Sportbiochemie*, Barth, Leipzig, 1977.
5. **Yakovlev, N.N.**, Biochemische and Morphologishe Veränderungen der Muskelfasern in Abhängigkeit von der Art des Training, *Med. Sport*, 18, 161, 1978.
6. **Morpurgo, B.**, Ueber Activitatis-Hypertrophie der willkürlichen Muskeln, *Virchows Arch. Pathol. Anat.*, 150, 522, 1897.
7. **Hettinger, F.**, *Physiology of Strength*, Charles C. Thomas, Springfield, 1961.
8. **Hollmann, W., and Hettinger, T.**, *Sportmedizin — Arbeits and Trainingsgrundlagen*, F.K. Schattauer, Stuttgart, 1976.
9. **Booth, F.W.**,Perspectives on molecular and cellular exercise physiology, *J. Appl. Physiol.*, 65, 1461, 1988.
10. **Pipes, T.V.**, Physiologic characteristic of elite bodybuilders, *Physician Sportmed.*, 7, 116, 1979.
11. **Katch, V.L., Katch, F.I., Moffatt, R., and Gittlesen, M.**, Muscular development and lean body weight in body builders and weight lifters, *Med. Sci. Sports Exerc.*, 12, 240, 1980.
12. **Häkkinen, K., Alén M., and Komi, P.V.**, Neuromuscular, anaerobic, and aerobic performance characteristics of elite power athletes, *Eur. J. Appl. Physiol.*, 53, 97, 1984.
13. **Tesch, P.A., and Larsson, L.**, Muscle hypertrophy in bodybuilders, *Eur. J. Appl. Physiol.*, 49, 301, 1982.
14. **Prince, E.P., Hikida, R.S., and Hagerman, F.C.**, Human muscle fiber types in power lifters, distance runners and untrained subjects, *Pflügers Arch. ges. Physiol.*, 363, 19, 1976.
15. **Thorstensson, A., Hulrén, B., von Döblen W., and Karlsson, J.**, Effect of strength training on enzyme activities and fibre characteristics in human skeletal muscle, *Acta Physiol. Scand.*, 96, 392, 1976.
16. **Dons, B., Bollerup. K., Bonde-Peterson, F., and Hancke, S.**, The effect of weight-lifting exercises related to muscle fiber composition and muscle cross-sectional area in humans, *Eur. J. Appl. Physiol.*, 40, 95, 1978.

17. **Häggmark, T., Jansson, E., and Svane, B.,** Cross-sectional area of the thigh muscle in man measured by computed tomography, *Scand. J. Clin. Lab. Invest.,* 38, 355, 1978.
18. **Häkkinen, K., Komi, P.V., and Tesch, P.A.,** Effect of combined concentric and eccentric strength training and detraining on force-time, muscle fiber and metabolic characteristics of leg extensor muscles, *Scand. J. Sports Sci.,* 3, 50, 1981.
19. **Young, A., Stokes, M., Round, J.M., and Edwards R.H.T.,** The effect of high-resistance training on the strength and cross-sectional area of the human quadriceps, *Eur. J. Clin. Invest.,* 13, 411, 1983.
20. **MacDoughall, J.D., Elder, G.C.B., Sale, D.G., Moroz, J.R., and Sutton, J.R.,** Effects of strength training and immobilization on human muscle fibers, *Eur. J. Appl. Physiol.,* 43, 25, 1980.
21. **Yakovleva, E.S.,** Micromorphological changes in skeletal muscle fibers of white rats in working strain, *Arch. Anat. Khistol. Embriol.,* 17, 519, 1968 (in Russian).
22. **Lüthi, J.M., Howald, H., Claasen, H., Rösler, K. Vock, P., and Hoppler, H.,** Structural changes in skeletal muscle tissue with heavy-resistance exercise, *Int. J. Sports Med.,* 7, 123, 1986.
23. **Helander, E.A.S.,** Influence of exercise and restricted activity on the protein composition of skeletal muscle, *Biochem. J.,* 78, 478, 1961.
24. **McDonagh, M.J.M., and Davies, C.T.M.,** Adaptive response of mammalian muscle to exercise with high loads, *Eur. J. Appl. Physiol.,* 52, 139, 1984.
25. **Goldspink, G.,** The combined effects of exercise and reduced food intake on skeletal muscle fibers, *J. Cell. Comp. Physiol.,* 63, 309, 1964.
26. **Gudz, P.,** Reforming of muscular structure, their innervation and blood supply under the influence of intensive physical loads, in *Abstr. Pap. Presented Int. Congr. Sports Sci.,* Tokyo, 1964, 142.
27. **Gudz, P.,** Adaptive transformations of structures of the organism as material foundation for endurance in conditions of enhanced muscular activity, in *Physiological Characteristics of Endurance and Methods of Its Estimation in Sports,* Zimkin, N.V., Ed., FiS, Moscow, 1972, 41 (in Russian).
28. **Hamosh, M., Lesch, M., Baron, J., and Kaufman, S.,** Enhanced protein synthesis in a cell-free system from hypertrophied skeletal muscle, *Science,* 157, 935, 1967.
29. **Goldberg, A.L.,** Protein synthesis during work-induced growth of skeletal muscle, *J. Cell. Biol.,* 36, 653, 1968.
30. **Gollnick, P.D.,** Cellular adaptation to exercise, in *Frontiers of Fitness,* Shephard, R.J., Ed., Charles C. Thomas, Springfield, 1971, 112.
31. **Hoppeler, H.,** Exercise-induced changes in skeletal muscle, *Int. J. Sports Med.,* 7, 187, 1986.
32. **Pehme, A., and Seene, T.,** Importance of the relation of power to total volume of work on the protein synthesis in different types of skeletal muscles during strength training of rats, *Acta Comment. Univ. Tartuensis,* 814, 15, 1988.
33. **Yakovlev, N.N., and Yakovleva, E.S.,** Influence of various kinds of training on 'white' and 'red' muscles of animals, *Sechenov Physiol. J. USSR,* 57, 1287, 1971 (in Russian).
34. **Edström, L., and Ekblom, B.,** Differences in sizes of red and white muscle fibers in vastus lateralis of musculus quadriceps femoris of normal individuals and athletes. Relation to physical performance, *Scand. J. Clin. Lab. Invest.,* 30, 175, 1972.
35. **Costill, D.L., Coyle, E.F., Fink, W.F., Lesmes, G.R., and Witzman, F.A.,** Adaptations in skeletal muscle following strength training, *J. Appl. Physiol.,* 46, 96, 1979.
36. **Komi, P.V.,** Training of muscle strength and power: interaction of neuromotoric, hypertrophic, and mechanical factors, *Int. J. Sports Med.,* 7 (Suppl. 1), 10, 1986.
37. **Tesch, P.A., and Karlsson, J.,** Muscle fiber types and size in trained and untrained muscles of elite athletes, *J. Appl. Physiol.,* 59, 1716, 1985.
38. **Tesch, P.A.,** Skeletal muscle adaptations consequent to long-term heavy resistance exercise, *Med. Sci. Sport Exerc.,* 20, S132, 1988.
39. **Salmons, S., and Henriksson, J.,** The adaptive response of skeletal muscle to increased use, *Muscle Nerve,* 4, 94, 1981.
40. **Hoppeler, H., Howald, H., Conley, K.E., Lindstedt, S.L., Claasen, H., Vock, P., and Weibel, E.R.,** Endurance training in humans: aerobic capacity and structure of skeletal muscle, *J. Appl. Physiol.,* 59, 320, 1985.
41. **Rösler, K., Conley, E.K., Claasen, H., Howald, H., and Hoppeler, H.,** Transfer effects in endurance exercise: Adaptations in trained and untrained muscles, *Eur. J. Appl. Physiol.,* 54, 355, 1985.
42. **Gollnick, P.D., Armstrong, R.B., Saltin, B., Sauber, C.W., Sembrowich, W.L., and Shephard, E.R.,** Effect of training on enzyme activity and fiber composition of human skeletal muscle, *J. Appl. Physiol.,* 34, 107, 1973.
43. **Bylund, A.-C., Bjurö, T., Cederblad, G., Holm, J., Lundholm, K., Sjöström, M., Angquist, K.A., and Scherstén, T.,** Physical training in man. Skeletal muscle metabolism in relation to muscle morphology and running ability, *Eur. J. Appl. Physiol.,* 36, 151, 1977.
44. **Howald, H., Hoppeler, H., Claasen, H., Mathieu, O., and Straub, R.,** Influences of endurance training on the ultrastructural composition of the different muscle fiber types in humans, *Pflügers Arch. ges. Physiol.,* 403, 369, 1985.

45. **James, D.E., and Kraegen, E.W.,** The effect of exercise training on glycogen, glycogen synthase, and phosphorylase in muscle and liver, *Eur. J. Appl. Physiol.*, 52, 276, 1984.
46. **Seene, T., and Alev, K.,** Effect of muscular activity on the turnover rate of actin and myosin heavy and light chains in different types of skeletal muscle, *Int. J. Sports Med.*, 12, 204, 1991.
47. **Macková, E., Melichna, J., Havlickova, L., Placheta, Z., Blahová, D., and Semiginovsky, B.,** Skeletal muscle characteristics of sprint-cyclists and nonathletes, *Int. J. Sports Med.*, 7, 295, 1986.
48. **Saltin, B., Nazar, K., Costill, D.L., Stein, E., Jansson, E., Essèn, B., and Gollnick, P.D.,** The nature of the training response, peripheral and central adaptations to one-legged exercise, *Acta Physiol. Scand.*, 96, 289, 1976.
49. **Costill, D.L., Daniels, J., Evans, W., Fink, W., Krahenbuhl, G., and Saltin, B.,** Skeletal muscle enzymes and fiber composition in male and female track athletes, *J. Appl. Physiol.*, 40, 149, 1976.
50. **Costill, D.L., Fink, W.J., and Pollock, M.L.,** Muscle fiber composition and enzyme activities of elite distance runners, *Med. Sci. Sports*, 8, 96, 1976.
51. **Cabric, M., and James, N.T.,** Morphometric analysis on the muscles of exercise trained and untrained dogs, *Am. J. Anat.*, 166, 359, 1983.
52. **Andokian, M.H., and Fahim, M.I.,** Endurance exercise alters the morphology of fast- and slow-twitch rat neuromuscular junctions, *Int. J. Sports Med.*, 9, 218, 1988.
53. **Yakovleva, E.S.,** Morphological changes of motor nerve terminals of striated muscles in physical activity of various character, *Proc. P. Leshaft Res. Inst.,* Leningrad, 26, 208, 1954 (in Russian).
54. **Van Longe, B.,** The response of muscle to strenuous exercise, *J. Bone Joint Surg.*, 44B, 711, 1962.
55. **Reitsma, W.,** Skeletal muscle hypertrophy after heavy exercise in rats with surgically reduced muscle function, *Am. J. Phys. Med.*, 48, 237, 1969.
56. **Edgerton, V.R.,** Morphology and histochemistry of the soleus muscle from normal and exercised rats, *Am. J. Anat.*, 127, 81, 1970.
57. **Gonyea, W., Ericson, C., and Bonde-Petersen, F.,** Skeletal muscle fiber splitting induced by weight-lifting exercise in cats, *Acta Physiol. Scand.*, 99, 105, 1977.
58. **Gonyes, W.,** Role of exercise in inducing increases in skeletal muscle fiber number, *J. Appl. Physiol.*, 48, 421, 1980.
59. **Gudz, P.Z.,** Adaptational, pathological, and compensatory processes in skeletal muscles under great physical stresses, in *Physical Activity and Human Well-Being.* Int. Congr. Phys. Act. Sci., Abstr., Quebec City, 1976, 100.
60. **Nygaard, E.,** Number of fibers in skeletal muscle of man, *Muscle Nerve,* 3, 268, 1980.
61. **Nygaard, E.,** Skeletal muscle fibre characteristics in young women, *Acta Physiol. Scand.*, 112, 299, 1982.
62. **Gollnick, P.D., Timson, B.F., Moore, R.L., and Riedy, M.,** Muscular enlargement and number of fibers in skeletal muscles of rats, *J. Appl. Physiol.*, 50, 936, 1981.
63. **Saltin, B., and Gollnick, P.D.,** Skeletal muscle adaptability: significance for metabolism and performance, in *Handbook of Physiology. Section 10: Skeletal Muscle*, Peachy, L.D., Adrian, R.H., and Geiger, S.R., Eds., Williams and Wilkins, Baltimore, 1983, 555.
64. **Hubbard, R.W., Ianuzzo, C.D., Matthew, W.T., and Linduska, J.D.,** Compensatory adaptation of skeletal muscle composition to a long-term functional overload, *Growth,* 39, 85, 1975.
65. **Kelly, F.J., Watt, P.W., Goldspink, D.F., and Goldspink, G.,** Exercise-induced changes in skeletal muscle in the rat, *Biochem. Soc. Trans.*, 10, 174, 1982.
66. **Jablecki, C.K., Heuser, J.E., and Kaufman, S.,** Autoradiographic localization of new RNA synthesis in hypertrophying skeletal muscle, *J. Cell. Biol.*, 57, 743, 1973.
67. **Moss, F.P., and Leblond, C.P.,** Nature of dividing nuclei in skeletal muscle of growing rats, *J. Cell. Biol.*, 44, 459, 1970.
68. **Schiaffino, S., Bormioli, P., and Aloisi, M.,** Cell proliferation in rat skeletal muscle during early stages of compensatory hypertrophy, *Virchows Arch.,* B11, 266, 1972.
69. **Fleckman, P., Bailyn, R.S., and Kaufman, S.,** Effects of the inhibition of DNA synthesis on hypertrophying skeletal muscle, *J. Biol. Chem.*, 253, 3320, 1978.
70. **Tibbits, G.F.,** Role of the sarcolemma in muscle fatigue, in *Biochemistry of Exercise VII*, Taylor, A.W. et al., Eds., Human Kinetics Books, Champaign, 1990, 37.
71. **Alession, H.M., and Goldfarb, A.H.,** Lipid peroxidation and scavenger enzymes during exercise: Adaptive response to training, *J. Appl. Physiol.*, 64, 1333, 1988.
72. **Byrd, S.K.,** Alterations in the sarcoplasmic reticulum: a possible link to exercise-induced muscle damage, *Med. Sci. Sports Exerc.*, 24, 531, 1992.
73. **Kôrge, P., Roosson, S., and Oks, M.,** Heart adaptation to physical exertion in relation to work duration, *Acta Cardiol.*, 29, 303, 1974.
74. **Kôrge, P., Viru, A., and Rosson, S.,** The effect of chronic physical overload on skeletal muscle metabolism and adrenocortical activity, *Acta Physiol. Acad. Sci. Hung.*, 45, 41, 1974.
75. **Tibbits, G.F., Barnard, R.J., Baldwin, K.M., Cugalj, N., and Roberts, N.K.,** Influence of exercise on excitation-contraction coupling in rat myocardium, *Am. J. Physiol.*, 240, H472, 1981.

76. **Klitgaard, H., and Clausen, T.**, Increased total concentration of Na,K-pump in vastus lateralis muscle of old trained human subjects, *J. Appl. Physiol.*, 67, 2491, 1989.

77. **McKenna, M.J., Schmidt, T.A., Jargreaves, M., Cameron, L., Skinner, S.L., and Kjeldsen, K.**, Sprint training increases human skeletal muscle ^{3}H-ouabain binding site concentration, improves K^+ regulation and reduces muscular fatigue during maximal intermittent exercise, *8th Int. Biochem. Exerc. Conf.*, Nagoya, 1991, 75.

78. **Kjeldsen, K., Richter, E.A., Galbo, H., Lortie, G., and Clausen, T.**, Training increases the concentration of [^{3}H] ouabain-binding sites in rat skeletal muscle, *Biochim. Biophys. Acta*, 860, 708, 1986.

79. **Knochel, J.P., Blachley, J.C., Johnson, J.H., and Carter, W.W.**, Muscle cell electrical hyperpolarization and reduced exercise hyperkalemia in physically conditioned dogs, *J. Clin. Invest.*, 75, 740, 1985.

80. **Tibes, U., Hemmer, B., Boning, D., and Schweigart, U.**, Relationships of femoral venous [K^+], [H^+], PO_2, osmolality and ortophosphate with heart rate, ventilation, and leg blood flow during bicycle exercise in athletes and nonathletes, *Eur. J. Appl. Physiol.*, 35, 201, 1976.

81. **Sembrowich, W.L., Kley, G.A., and Gollnick, P.D.**, The effects of endurance training on calcium uptake by rat heart and skeletal muscle sarcoplasmic reticulum, *Med. Sci. Sports,* 10, 42, 1978.

82. **Kim, D.H., Wible, G.S., Witzman, F.A., and Fitts, R.H.**, The effect of exercise-training on sarcoplasmatic reticulum function in fast and slow skeletal muscle, *Life Sci.*, 28, 2671, 1981.

83. **Viru, M.**, Differences in effects of various training regimes on metabolism of skeletal muscles, *J. Sports Med. Phys. Fitness*, 1994 (accepted for publication).

84. **Studitsky, A.K., Seene, T.P., and Umnova, M.M.**, Ultrastructure changes in red muscle fibers of the quadriceps femoris muscle in increased motor activity, *Byull. Eksp. Biol. Med.*, 100, 492, 1985 (in Russian).

85. **Hoppeler, H., Lüthi, P., Claasen, H., Weibel, E.R., and Howald, H.**, The ultrastructure of the normal human skeletal muscle. A morphometric analysis on untrained men, women and well-trained volunteers, *Pflügers Arch. ges. Physiol.*, 344, 217, 1973.

86. **Hashimoto, Y., and Yamaguchi, M.**, Effect of exercise training on tropomyosin isoforms in the hind limb skeletal muscle of growing rats, *8th Int. Biochem. Exerc. Conf.*, Nagoya, 1991, 105.

87. **Wilkerson, J.E., and Evonuk, E.**, Changes in cardiac and skeletal muscle myosin ATPase activities after exercise, *J. Appl. Physiol.*, 30, 328, 1971.

88. **Syrovy, L., Gutman, E., and Melichna, J.**, Effect of exercise on skeletal muscle myosin ATPase activity, *Physiol. Bohemoslov.*, 21, 633, 1972.

89. **Bagby, G.J., Sembrowich, W.L., and Gollnick, P.D.**, Myosin ATPase and fiber composition from trained and untrained rat skeletal muscle, *Am. J. Physiol.*, 223, 1415, 1972.

90. **Edgerton, V.R., Barnard, R.J., Peter, J.B., Gillespie, C.A., and Simpson, D.K.**, Overloaded skeletal muscles of a nonhuman primate (*Galage renegalenis*), *Exp. Neurol.*, 37, 322, 1972.

91. **Baldwin, K.M., Winder, W.W., and Holloszy, J.O.**, Adaptation of actomyosin ATPase in different types of muscle to endurance exercise, *Am. J.Physiol.*, 229, 422, 1975.

92. **Thornstensson, A., Sjödin, B., and Karlsson, J.**, Enzyme activities and muscle strength after 'sprint training' in man, *Acta Physiol. Scand.*, 94, 313, 1975.

93. **Hildebrand, R.**, Influence of intermittent long-term stimulation on contractile, histochemical, and metabolic properties of fibre population in fat and slow rabbit muscle, *Pflügers Arch. ges. Physiol.*, 361, 1, 1975.

94. **Tesch, P.A., Komi, P.V., and Häkkinen, K.**, Enzymatic adaptation consequent to long-term strength training, *Int. J. Sports Med.*, 8 (Suppl.), 66, 1987.

95. **Tesch, P.A., Thorsson, A., and Colleander, E.B.**, Effects of eccentric and concentric resistance training on skeletal muscle substrates, enzyme activities and capillary supply, *Acta Physiol. Scand.*, 140, 575, 1990.

96. **Häkkinen, K.**, Neuromuscular and hormonal adaptations during strength and power training, *J. Sports Med. Phys. Fitness*, 29, 9, 1989.

97. **Caiozzo, V., Perinne, J., and Edgerton, V.**, Training-induced alterations of the *in vivo* force-velocity relationship of human muscle, *J. Appl. Physiol.*, 51, 750, 1981.

98. **Coyle, E., Feiring, C., and Rotkis, T.**, Specificity of power improvements through slow and fast isokinetic training, *J. Appl. Physiol.*, 51, 1437, 1981.

99. **Häkkinen, K., and Komi, P.V.**, Changes in electrical and mechanical behaviour of leg extensor muscles during heavy resistance strength training, *Scand. J. Sports Sci.*, 7, 55, 1985.

100. **Häkkinen, K., and Komi, P.V.**, Effect of explosive type strength training on electromyographic and force production characteristics of leg extensor muscles during concentric and various stretch-shortening cycle exercises, *Scand. J. Sports Sci.*, 7, 65, 1985.

101. **MacDoughall, J.D., Ward, D., Sale, G., and Sutton, J.R.**, Biochemical adaptation of human skeletal muscle to heavy resistance training and immobilization, *J. Appl. Physiol.*, 43, 700, 1977.

102. **Gonyea, W., and Bonde-Petersen, F.**, Alterations in muscle contractile properties and fiber composition after weight-lifting exercise in cats, *Exp. Neurol.*, 59, 75, 1978.

103. **Staude, H.W., Exner, G.U., and Pette, D.**, Effects of short-term, high intensity (sprint) training on some contractile and metabolic characteristics of fast and slow muscle of the rat, *Pflügers Arch. ges. Physiol.*, 344, 159, 1973.

104. **Fitts, R.H., and Holloszy, J.O.**, Contractile properties of rat soleus muscle effects of training and fatigue, *Am. J. Physiol.*, 233, 86, 1977.

105. **Barnard, R.J., Edgerton, V.R., and Peter, J.B.**, Effect of exercise on skeletal muscle. II. Contractile properties, *J. Appl. Physiol.*, 28, 767, 1970.

106. **Gollnick, P.D., and King, D.W.**, Effect of exercise and training on mitochondria of rat skeletal muscle, *Am. J. Physiol.*, 216, 1502, 1969.

107. **Kraus, H., Kirsten, R., and Wolff, J.R.**, Die Wirkung von Schwimm- and Lauftraining auf die celluläre Funktion and Struktur des Muskels, *Pflügers Arch. ges. Physiol.*, 308, 57, 1969.

108. **Yakovlev, N.N., Krasnova, A.F., Lenkova, P.I., Leshkevich, L.G., Samodanova, G.I., and Chagovets, N.R.**, Effect of the adaptation to intensive muscle activity on the functional state of skeletal muscle mitochondria, *Cytologia*, 19, 197, 1972 (in Russian).

109. **Howald, H.**, Ultrastructure and biochemical function of skeletal muscle in twins, *Ann. Hum. Biol.*, 3, 455, 1976.

110. **Holloszy, J.O.**, Biochemical adaptations in muscle. Effects of exercise on mitochondrial oxygen uptake and respiratory enzyme activity in skeletal muscle, *J. Biol. Chem.*, 242, 2278, 1967.

111. **Holloszy, J.O., Oscai, L.B., Don, I.J., and Mole, P.A.**, Mitochondrial citric acid cycle and related enzymes: adaptive response to exercise, *Biochem. Biophys. Res. Comm.*, 40, 1368, 1970.

112. **Baldwin, K.M., Klinkerfuss, G.H., Terjung, R.L., Mole, P.A., and Holloszy, J.O.**, Respiratory capacity of white, red, and intermediate muscle adaptive response to exercise, *Am. J. Physiol.*, 222, 373, 1972.

113. **Gollnick, P.D., Armstrong, R.B., Saubert, C.W., Piehl, K., and Saltin, B.**, Enzyme activity and fiber composition in skeletal muscle of untrained and trained man, *J. Appl. Physiol.*, 33, 312, 1972.

114. **Holloszy, J.O.**, Biochemical adaptations to exercise: aerobic metabolism, *Exerc. Sport Sci. Rev.*, 1, 45, 1973.

115. **Fitts, R.H., Booth, F.W., Winder, W.W., and Holloszy, J.O.**, Skeletal muscle respiratory capacity, endurance and glycogen utilization, *Am. J. Physiol.*, 228, 1029, 1975.

116. **Holloszy, J.O., and Booth, F.W.**, Biochemical adaptations to endurance exercise in muscle, *Annu. Rev. Physiol.*, 38, 273, 1976.

117. **Jansson, E., and Kaijser, L.**, Muscle adaptation to extreme endurance training in man, *Acta Physiol. Scand.*, 100, 315, 1977.

118. **Saltin, B., Henriksson, J., Nygaard, E., Jansson, E., and Andersen, F.**, Fiber types and metabolic potentials of skeletal muscles in sedentary man and endurance runners, *Ann. N.Y. Acad. Sci.*, 301, 3, 1977.

119. **Green, H.J., Thomson, J.A., Daub, W.D., Houston, M.E., and Ranney, D.A.**, Fiber composition, fiber size and enzyme activities in vastus lateralis of elite athletes involved in high intensity exercise, *Eur. J. Appl. Physiol.*, 41, 109, 1979.

120. **Palladin, A.V.**, Studies on biochemistry of muscular training, *Sechenov Physiol. J. USSR*, 19, 277, 1935 (in Russian).

121. **Matoba, H., and Gollnick, P.D.**, Response of skeletal muscle to training, *Sports Med.*, 1, 240, 1984.

122. **Müller, W.**, Subsarcolemmal mitochondria and capillarization of soleus muscle fibers in young rats subjected to an endurance training. A morphometric study of semithin sections, *Cell. Tissue Res.*, 174, 367, 1976.

123. **Costill, D.L., Funk, W.J., Getschell, L.H., Ivy, J.H., and Witzman, F.A.**, Lipid metabolism in skeletal muscle of endurance-trained males and females, *J. Appl. Physiol.*, 47, 787, 1979.

124. **Schantz, P., Henriksson, J., and Jansson, E.**, Adaptation of human skeletal muscle to endurance training of long duration, *Clin. Physiol.*, 3, 141, 1983.

125. **Holloszy, J.O., and Coyle, E.F.**, Adaptation of skeletal muscle to endurance exercise and their metabolic consequences, *J. Appl. Physiol.*, 56, 831, 1984.

126. **Gollnick, P.D., and Saltin, B.**, Significance of skeletal muscle oxidative enzyme enhancement with endurance training, *Clin. Physiol.*, 2, 1, 1982.

127. **Gollnick, P.D., Riedy, M., Quintiskie, J.J., and Bertocci, L.A.**, Differences in metabolic potential of skeletal muscle fibres and their significance for metabolic control, *J. Exp. Biol.*, 115, 191, 1985.

128. **Saks, V.A., Rosenstrukh, L.V., Smirnov, V.N., and Chazov, E.I.**, Role of creatine phosphokinase in cellular function and metabolism, *Can. J. Physiol. Pharmacol.*, 56, 691, 1978.

129. **Saks, V.A., Kupriyanov, V.V., Elizarova, G., and Jacobus, W.E.**, Studies of energy transport in heart cells. The importance of creatine kinase localization for the coupling of mitochondrial phosphorylcreatine production to oxidative phosphorylation, *J. Biol. Chem.*, 255, 755, 1980.

130. **Oscai, L.B., and Holloszy, J.O.**, Biochemical adaptations in muscle. II. Response of mitochondrial adenosine triphosphate, creatine phosphokinase, and adenylate kinase activities in skeletal muscle to exercise, *J. Biol. Chem.*, 246, 6968, 1971.

131. **Lenkova, R.J., Usik, S.V., and Chumakova, M.G.**, A role of creatinekinase system in energy of physical exercise, *8th Int. Biochem. Exerc. Conf.*, Nagoya, 1991, 147.

132. **Terjung, R.L.**, Muscle fiber involvement during training of different intensities and duration, *Am. J. Physiol.*, 230, 946, 1976.

133. **Gollnick, P.D., Armstrong, R.B., Saubert, C.W., Semberowich, W.S., Shephard, R.E., and Saltin, B.,** Glycogen depletion pattern in human skeletal muscle fibers during prolonged work, *Pflügers Arch. ges. Physiol.*, 344, 1, 1973.

134. **Gollnick, P.D., Piehl, K., and Saltin, B.,** Selective glycogen depletion pattern in human muscle fibers after exercise of varying intensity and at varying pedalling rates, *J. Physiol.*, 241, 45, 1974.

135. **Winder, W.W, Baldwin, K.M., and Holloszy, J.O.,** Enzymes involved in ketone utilization in different types of muscles: adaptation to exercise, *Eur. J. Biochem.*, 47, 461, 1974.

136. **Tikkanen, H., and Härkönen, M.,** Regulatory enzyme activity adaptations in FT- and ST-muscle fibers of endurance trained rats, *Paavo Nurmi Congress*, Turku, 1989.

137. **MacDoughall, J.D., Sale, D.G., Moroz, J.R., Elder, C.B., Sutton, J.R., and Howald, H.,** Mitochondrial volume density in human skeletal muscle following heavy resistance training, *Med. Sci. Sports*, 11, 164, 1979.

138. **Howald, H.,** Training-induced morphological and functional changes in skeletal muscle, *Int. J. Sports Med.*, 3, 1, 1982.

139. **MacDoughall, J.D., Sale, D.G., Elder, G.C.B., and Sutton, J.R.,** Muscle ultrastructural characteristics of elite powerlifters and bodybuilders, *Eur. J. Appl. Physiol.*, 48, 117, 1982.

140. **Komi, P.V., Viitasalo, J., Rauramaa, R., and Vihko, V.,** Effect of isometric strength training on mechanical, electrical and metabolic aspects of muscle function, *Eur. J. Appl. Physiol.*, 40, 45, 1978.

141. **Houston, M.E., Froese, E.A., Valeriete, St. P., Green, H.J., and Ranney, D.A.,** Muscle performance, morphology and metabolic capacity during strength training and detraining: a one leg model, *Eur. J. Appl. Physiol.*, 51, 25, 1983.

142. **Brzank, K.-D., and Pieper, K.-S.,** Mitochondrienverfeilung, Ausfauschstrecken and O_2-Versordungsbedingungen im Skelettmuskel von Ausdauer, Kraftausdauer sowie Schnellkrafttrainierten, *Med. Sport*, 27, 65, 1987.

143. **Dudley, G.A., Abraham, W.M., and Terjung, R.L.,** Influence of exercise intensity and duration on biochemical adaptatons in skeletal muscle, *J. Appl. Physiol.*, 53, 844, 1982.

144. **Shephard, E.R., and Gollnick, P.D.,** Oxygen uptake of rats at different work intensities, *Pflügers Arch. ges. Physiol.*, 362, 219, 1976.

145. **Volkov, N.I.,** The problems of biohemical assays in sport activities of man, in *Metabolism and Biochemical Evaluation of Sportsmen's Fitness*, Yakovlev, N.N., Ed., Leningrad Research Institute of Physical Culture, Leningrad, 1974, 213 (in Russian).

146. **Hickson, R.G.,** Skeletal muscle cytochrome c and myoglobin endurance and frequency of training, *J. Appl. Physiol.*, 51, 746, 1981.

147. **Hickson, R.C., Heusner, W.W., and Van Huss, W.D.,** Skeletal muscle enzyme alterations after sprint and endurance training, *J. Appl. Physiol.*, 40, 868, 1975.

148. **Fournier, M., Ricci, J., Taylor, A.W., Fergusen, R.J., Montpetit, R.R., and Chaitman, B.R.,** Skeletal muscle adaptation in adolescent boys: sprint endurance training and detraining, *Med. Sci. Sports Exerc.*, 14, 453, 1982.

149. **Sharp, R.L., Costill, D.L., Fink, W.J., and King, D.S.,** Effects of eight weeks of bicycle ergometer sprint training on human muscle buffer capacity, *Int. J. Sports Med.*, 7, 13, 1986.

150. **Jacobs, I., Esbjörsson, M., Sylven, C., Holm, I., and Jansson, E.,** Sprint training effects on muscle myoglobin, enzymes, fiber types, and blood lactate, *Med. Sci. Sports Exerc.*, 19, 368, 1987.

151. **Saubert, C.W., Armstrong, R.B., Shephard, R.E., and Gollnick, P.D.,** Anaerobic enzyme adaptations to sprint training in rats, *Pflügers Arch. ges. Physiol.*, 341, 305, 1973.

152. **Gillespie, A.C., Fox, L.E., and Merola, A.J.,** Enzyme adaptations in rat skeletal muscle after two intensities of treadmill training, *Med. Sci. Sports Exerc.*, 14, 461, 1982.

153. **Pfister, M., Moesch, H., and Howald, H.,** Beeinflussung glykolytischer und oxidativer Skelettmuskelenzyme des Meschen durch anaerobes Training oder anabols Steroide, *Schweiz. Z. Sportmed.*, 29, 45, 1981.

154. **Donovan, C.M., and Brooks, G.A.,** Endurance training affects lactate clearance, not lactate production, *Am. J. Physiol.*, 244, E83, 1983.

155. **Hochacka, P.W., and Somero, G.N.,** *Biochemical Adaptation*, Princeton University Press, Princeton, 1984.

156. **Thorstensson, A., Hulten, B., Döberln von W., and Karlsson, J.,** Effect of strength training on enzyme activities and fibre characteristics in human skeletal muscle, *Acta Physiol. Scand.* 96, 392, 1976.

157. **Thorstensson, A.,** Muscle strength, fibre type and enzyme activities in man, *Acta Physiol. Scand.*, *Suppl.* 443, 1976.

158. **Yamashita, K., and Yoshicka, T.,** The physiological significance of creatine kinase in muscle cells, *8th Int. Biochem. Exerc. Conf.*, Nagoya, 1991, 96.

159. **Apple, F.S., and Tesch, P.A.,** CK and LD isozymes in human single muscle fibers in trained athletes, *J. Appl. Physiol.*, 66, 2717, 1989.

160. **Jansson, E., and Sylvén, C.,** Creatine kinase MB and citrate synthetase in type I and type II muscle fibers in trained and untrained men, *Eur. J. Appl. Physiol.*, 54, 207, 1985.

161. **Komi, P.V., Rusko, H., Vos, J., and Vihko, V.,** Anaerobic performance capacity in athletes, *Acta Physiol. Scand.*, 100, 107, 1977.

162. **Roberts, A.D., Balleter, R., and Howald, H.,** Anaerobic muscle enzyme changes after interval training, *Int. J. Sports Med.*, 3, 18, 1982.

163. **Baldwin, K.M., Cooke, D.A., and Cheadle, W.G.,** Time course of adaptations in cardiac and skeletal muscle to different running programs, *J. Appl. Physiol.*, 42, 267, 1977.

164. **Baldwin, K.M., Winder, W.W., Terjung, R.L., and Holloszy, J.O.,** Glycolytic enzymes in different types of skeletal muscle: adaptation to exercise, *Am. J. Physiol.*, 255, 962, 1973.

165. **Bernard, R.J., and Peter, J.B.,** Effect of training and exhaustion on hexokinase activity of skeletal muscle, *J. Appl. Physiol.*, 27, 691, 1969.

166. **Guy, P.S., and Snow, D.H.,** The effect of training and detraining on lactate dehydrogenase in the horse, *Biochem. Biophys. Res. Comm.*, 75, 863, 1977.

167. **Sjödin, B.,** Lactate dehydrogenase in human skeletal muscle, *Acta Physiol. Scand.*, 436, 5, 1976.

168. **Sjödin, B., Thorstensson, A., Frith, K., and Karlsson, J.,** Effect of physical training on LDH activity and LDH isozyme pattern in human skeletal muscle, *Acta Physiol. Scand.*, 97, 150, 1976.

169. **Apple, F.S., and Rogers, M.A.,** Skeletal muscle lactate dehydrogenase isozyme alterations in men and women marathon runners, *J. Appl. Physiol.*, 61, 477, 1986.

170. **Morgan, T.E., Cobb, L.A., Short, F.A., Ross, R., and Gunn, D.R.,** Effects of long-term exercise on human muscle mitochondria, in *Muscle Metabolism During Exercise,* Pernow, B. and Saltin, B., Eds., Plenum Press, New York, 1971, 87.

171. **Erikson, B.O., Gollnick, P.D., and Saltin, B.,** Muscle metabolism and enzyme activities after training in boys 11–13 years old, *Acta Physiol. Scand.*, 87, 485, 1973.

172. **Illg, D., and Pette, D.,** Turnover rates of hexokinase I, phosphofructokinase, pyruvate kinase, and creatinine kinase in slow-twitch soleus muscle and heart of the rabbit, *Eur. J. Biochem.*, 97, 267, 1979.

173. **Thornheim, K., and Lowenstein, J.M.,** Control of PFK from rat skeletal muscle, *J. Biol. Chem.*, 251, 7322, 1976.

174. **Trivedi, B., and Danforth, W.H.,** Effects of pH on the kinetics of frog muscle PFK, *J. Biol. Chem.*, 241, 4110, 1966.

175. **Bosca, L., Aragon, J.J., and Sols, A.,** Modulation of muscle PFK at physiological concentration of enzyme, *J. Biol. Chem.*, 260, 2100, 1985.

176. **Newsholme, E.A.,** Application of principles of metabolic control to the problem of metabolic limitation in sprinting, middle-distance, and marathon running, *Int. J. Sports Med.,* 7 (Suppl.), 66, 1986.

177. **Challiss, R.A.J., Arch, J.R.S., and Newsholme, E.A.,** The role of substrate cycling between fructose-6-phosphate and fructose 1,6-biphosphate in skeletal muscle, *Biochem. J.*, 221, 153, 1984.

178. **Yakovlev, N.N.,** The role of sympathetic nervous system in the adaptation of skeletal muscles to increased activity, in *Metabolic Adaptation to Prolonged Physical Exercise,* Howald, H. and Poortmans, J., Eds., Birkhäuser, Basel, 1975, 293.

179. **Goldberg, N.D.,** Changes of activity and isozyme spectra of hexokinase of skeletal muscles and brain in adaptation to intensive physical exercises, *Ukr. Biokhim. Zh.*, 57(2), 46, 1985.

180. **Parkhouse, W.S., and McKenzie, D.C.,** Possible contribution of skeletal muscle buffers to enhanced anaerobic performance: a brief review, *Med. Sci. Sports Exerc.*, 16, 328, 1989.

181. **Gollnick, P.D., and Hermansen, L.,** Biochemical adaptaion to exercise: anaerobic metabolism, *Exerc. Sport Sci. Rev.*, 1, 1, 1973.

182. **Viru, A., Jürgenstein, J., and Pisuke, A.,** Influence of training methods on endurance, *Track Tech.*, 47, 1494, 1972.

183. **McKenzie, D.C., Parkhouse, W.S., Rhodes, E.C., Hochacka, P.W., Ovalle, W.K., Monsensen, T.P., and Shinn, S.L.,** Skeletal muscle buffering capacity in elite athletes, in *Biochemistry of Exercise,* Knuttgen, H.G., Vogel, J.A., and Poortmans, J., Eds., Human Kinetics, Champaign, 1983, 584.

184. **Sharp, R.L., Armstrong, L.E., King, D.S., and Costill, D.L.,** Buffer capacity of blood in trained and untrained males, in *Biochemistry of Exercise,* Knuttgen, H.G., Vogel, J.A., and Poortmans, J., Human Kinetics, Champaign, 1983, 595.

185. **Parkhouse, W.S., McKenzie, D.C., Hockachka, P.W., Mommsen, T.B., Ovalle, W.K., Chinn, S.L., and Rhodes, E.C.,** The relationship between carnosine levels, buffering capacity, fiber types, and anaerobic capacity in elite athletes, in *Biochemistry of Exercise,* Knuttgen, H., Vogel, J., and Poortmans, J., Eds., Human Kinetics, Champaign, 1983, 590.

186. **Castelini, M.A., and Somero, G.N.,** Buffering capacity of vertebrate muscle: correlations with potentials for anaerobic function, *J. Comp. Physiol.*, 143, 191, 1981.

187. **Burton, R.F.,** Intracellular buffering, *Respir. Physiol.,* 33, 51, 1978.

188. **Nevill, M.E., Boabis, L.H., Brooks, S., and Williams, C.,** Effect of training on muscle metabolism during treadmill sprinting, *J. Appl. Physiol.*, 67, 237, 1989.

189. **Houston, M.E., Wilson, D.M., Green, H.J., Thomson, J.A., and Ranney, D.A.,** Physiological and muscle enzyme adaptations to two different intensities of swim training, *Eur. J. Appl. Physiol.*, 46, 283, 1981.

190. **Kindermann, W., and Keul, J.** *Anaerobe Energiebereitstellung im Hochleistungssport,* Verlag K. Hofmann, Schorndorf, 1977.

191. **Karlsson, J., Diament, B., and Saltin, B.**, Muscle metabolites during submaximal and maximal exercise in man, *Scand. J. Clin. Lab. Invest.*, 26, 358, 1971.

192. **Karlsson, G., Nordesjö, L.-O., Jorfeldt, L., and Saltin, B.**, Muscle lactate, ATP and CP levels during exercise after physical training in man, *J. Appl. Physiol.*, 33, 199, 1972.

193. **MacDoughall, J.D., Ward, G.R., Sale, D.G., and Sutton, J.R.**, Biochemical adaptation of human skeletal muscle to heavy resistance training and immobilization, *J. Appl. Physiol.*, 43, 700, 1977.

194. **Palladin, A., and Ferdmann, D.**, Über den Einfluss der Trainings der Muskeln auf ihren Kreatingehalt, *Hoppe-Seyler's Z. Physiol. Chem.*, 174, 284, 1928.

195. **Ferdmann, D., and Feinschmidt, O.**, Über den Einfluss des Trainierens des Muskels auf seinen Gehalt and Phosphoverbindungen, *Hoppe-Seyler's Z. Physiol. Chem.,* 183, 216, 1929.

196. **Embden, G.E., and Habs, H.**, Über chemische and biologische Veränderungen der Muskulatur nach öften wiederhalter faradischer Reizung, *Hoppe-Seyler's Z. Physiol. Chem.,* 171, 16, 1927.

197. **Hermansen, L., Hultman, E., and Saltin, B.**, Muscle glycogen during prolonged severe exercise, *Acta Physiol. Scand.*, 71, 129, 1967.

198. **Hultman, E.**, Studies on muscle metabolism of glycogen and active phosphate in man with special reference to exercise and diet, *Scand. J. Clin. Lab. Invest.*, 19, Suppl. 94, 1967.

199. **Taylor, A.W., Thayer, R., and Rao, S.**, Human skeletal muscle glycogen synthetase activities with exercise and training, *Can. J. Physiol. Pharmacol.*, 50, 411, 1972.

200. **Piehl, K., Adolfsson, S., and Nazar, K.**, Glycogen storage and glycogen synthase activity in trained and untrained muscle of man, *Acta Physiol. Scand.*, 90, 779, 1974.

201. **Tesch, P., Piehl, K., Wilson, G., and Karlsson, J.**, Physiological investigations of Swedish elite canoe competitors, *Med. Sci. Sports*, 8, 214, 1976.

202. **Burke, E., Carny, F., Costill, D., and Fink, W.**, Characteristics of skeletal muscle in competitive cyclists, *Med. Sci. Sports*, 9, 109, 1977.

203. **Morgan, T.E., Short, F.A., and Cobb, L.A.**, Effect of long-term exercise on skeletal muscle lipid composition, *Am. J. Physiol.*, 216, 82, 1969.

204. **Henriksson, J.**, Training-induced adaptation of skeletal muscle and metabolism during submaximal exercise, *J. Physiol.*, 270, 677, 1977.

205. **Förberg, S.O.**, Effect of training and of acute exercise in trained rats, *Metabolism*, 20, 1034, 1971.

206. **Lawrie, R.A.**, Effect of enforced exercise on myoglobin concentration in muscle, *Nature*, 171, 1069, 1983.

207. **Pattengale, P.K., and Holloszy, J.O.**, Augmentation of skeletal muscle myoglobin by a program of treadmill running, *Am. J. Physiol.*, 213, 783, 1967.

208. **Jansson, E., Sylván, C., and Nordevang, E.**, Myoglobin in the quadriceps femoris muscle of competitive cyclists and untrained men, *Acta Physiol. Scand.*, 114, 627, 1982.

209. **Svedenhag, J., Henriksson, J., and Sylván, C.**, Dissociation of training effects on skeletal muscle mitochondrial enzymes and myoglobin in man, *Acta Physiol. Scand.*, 117, 213, 1983.

210. **Vannotti, H., and Magiday, M.**, Untersuchungen zum Studium des Trainertseins. V Über die Kapillarisierung der trainierten Muskulatur, *Arbeitsphysiologie*, 7, 615, 1934.

211. **Petrén, T., Sjöstrand, T., and Sylven, B.**, Der Einfluss des Trainings auf die Häufigkeit der Capillaren in Herz- and Skeletmusculatur, *Arbeitsphysiolgie*, 9, 376, 1936.

212. **Hermansen, L., and Wachtlova, M.**, Capillary density of skeletal muscle in well-trained and untrained men, *J. Appl. Physiol.*, 30, 860, 1971.

213. **Andersen, P., and Henrikson, J.**, Capillary supply of the quadriceps femoris muscle of man: adaptive response to exercise, *J. Physiol.*, 270, 677, 1977.

214. **Brodal, P., Ingjer, F., and Hermansen, L.**, Capillary supply of skeletal muscle fibres in untrained and endurance-trained men, *Am. J. Physiol.*, 232, H705, 1977.

215. **Ingjer, F., and Brodal, P.**, Capillary supply of skeletal muscle fibers in untrained and endurance-trained women, *Eur. J. Appl. Physiol.*, 38, 291, 1978.

216. **Ingjer, F.**, Capillary supply and mitochondrial content of different skeletal muscle fiber types in untrained and endurance-trained men, *Eur. J. Appl. Physiol.*, 40, 197, 1979.

217. **Kuzon, W.M., Rosenblatt, J.D., Huebel, S.C., Leatt, P., Plyley, M.J., McKee, N.H., and Jacobs, I.**, Skeletal muscle fiber type, fiber size and capillary supply in elite soccer players, *Int. J. Sports Med.*, 11, 99, 1990.

218. **Ingjer, F.**, Maximal aerobic power related to the capillary supply of the quadriceps femoris muscle in man, *Acta Physiol. Scand.*, 104, 238, 1978.

219. **Nygaard, E., and Nielsen, E.**, Skeletal muscle fiber capillarization with extreme endurance training in man, in *Swimming Medicine IV*, Eriksson, B. and Furberg, B., Eds., University Park, Baltimore, 1978, 282.

220. **Hudlicka, O.**, Effect of training on macro- and microcirculatory changes in exercise, *Exerc. Sport Sci. Rev.*, 6, 181, 1980.

221. **Adolfson, J., Ljungquist, A., Tornling, G., and Unge, G.**, Capillary increase in the skeletal muscle of trained young and adult rats, *J. Physiol.*, 310, 259, 1981.

222. **Mai, J.V., Edgerton, V.R., and Barnard, R.J.,** Capillarity of red, white, and intermediate muscle fibres in trained and untrained guinea-pig, *Experimentia*, 26, 1222, 1970.

223. **Romunul, F.C.A.,** Capillary supply and metabolism of muscle fibers, *Arch. Neurol.*, 12, 497, 1965.

224. **Romunul, F.C.A., and Pollack, M.,** The parallelism of changes in oxidative metabolism and capillary supply of skeletal muscle fibers, in *Modern Neurology*, Locke, S., Ed., Little, Brown, Boston, 1969, 203.

225. **Tesch, P.A., Thorsson, A., and Kaiser, P.,** Muscle capillary supply and fiber type characteristics in weight and power lifters, *J. Appl. Physiol.*, 56, 35, 1984.

226. **Sjøgaard, G.,** Changes in skeletalmuscle capillarity and enzyme activity with training and detraining, in *Physiological Chemistry of Training and Detraining,* Marconnet, P., Poartmans, J., and Kermansur, L., Eds., Karger, Basel, 1984, 202.

227. **Burton, H.W., and Barclay, J.K.,** Metabolic factors from exercising muscle and the proliferation of endothelial cells, *Med. Sci. Sports Exerc.*, 18, 390, 1986.

228. **Appell, H.J.,** Morphological studies on skeletal muscle capillaries under conditions of high altitude training, *Int. J. Sports Med.*, 1, 103, 1980.

229. **Poole, D.C., Mathieu-Costello, O., and West, J.B.,** Capillary tortuosity in rat soleus muscle is not affected by endurance training, *Am. J. Physiol.*, 256, H1110, 1989.

230. **Saltin, B., Nygaard, E., and Rasmussen, B.,** Skeletal muscle adaptation in man following prolonged exposure to high altitude, *Acta Physiol. Scand.*, 109, 31A, 1980.

231. **Laughlin, M.H., and Ripperger, A.J.,** Vascular transport capacity of hind limb muscles of exercise-trained rats, *J. Appl. Physiol.*, 62, 438, 1987.

232. **Pette, D., and Schruez, U.,** Myosin light chain patterns of individual fast and slow-twitch fibers of rabbit muscles, *Histochemistry*, 54, 97, 1977.

233. **Lutz, H., Weber, H., Billeter, R., and Jenny, E.,** Fast and slow myosin within single skeletal muscle fibers of adult rabbits, *Nature,* 281, 142, 1979.

234. **Rapp, G., and Weicker, H.,** Comparative studies on fast muscle myosin light chains after different training programs, *Int. J. Sports Med.*, 3, 58, 1982.

235. **Drachman, D.B., and Jonhnsten, D.M.,** Development of mammalian fast muscle: dynamic and biochemical properties correlated, *J. Physiol.*, 234, 29, 1973.

236. **Whalen, R.G., Sell, S.M., Butler-Browne, G.S., Schwartz, K., Bouveret, P., and Plnset-Harstrom, I.,** Three myosin heavy-chain isozymes appear sequentially in rat muscle development, *Nature*, 292, 805, 1981.

237. **Salmons, S., and Vrbova, G.,** The influence of activity on some contractile characteristics of mammalian fast and slow muscles, *J. Physiol.*, 201, 535, 1969.

238. **Pette, D., Ramirez, B.A., Müller, W., Simon, R., Exner, G.U., and Hildebrand, R.,** Influence of intermittent long-term stimulation of contractile histochemical and metabolic properties of fibre populations in fast and slow rabbit muscles, *Pflügers Arch. ges. Physiol.*, 361, 1, 1975.

239. **Hudlicka, O., Brown, M., Catter, M., Smith, M., and Vrbova, G.,** The effect of long-term stimulation of fast muscle on their blood flow, metabolism, and ability to withstand fatigue, *Pflügers Arch. ges. Physiol.*, 369, 141, 1977.

240. **Pette, D.,** Activity-induced fast to slow transitions in mammalian muscle, *Med. Sci. Sports Exerc.*, 16, 517, 1984.

241. **Fitsimons, D.P., Diffee, G.M., Herrick, R.E., and Baldwin, K.M.,** Effects of endurance exercise on isomyosin patterns in fast- and slow-twitch skeletal muscles, *J. Appl. Physiol.*, 68, 1950, 1990.

242. **Sugiura, T., Morimoto, A., Sakata, Y., Watenabl, T., and Murakami, N.,** Myosin heavy chain isoform changes in rat diaphragm are induced by endurance training, *Jpn. J. Physiol.*, 40, 759, 1990.

243. **Jansson, E., Sjödin, B., Thorstensson, A., Hultèn, B., and Frith, K.,** Changes in muscle fibre type distribution in man after physical exercise. A sign of fibre type transformation?, *Acta Physiol. Scand.*, 104, 235, 1978.

244. **Andersen, P., and Hendriksson, J.,** Training induced changes in the subgroups of human type II skeletal muscle fibers, *Acta Physiol. Scand.*, 99, 123, 1977.

245. **Schantz, P.G., and Dhoot, G.K.,** Coexistance of slow and fast isoforms of contractile and regulatory proteins in human muscle fibres induced by endurance training, *Acta Physiol. Scand.,* 131, 147, 1987.

246. **Simoneau, J.-A., Lortie, G., Boulay, M.R., Marcotte, M., Thibault, M.-C., and Bouchard, C.,** Human skeletal muscle fiber alteration with high-intensity intermittent training, *Eur. J. Appl. Physiol.*, 54, 250, 1985.

247. **Schantz, P., Billeter, R., Hendriksson, J., and Jansson, E.,** Training-induced increase in myofibrillar ATPase intermediate fibers in human skeletal muscle, *Muscle Nerve,* 5, 628, 1982.

248. **Jansson, E., Esbjörnsson, M., Holm, I., and Jacobs, I.,** Increase in the proportion of fast-twitch muscle fibers by sprint in males, *Acta Physiol. Scand.*, 140, 359, 1990.

249. **Ciriella, V.M., Holden, W.L., and Evans, W.J.,** The effect of two isokinetic training regimes on muscle strength and fiber composition, in *Biochemistry of Exercise,* Knuttgen, H.G., Vogel, J.A., and Poortmans, J., Eds., Human Kinetics, Champaign, 1983, 787.

250. **Harmon, M., and Nimmo, M.A.,** Quantitative histochemical analysis of skeletal muscle adaptation to endurance training in man, *J. Physiol.*, 394, 72R, 1987.

251. **Bagby, G.J., Semberowich, W.L., and Gollnick, P.D.,** Myosin ATPase and fiber composition from trained and untrained rat skeletal muscle, *Am. J. Physiol.*, 223, 1415, 1972.

252. **Green, H.J., Klug, G.A., Reichmann, H., Seedorf, U., Wiehren, W., and Pette, D.,** Exercise induced fibre type transition with regard to myosin parvalbumin and sarcoplasmatic reticulum in muscles of the rat, *Pflügers Arch. ges. Physiol.*, 400, 432, 1984.

253. **Green, H.J., Reichmann, H., and Pette, D.,** Fibre type specific transformations in the enzyme activity pattern of rat vastus lateralis muscle by prolonged endurance training, *Pflügers Arch. ges. Physiol.*, 339, 216, 1983.

254. **Yarasheski, K.E., Lemon, P.W.P., and Gilloteaux, J.,** Effect of heavy-resistance exercise training on muscle fiber composition in young rats, *J. Appl. Physiol.*, 69, 434, 1990.

Chapter 6

SPECIFICITY OF TRAINING EFFECTS ON AEROBIC WORKING CAPACITY AND THE CARDIOVASCULAR SYSTEM

TRAINING EFFECTS ON ANAEROBIC THRESHOLD AND MAXIMAL OXYGEN UPTAKE

ANAEROBIC THRESHOLD

Training effects on the mitochondria enable the use of oxidative phosphorylation for ATP resynthesis during performance of more and more intensive exercises. The so-called anaerobic threshold is very likely a qualitative measure of the highest exercise intensity performed on the basis of oxidative phosphorylation without an extended use of anaerobic energy mechanisms. To put it more precisely, the anaerobic threshold expresses the highest exercise intensity during performance in which the pyruvate formation rate still does not exceed the maximal rate of oxidative phosphorylation. Accordingly, the formed lactate can be oxidized or used for gluconeogenesis by nonworking muscles, heart, and liver. Up to this qualitative point an equilibrium exists between lactate formation and elimination.[1,2]

Since the maximal oxygen uptake is obtained in exercise level, causing a pronounced lactate accumulation, exercise intensity at VO_2max does not indicate maximal performance on the basis of aerobic resynthesis of ATP. Actually, it was found that there is no close coupling between the whole body VO_2max and the oxidative capacity of a local muscle group in elite road cyclists during a session.[3] There is a close relationship of these variables over the first 3 to 4 weeks of training. Thereafter, the increase in VO_2max levels off, but the activity of mitochondrial enzymes continues to rise.[4] The VO_2max of athletes may be twice that of untrained persons, whereas their activity of mitochondrial enzymes of the muscle is three- to fourfold higher than that of sedentary individuals.[5] When training was discontinued, the activity of oxidative enzymes dropped to the initial level within 2 to 4 weeks. However, VO_2max remained high for 6 weeks.[4]

The anaerobic threshold is a variable rather accurately predicting athletic endurance performance, particularly in running races of 10 to 42 km.[6-23] In male and female marathon runners, elevated relationships were found between the running velocities determined at 2.5, 3, and 4 mmol·l⁻¹ of blood lactate and marathon running velocity. Running at marathon velocity did not cause a change in pH; the blood lactate rose up to 2.2 to 3.5 mmol·l⁻¹.[24] Anaerobic threshold correlates closely to performance in race-walkers. The factor of submaximal economy, which partly determines the velocity at anaerobic threshold, is related to performance ability in race-walking[25] more than in running.[26] In 21 endurance-trained runners longitudinal changes in the anaerobic threshold and distance-running performance were in consistently high correlation over a 9-month training period.[26]

The anaerobic threshold appears at an exercise intensity of 75 to 90% VO_2max. At 75 to 80% VO_2max the ATP turnover rate is high enough to elevate ADP, AMP, P_i, and H° concentrations stimulating glycolysis. Therefore, at 75% VO_2max, lactate begins to accumulate in muscles (most of all in type II fibers) and blood.[27] A study of 25 members of the U.S. Olympic rowing team showed that a mean anaerobic threshold of 83% VO_2max attests to the high aerobic capacity of oarsmen. Power output data indicated that 72% of total power is generated at the anaerobic threshold.[28] In top class long-distance runners the anaerobic threshold is as high as 85 to 90% VO_2max and in skiers, 75 to 80% VO_2max. The difference is related to the higher VO_2max in skiers.[29] However, for predicting the endurance performance level, exercise intensity at the anaerobic threshold is more important (Figure 6-1) than the percent of VO_2max at this exercise intensity. The highest running velocity at blood lactate 4 mmol·l^{-1} was found in 10,000-m or marathon runners[67] (Figure 6-2).

In athletes the percent of ST was significantly related to running velocity corresponding to the onset of blood lactate accumulation, the average speed of the marathon race, and the average mechanical power output during running at the velocity corresponding to the onset of blood lactate accumulation.[30] Analogous relationships were found in a group of persons tested by their cycling time to exhaustion.[21]

An effective tool for improvement of the anaerobic threshold is aerobic endurance training.[17,31-33] Aerobic training is most effective at intensities of exercises corresponding to the anaerobic threshold[31,34,35] or at an intensity slightly higher than the anaerobic threshold.[34] Training for 40 weeks at the anaerobic threshold (80 to 85% VO_2max, 1 h/day, 3 days/week) resulted in pronounced increases in the anaerobic threshold, maximal working capacity at 80 to 85% VO_2max, and net efficiency of muscular work. However, there was no significant increase in VO_2max.[36]

According to differences in anaerobic and aerobic training effects, the anaerobic threshold constituted $65.9 \pm 0.3\%$ of VO_2max in swimmers-sprinters, compared to $90.4 \pm 0.1\%$ in swimmers-skiers.[37] The specificity of the training effect on the anaerobic threshold was confirmed in various studies.[31,36,38] In case of a similar training protocol, running resulted in large improvements in the anaerobic threshold for both cycling and running, with a larger improvement in the running anaerobic threshold. Cyclic training resulted in an improvement in the cycling anaerobic threshold with no change in the running anaerobic threshold[39] (Figure 6-3).

EXERCISE ECONOMY

The increased oxidative capacity of working muscles warrants a possibility of utilizing a smaller fraction of it for performance of exercises of moderate intensity. Accordingly, it is affirmed that successful distance running is dependent on the economical utilization of a highly developed aerobic capacity and the ability to employ a large fraction of that capacity with minimal accumulation of lactic acid.[40] This specific effect of training has been considered in a number of papers, and its significance for endurance performance has been confirmed.[9,41-50] Among Sweden's best runners the lowest VO_2 during running at 15 m·h^{-1} was found in those who were specialized for 10,000 m or marathon[67] (Figure 6-2). However, in a number of studies no good accordance was found between running economy and endurance performance.[10,16,51] In female athletes correlation coefficients between the running pace for 5 km, 10 km, and 10 mile distances on the one hand, and maximal oxygen uptake, speed at 2.0, as well as at 4.0 mmol·l^{-1} of plasma lactate, on the other hand, ranged between 0.84 and 0.94. The oxygen costs of running at each of the three distances moderately correlated with the pace of each race (r = –0.40 to 0.63).[52]

Exercise economy and correspondingly the employed fractions of aerobic capacity are specifically related to training exercises in two ways: (1) the specific effect of exercises on the oxidative enzymes of related muscles, and (2) the specific improvement of muscle coordination that warrants the more accomplished biomechanical utilization of muscle forces and thereby, an increased mechanical efficiency.

MAXIMAL OXYGEN UPTAKE

An integral index of the aerobic capacity of the organism is maximal oxygen uptake. This index only partly depends on the oxidative capacity of muscles. VO_2max depends also on oxygen binding in erythrocytes. Moreover, fundamental studies have established that VO_2max is mainly set by cardiovascular determinants.[5,53-58]

It is possible to find a great number of studies indicating the relation of individual VO_2max values to endurance performance (for instance, Reference 59-68). The high performance capacity in sprint, power, strength, and skill events is not related to VO_2max. The usual finding in endurance athletes is that the longer the main distance, the higher is the maximal oxygen uptake (Figure 6-2). In this regard an exception is revealed when marathon runners are compared with runners of 5000 to 10,000 m.[67] However, changes in running performance with training may occur without equivalent changes in VO_2max.[69]

VO_2max was found to be a good interpreter of endurance performance when a heterogenous group of persons with quite different athletic abilities were studied.[26,40,51,61,70-76] However, it is a relatively poor predictor when athletes of similar ability are evaluated.[16,48,61,66,76] When two athletes with the same VO_2max were compared, the runner with a higher running economy was faster.[77] Cases are possible where runners with quite different VO_2max values have the same running ability.[69] It was also found that in runners with the best marathon result, within 2 h 30 min to 2 h 35 min, running economy was quite different, and in runners with similar VO_2max values of 65 to 71 $ml \cdot min^{-1} \cdot kg^{-1}$, the best marathon result ranged from 3 h 12 min to 2 h 8 min.[69]

Furthermore, the factor predicting endurance performance may be related to 'muscle power', measured as the peak workload reached during maximum treadmill running[78] or isokinetic muscle power measured in swimmers.[79] A relationship was found between VO_2max and total work output during maximal isokinetic exercise of 30 s duration.[80] However, a question remains whether the increased 'muscle power' is a result of specific aerobic exercises, or whether special exercises are necessary for developing 'muscle power'. Strength training in prepubertal boys[81] as well as sprint training in rats[82] increased VO_2max without increasing muscle oxidative capacity. These findings were explained on the basis of training-induced increases in muscle power, enabling exercise at higher work loads.[76] This explanation disagrees with the main role of the heart and the circulating function limiting VO_2max. Both strength and sprint training are also ineffective in increasing the functional capacity of the cardiovascular system (see below). However, these results agree with the suggestion that the possibilities for oxygen transport system can be measured only in sufficiently intense exercises.

The highest peak VO_2 for each athlete was measured in performing the exercise for which he was specifically trained.[83]

The 'specificity of training' concept has been supported by researchers on training-induced changes in VO_2max measured in various exercises. Significant differences were found when VO_2max was compared in running vs. swimming,[84,85] running vs. cycling,[86,87] running vs. rowing,[88] and kayaking vs. cycling.[89] The specificity of training response appears also to be present in regard to muscle groups utilized in training vs. test exercises.[90] The comparison of training on a standard swim-bench pulley system and swim training supports the specificity of aerobic improvement with training and suggests that local adaptations significantly contribute to improvement in peak VO_2.[91]

A specific effect of aerobic endurance training may be not only the improvement of maximal aerobic power, measured as VO_2max, but also increased capacity to perform prolonged aerobic exercise (maximal aerobic capacity). Aerobic training during a 20-week period enhanced the mean maximal aerobic power by 33% and maximal aerobic capacity by 51%. The latter was computed as the total work output accomplished during a 90-min maximal ergocycle test.[92]

Cycling exercises lasting 18 weeks and performed 3 times weekly increased maximal oxygen uptake both in case of 25-min exercise at 80 to 85% VO_2max and in case of 50-min exercise at 45% VO_2max.[93] Thus, VO_2max increases as a result of exercise performed at levels both above and below the anaerobic threshold. When 8-week training was performed with continuous running[94,95] or aerobic gymnastics[96] at intensities causing increases in heart rate up

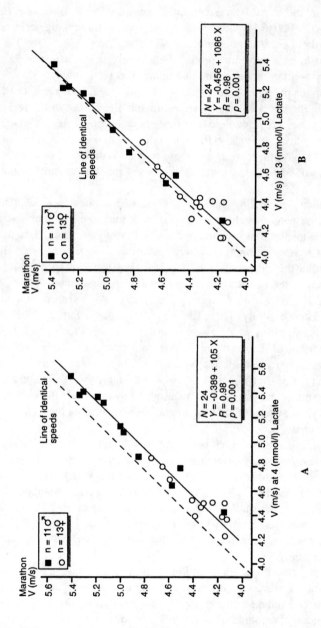

FIGURE 6-1. Correlations of the marathon velocity with running velocities at lactate levels of 4 mmol·l⁻¹ (A), 3 mmol·l⁻¹ (B), and 2.5 mmol·l⁻¹ (C), determined in the incremental field test in female (open circles) and male (closed circles) runners. (D) Individual lactate-running velocity relationship in female (open symbols) and male (closed symbols) marathon runners. The average marathon velocity (vertical arrows) corresponds to the lactate-running velocity relationship determined in the incremental field test in the range 2 to 3 mmol·l⁻¹ lactate. (From Mader, A., *J. Sports Med. Phys. Fitness*, 31, 1, 1991, With permission.)

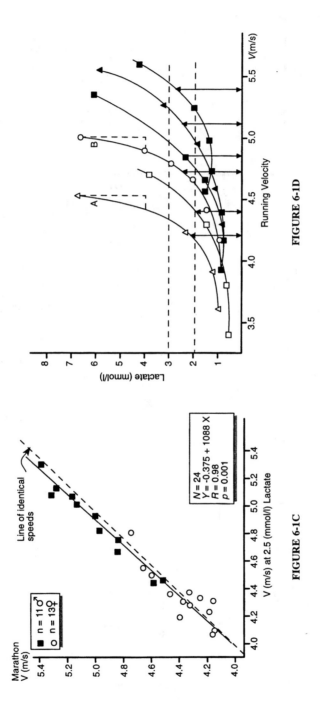

FIGURE 6-1D

FIGURE 6-1C

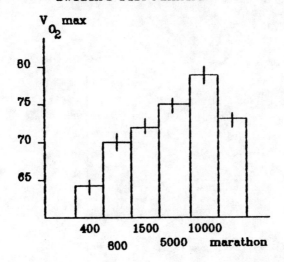

Sweden's best runners

	n	The personal best	
		mean	limits
400 m	2	46.96	45.63—48.33
800 m	6	1.46.41	1.47.64—1.50.42
800—1500 m	5	1.49.68	1.49.07—1.50.66
		3.41.86	3.38.51—3.46.43
1500—5000 m	6	3.44.7	3.41.9—3.48.1
		13.56.6	13.57.1—14.00.4
5000—10000	5	13.49.9	13.44.7—13.59.1
		26.57.9	28.36.6—29.21.0
1000-marathon	5	29.22.7	26.56.6—29.48.8
		2.16.18	2.12.07—2.21.04

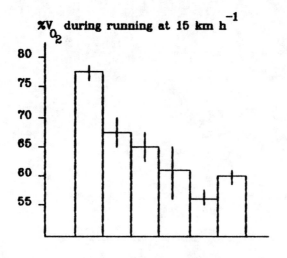

FIGURE 6-2 (left)

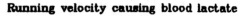

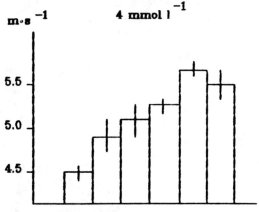

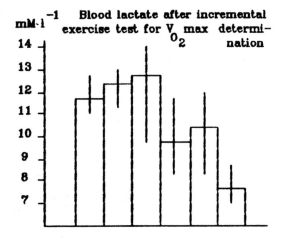

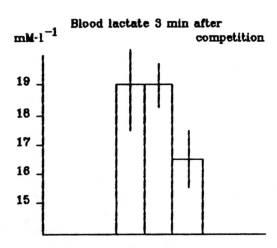

FIGURE 6-2. VO$_2$max, % VO$_2$max during swimming at 15 km·h^{-1}, running velocity causing a blood lactate level of 4 mmol·l^{-1} and blood lactate levels after incremental test exercise for VO$_2$max determination, blood lactate levels at the finish of competition in best Swedish runners. Constructed by results of J. Svedenhag and B. Sjödin.[67]

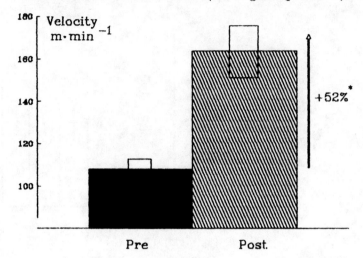

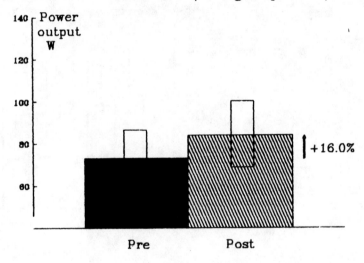

FIGURE 6-3. Effect of 10 weeks (four training sessions per week) of aerobic training in running or in cycling on the lactate threshold determined by incremental exercises on treadmill or on bicycle ergometer. Mean ± SEM are indicated. Asterisk denotes statistically significant difference between pre- and post-training values. Constructed by results of E.F. Pierce et al.[39]

to 140 to 150 or 165 to 175 beats/min, significant increases in VO_2max were found at both intensities of aerobic gymnastics and at the higher running intensity. Running training at the lower intensity as well as anaerobic exercise regimes (interval running or aerobic gymnastics with periodic use of exercises of anaerobic intensities) were ineffective. However, when the training program consisted of low- intensity continuous running during the first 3 weeks, then continuous running at a higher intensity (during 2 weeks) and finally 2 weeks of interval training, a significant increase was detected both in male[94] and female[97] university students. These results indicate: (1) the existence of optimal limits of exercise intensity for improvement of VO_2max, and (2) that anaerobic regimes of exercises are effective only after prior 'preparation' with the help of aerobic exercises. Further, it was found that female students with low initial values of VO_2max (25 ± 3.5 ml·min^{-1}·kg^{-1}) exhibited a greater increase in aerobic

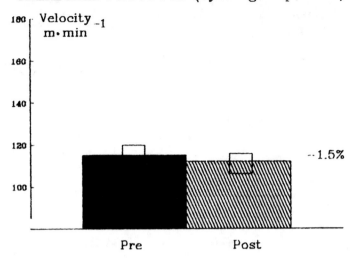

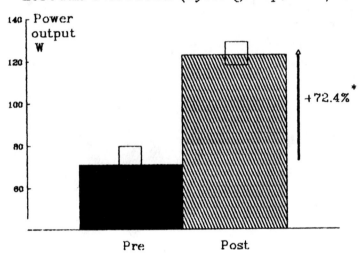

FIGURE 6-3 (continued).

power than those with higher initial values (32 ± 1.6 ml·min^{-1}·kg^{-1}). In a group with the initial level of VO$_2$max of 38 ± 2.5 ml·min^{-1}·kg^{-1} the training regime used was ineffective.[97]

A number of studies indicate the effectiveness of interval training for improvement of VO$_2$max. Obviously, the exercise intensities used and the previous fitness level of the persons were in necessary accordance. It was established that in anaerobic interval training the exercise intensity, rather than the distance, is the most important factor in improving VO$_2$max.[98,99] The gains in VO$_2$max were independent of training frequency both in men[100] and women.[101] During a 2-month interval training period (three times per week) VO$_2$max increased. The training regimes based on 3-min periods were more effective than 15-s periods.[102] Interval training programs lasting 8 weeks (3 days/week) induced equal increases in VO$_2$max for 30-s runs with 19 repetitions at treadmill speed of 15 to 17 km·h^{-1} or 120-s runs with 7 repetitions at 10 to 12 km·h^{-1} (incline 5 to 12° in both cases, rest intervals until heart rate decreased to 120 to 140 beats/min). In neither case were there changes in the amount of lactate accumulated in the blood during 4- to 8-min runs to exhaustion.[99,103] However, taking into consideration the experience of sports practice, there can be no doubt about the effect of interval training on

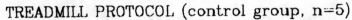

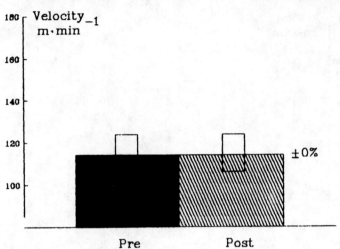

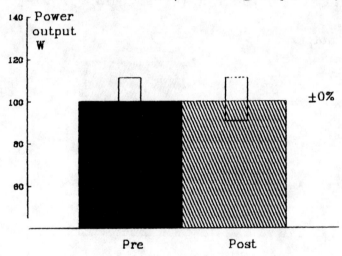

FIGURE 6-3 (continued).

capacity for anaerobic performance. In runners, an interval training period improved the results in middle-distance more than other tools improved endurance.[104,105] Increases in blood lactate levels up to 20 mmol·l[-1] or more and drops in pH to 7.0 during an interval training session evidence a great strain on anaerobic metabolism.[106,107] In turn, the lactate accumulation depends on the duration of both the exercise bout and the rest intervals between repetitions.[108]

Repeated uphill running gives a combined improvement of VO_2max, leg muscle power, and indices of anaerobic performance capacity.[109]

Endurance training effect on the maximal oxygen uptake was also confirmed in an experiment with rats.[110]

In contrast to aerobic and anaerobic endurance training, high-resistance strength training induces no increases in maximal oxygen uptake.[111] Olympic weight-lifters and body-builders show VO_2max values similar or slightly above those of untrained individuals.[60,112] Concurrent performance of endurance and resistive training does not affect the magnitude of increase in aerobic power induced by endurance training only.[111,113,114] The situation may change in two cases: (1) when moderate resistance exercises are repeated over a prolonged period with short rest intervals between repetitions, and (2) when very intensive resistance exercises are used.

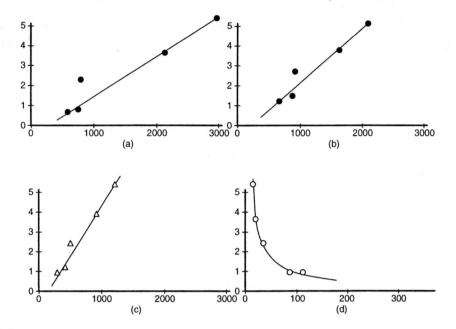

FIGURE 6-4. Dependence of VO$_2$max improvement (ml·min^{-1}·kg^{-1}) on volume of various training exercises per year in km. A — total volume of running exercises, B — volume of aerobic exercises, C — volume of aerobic-anaerobic exercises, D — volume of anaerobic exercises. Constructed by N. Volkov. (Human Bioenergetics in Strenuous Muscular Activity and Pathways of Improved Performance in Sportsmen, Anokin Res. Inst. Normal Physiol., Moscow, 1990).

In the latter case an increase in the blood lactate concentration up to 13[115] or 16 to 17 mmol·l^{-1} [116] was observed. However, 16 weeks of high-intensity, variable-resistance strength training did not change either VO$_2$max or hemodynamic responses to submaximal exercise. Muscle strength increased by 44% in one study.[115] Probably, to improve VO$_2$max, a considerable exercise duration and a sufficient intensity is necessary. Accordingly, the lack of effect of strength as well as sprint training can be explained by insufficient duration of exercise influence (exercise time plus recovery time at high oxygen uptake level).

In runners the VO$_2$max improvement correlated with the total volume of running exercises, the volume of aerobic exercises, as well as with the volume of anaerobic exercises during a training year. The relationship between VO$_2$max improvement and the volume of anaerobic exercises was inverted (Figure 6-4).

In any case, highly qualified decathlonists exhibited a VO$_2$max level of 55 ± 1.3 ml·min^{-1}·kg^{-1},[117] which is higher than usually found in power athletes.

Only minimal increases in aerobic power[118] and in the oxidative potential of the muscle cell[119] were found as a result of ice hockey training. When maximal or submaximal cycling was employed in hockey players, no training-induced alterations were found except for a reduced heart rate during submaximal cycling.[118] Thus, the adaptation process possesses specific peculiarities also in the case of ice hockey training.

SPECIFICITY OF TRAINING EFFECTS ON THE CARDIOVASCULAR SYSTEM: HEART HYPERTROPHY

The effect of endurance training is pronounced in regard to adaptive change in the structure and function of organs of the functional system responsible for oxygen intake and transport. As was affirmed by E.A. Newsholme,[121] except only for the 100-m sprint, it is enormously advantageous from a metabolic point of view to increase the blood flow to the working muscles.

Since the accurate chest percussion studies from the end of last century,[122] enlargement of the heart is known as a typical result of endurance training. Subsequent X-ray studies confirmed this fact.[123-130] The background for heart enlargement in endurance sportsmen is both myocardial hypertrophy as well as increase in heart cavities. Three variants of heart dilation were discriminated: (1) myogenic dilation due to damages in the myocardium, (2) tonogenic dilation caused by loss in myocardial tone, and (3) regulative dilation, expressed by low myocardial tone in the resting state and by high contractility and tone of myocardium in a strain situation caused by exercise or other factors.[127,128] The latter variant is the usual result of endurance training.[127,131] An expression of regulative dilation is the augmented residual blood volume in the heart during resting conditions and its almost maximal utilization for the increased stroke volume during exercise.[128,131] In the resting state, endurance athletes revealed a 3:1 ratio between residual and stroke volumes.[127]

In sprinters, field athletes, gymnasts, and fencers the heart volume, estimated from X-ray pictures, is close to values in untrained persons.[127,128,130] Heart enlargement was found in weight-lifters. However, differently from endurance athletes the enlargement was mainly on account of the right ventricle in these cases. More than half a century ago it was assumed that the increase in the right heart ventricle is caused by exercises connected with short-term but intensive muscular effort and with respiration stop in the inspiration phase.

An enlarged heart in endurance athletes was confirmed by autopsy material of sportsmen who had perished in accidents. Both increased volume of heart cavities and heart weight were detected. However, only in a single case did the weight of an athlete's heart exceed 500 g.[128] This heart mass was considered to be critical; larger human hearts were associated with cardiovascular efficiency.[132] Accordingly, myocardial fibers thickness of over 20 μm was considered to be critical.[133]

After 16 weeks of swim training the maximal duration of swimming was shorter in rats with an increase in heart mass by 18% or more, in comparison with rats who exhibited a less pronounced cardiac hypertrophy.[134]

A comprehensive study of training-induced cardiac hypertrophy showed that endurance exercises induced an increase in the diameter as well as cross-sectional area of myocardial fibers from both the left and right ventricles of the dog heart. This change was associated with an augmentation of the number of capillaries per myocardial fiber.[135] Instead of the increase in the number of myocardial fibers found in rats,[136] in dogs a slight decrease was observed.[135] In rats heart hypertrophy was also associated with an increased amount of sarcoplasma in individual myocardial fibers.[136] A 7% increase in heart weight with endurance training in rats was accompanied by a slight increase in sarcomere length and compositional changes in the sarcolemma.[137]

The increased capillarity and capillary-to-fiber ratio in the myocardium of endurance-trained animals has been evidenced by results of various studies.[138-143] Increased capillary diffusion capacity,[144] precapillary vascularity[145] and total size of the coronary tree,[146,147] development of extra coronary colletrals,[148,149] and increased coronary artery lumina[148] have also been found.

When heart rate, afterloads, and perfusion pressure were all kept constant in isolated hearts, the coronary blood flow was much greater in the hearts from trained animals. The coronary blood flow increased with a rise in heart rate in trained hearts, but not in hearts from untrained rats.[150]

A further specification of training effects on the human heart became possible with the use of the echocardiographic method. Cross-sectional echocardiographic studies demonstrated larger right[151-153] and left ventricular diameters[154-156] and calculated left ventricular masses[154-158] in endurance athletes as compared to sedentary persons.

Different patterns of left ventricular hypertrophy exist among different types of athletes, with mainly increased wall thickness in athletes trained primarily with static exercises (wrestlers) and increased volume in dynamically trained athletes (runners).[154,159]

In contrast, in regard to an old opinion, the echocardiographic studies show that resistance training increases absolute left ventricular wall thickness and left ventricular mass.[156,160,161] These increases are not as evident when expressed relative to body surface or lean body mass.[162,163] There is little or no change in the left ventricular internal dimensions in absolute terms or relative to body surface area,[163] resting heart rate and blood pressure,[156,160,164-166] and diastolic dimensions of the left ventricle[163,165,167] due to resistance training. No changes or slight positive effects are noted in systolic function of the left ventricle with strength training.[160,162,165,167] A group of nationally ranked U.S. weight-lifters had normal left ventricular mass/volume ratios in spite of an increased septal/free wall ratio.[162]

In long-distance runners and cycle racers the left ventricular mass is significantly increased as compared to sedentary subjects.[168] This resulted from thickening of the intraventricular septum and the left ventricular posterior wall as well as from enlargement of the left ventricular internal diameter.[168,169] Although the left ventricular wall was enlarged in weight-lifters, their left ventricular mass was not significantly increased as compared to sedentary persons.[168]

A study of 7- to 16-year-old boys showed that endurance training resulted in an increased volume of the left ventricle and stroke volume in association with a slight increase in the thickness of ventricular walls. Training in power events induced a pronounced myocardial hypertrophy, but changes in the left ventricular volume and stroke volume were insignificant.[170]

In adolescent boys VO$_2$max increased significantly together with a slight enlargement of calculated left ventricular mass as a result of endurance training. In a group that underwent sprint training these changes were insignificant. In a strength-trained group a less pronounced increase was found in the left ventricular mass in combination with a pronounced rise in muscular strength.[171]

In endurance-trained female athletes the aerobic capacities were 30 to 40% greater than in sedentary subjects. The athletes also exhibited trends toward higher left ventricular end-diastolic dimensions and volumes, stroke volume, left ventricular mass, and left atrial dimensions when data were standardized for body surface area.[172]

J. Morganroth et al.[154] considered the training effect on the heart in power athletes a concentric hypertrophy, as opposed to 'pure dilation' in endurance athletes, in regard to the increased pressure work during static or power exercises and to the predominant volume work during dynamic exercises, respectively. However, R. Rost[173] did not confirm concentric hypertrophy in power athletes. He found only some examples of such hypertrophy in power athletes, but for an unknown reason this could also be found in endurance athletes. He assumed that cardiac hypertrophy takes place in a uniform way as eccentric hypertrophy. The differences between the hearts of sportsmen of various events are only quantitative, according to his data. A common result of many years of training is the increased volume of the left ventricle at the end of diastole during exercise.[174]

According to the generalization by J. Keul and collaborators,[175] as a result of dynamic endurance training the reduction in the sympathoadrenal drive causes a decrease in heart rate, blood pressure, contractility, and oxygen and substrate consumption. The diastolic filling velocity accelerates and stroke volume increases. As a result of growth processes, the heart enlarges. These changes are the prerequisites for a high increase in cardiac output, and a higher efficiency of heart work can be achieved (Figure 6-5). As a result of strength training the muscle mass of the heart increases at the expense of the heart cavities. Cardiac output does not increase, and neither does the sympatho-adrenergic drive.

A study of arm vs. leg training indicated that in cardiovascular adaptation, specific and general training effects can be discriminated. The central circulatory function (stroke volume) plays a more dominant role in arm exercise after training, suggesting that the metabolic and circulatory responses during arm work become more like the responses observed during leg work.[176]

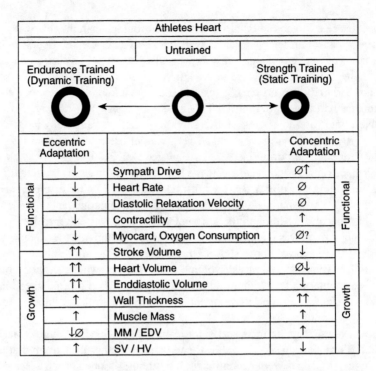

FIGURE 6-5. A schematized summary of the development of the athlete's heart. The modification to exercise is at first a functional one, followed by growth. As a result of the reduced sympathetic drive in endurance trained athletes the heart rate, the contractility, and the myocardial oxygen consumption all decrease; the diastolic filling velocity accelerates, and the stroke volume is moderately increased. These values remain unchanged as a result of static training, or even develop in the opposite direction. Growth, as a result of dynamic training, leads to an increase in the heart volume, the end diastolic volume and the muscle mass, at the expense of the end diastolic volume. In this way there is a favorable influence on the relationship of the muscle mass to the end diastolic volume, and the stroke volume to the heart volume in endurance trained athletes. Static training, on the other hand, has a negative effect on these relationships. (From Keul, J., Dickhuth, H.-H. Lehmann, M., and Staiger, J., Int. J. Sports Med., 3 (Suppl. 1), 33, 1982. With permission.)

Against the background of the results of echocardiographic studies, it was necessary to reevaluate the standpoint on the critical size of the athlete's heart. Corresponding analysis led to the conclusion that the physiological heart hypertrophy as a healthy process always remains within restricted borderlines. Even in a very early onset of top training in childhood, the limits of physiological hypertrophy are maintained. However, in contrast to the old hypothesis of 'critical heart size', the maximum of physiological hypertrophy cannot be considered a really critical limit: it seems to be an individual rather than absolute parameter, depending on the athlete's body size and heredity.[173] In regard to the body size, a relative maximum critical heart weight of 7.5 g·kg^{-1} b.w. was suggested.[177]

Myocardial hypertrophy is not an unavoidable result of endurance or other kinds of exercise training. For example, in a study of 271 members of the Italian Olympic Team, pronounced heart hypertrophy was detected only in 23 sportsmen (9 cyclists, 9 rowers, 2 basketball players, 1 volleyball player, and 2 weight-lifters).[178] More than 10 years ago it was concluded that the large heart of athletes is mainly caused genetically or by intensive training from an early age.[179]

CARDIAC PERFORMANCE

Endurance training increases the cardiac performance in both humans[180-183] and test animals.[184-186] The major adaptation to endurance training is the generation of a greater stroke volume at any given level of exercise as well as a greater maximal stroke volume (Figure 6-6).

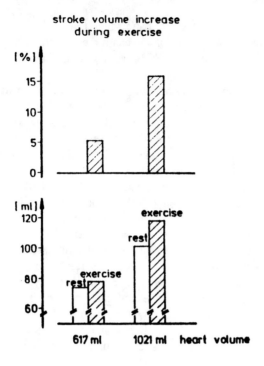

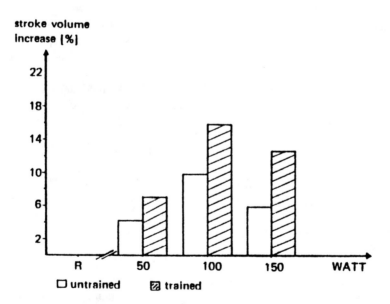

FIGURE 6-6. Stroke volume increase during exercise in untrained persons and in athletes. On the upper panel the stroke volume increase in sportsmen possessing enlarged athlete's heart is compared to the volume in untrained persons. On the lower panel the stroke volume increase during an incremental exercise is shown in untrained persons and trained subjects who have not increased the size of the heart. Constructed by J. Keul et al.[175]

This adaptation has been attributed to the Frank-Starling mechanism resulting from an increased end-diastolic volume, as well as from cardiac hypertrophy. In regard to the first mechanism, it was indicated that the larger stroke volume of the trained heart is related to the increase in blood volume,[187] actually caused by endurance training.[188,189] An experimental expansion of plasma volume by infusion of dextran solution increased the stroke volume by

11%. Any further increase in the volume of the circulating blood did not cause additional increase in stroke volume.[190] However, the stroke volume can increase with training without any increase in the heart or central blood volume.[191,192] This is accomplished by increasing the contractility of the myocardium to decrease the end-systolic volume.

The endurance-training effect on the myocardium contractility is proved in various kinds of experiments. The active tension is much greater in the strips of columna carnae taken from trained hearts.[193,194] Experiments on isolated papillary muscle preparation confirmed the training-induced improvement of the myocardial function.[195] Several studies have demonstrated an increase in the intrinsic contractile performance of isolated perfused hearts taken from exercise-trained rats as compared to untrained animals.[186,196,197] In the rat heart isolated after training with daily running, the increase in heart mass by 14% was accompanied by increases in maximal stroke volume (+67%), maximal stroke work (+111%), and in maximal power output by the left ventricle (+112%). However, in hearts exceeding the heart mass of sedentary animals by 30%, the maximal stroke volume was increased by only 45%, and maximal power output by the left ventricle by 36%.[198] Further experiments on isolated working heart preparations indicated increase with training in percent changes of systolic pressure, stroke work, ejection fraction, circumferential shortening velocity, and relaxation rate working at 20 cm H_2O of the atrial pressure.[199] The contractile performance appeared to be in relation with the magnitude of coronary blood flow generated by the preparation.[200] In a study, no enhanced performance was found in the hearts of female rats conditioned by running.[201] The papillary muscle contractile responses to calcium, noradrenaline, or hypoxia were not altered by training.[202]

Relatively small differences were seen in the left ventricular performance in trained and untrained animals investigated *in situ* under a variety of conditions such as increased afterload and/or inotropy stimulation.[203-206] However, the systolic tension at any given diastolic tension was greater in rats trained by swimming.[207] The maximal velocity of shortening is also increased in the trained myocardium.[194,198]

In dogs, endurance training improved the stroke volume potential in association with increased left ventricular relaxation rate.[208-210] In rats, training enhanced VO_2max by 16 to 20% on the background of an increase in stroke volume (11%) and O_2 extraction (8%).[211]

CONTRACTILE MECHANISM OF THE MYOCARDIUM

The ATPase activity of myosin,[212-215] actomyosin,[211,212] and myofibrils[215,216] is increased by 15 to 30% in male rats conditioned by swimming for 8 to 18 weeks. In female rats the response is similar, but its magnitude is not so great as compared to the results on male rats.[215] Significant changes were not found in a study.[217] The increase in ATPase activity has been attributed to conformational changes in the heavy meromyosin component of the myosin molecule.[214,218,219]

In contrast to swimming training there is a relatively small increase in ATPase activity of the cardiac contractile proteins of rodents in response to endurance treadmill running.[220,221] In some studies no changes in ATPase were detected after running training in rats,[217,222-224] dogs,[208,225] or guinea pigs.[204] In a study, a decrease in myosin ATPase activity was found in female rats after a running training.[204] On the other hand, a high-intensity interval running program resulted in a 15% increase in myofibrillar ATPase activity.[223]

The cardiac muscle can express three different isoforms of myosin. The predominance of the V_3 isoform has been associated with greater cross-bridge cycling economy at the expense of contraction intensity, whereas the predominance of the V_1 isoform has been associated with less economical but intensive contractions.[215] In running training of rats the myosin isozyme profile indicates a modest conversion to greater V_1 predominance.[214,216] The shift in isozyme forms induced with swimming is mediated through thyroid hormone influence, because the alteration was blocked in swim-trained, thyroid-deficient rats.[214] Controversially, endurance running training induced a greater V_3 expression without a compromise in exercise capacity.[226,227] It is noteworthy that this adaptation was enhanced if the involvement of the sympathetic nervous system was severely reduced by sympathectomy. At the same time, the maximal exercise capacity of trained sympathectomized rats was increased even though 50% of the cardiac myosin expressed in these animals was V_3. These changes were associated with reduction in the specific activity of myofibrillar Ca-ATPase and myosin Ca-ATPase.[227,228]

It was found that myosin light chain phosphorylation decreased the ATPase activity of cardiac myofibrils[229] and increased the myosin affinity for actin.[230] These findings suggest a possible link between myosin phosphorylation and the level of mechanical activity of the heart.[227] Further, it was demonstrated that training induced alterations in cardiac sarcolemma composition and functional properties. As a result, an increased calcium influx appears, which can potentially enhance activation of the contractile machinery.[231] These adaptations can contribute to the higher level of cardiac performance that is achieved with training.

The maximal force of the papillary muscle, studied *in vitro* as a function of external calcium concentration, improved in female rats with running training in association with decreased affinity of calcium binding sites on the sarcolemmal membrane.[231] The specific content of sarcolemmal phosphatidyl serine (a sarcolemmal phospholipid, critical for sarcolemmal calcium binding moiety) increased by approximately 50% in the trained myocardium.[232] These data provide a possible mechanism by which more externally bound calcium could be made available to the interior of the cell during the action potential.[215]

The cardiac sarcoplasmic reticulum has a greater capacity to sequester and bind calcium in swim-trained vs. control rats.[217,224] However, calcium sequestering and binding capacity of the cardiac sarcoplasmic reticulum did not improve after running training.[209,220] Within great limits of heart rate the heart of a trained rat exerts a greater level of left ventricular pressure than that of an untrained rat.[227] Consequently, adaptive mechanisms to economize cross-bridge cycling may be necessary to buffer the high degrees of contractile activation that can be achieved at high-intensity levels of exercise in the trained state.[227] In dogs, an improvement of the contractile state of myocardium occurred during exercise following training in spite of the lack of change in contractile protein ATPase.[208,210] Eleven weeks of progressive treadmill running for 1 h daily did not increase the concentration of myofibrillar protein, nor the myofibrillar ATPase activity. The time course of isometric twitch of the papillary muscle did not change. However, tension output per unit area increased and this appeared to be due to a greater amount of Ca^{2+} being made available to the contractile apparatus.[233] In the context of the specificity of training effects, it is important to emphasize that in this experiment as well as in other investigations[222,223,234] the use of similar training programs did not produce marked degrees of cardiac hypertrophy. Consequently, there are two versions of heart adaptation to training. One of them is connected with myocardial hypertrophy. In rats this version appears mainly as a result of swimming training. The other version of cardiac adaptation is connected to adjustments that do not necessarily include heart muscle hypertrophy, increased amount of contractile protein, and elevated activity of ATPase in myofibrils. The other version of adaptation is revealed mainly as a result of running training and seems to be related to adjustment on the level of intracellular Ca^{2+} metabolism. At the same time these training programs induce a pronounced enhancement of oxidation potential in skeletal muscles.[233] In dogs also, running training increased the maximal rate of the left ventricular pressure development but not the content of myofibrillar proteins and ATPase activity.[208]

ENERGETICS OF THE MYOCARDIUM

With the exception of some earlier studies,[235,236] a common result is that neither endurance nor other kinds of training increase the amount of cardiac mitochondrial protein per gram wet tissue or the activity of mitochondrial enzymes.[223,237-242] In rats the activity of oxidation enzymes increased neither with swimming nor running training. In the untrained organism the oxidative capacity of the heart already exceeds that of the oxidative skeletal muscles by approximately three times.[243] With training, the skeletal muscle can approximately double its oxidative capacity (see above), while that of the heart remains unaffected under intense training regimes.[223,227] It is suggested that the myocardial mitochondria is chronically maintained in a maximal 'up-regulated' state. This property permits the heart to maintain a positive energy balance in the face of a constantly changing availability of substrates. Hence, the endurance training effect on skeletal muscle mitochondria implies the reduction of differences between skeletal and heart muscles' oxidative capacities. In regard to the heart muscle, it was assumed that training induced a proportional increase in myofibrillar and mitochondrial protein.[239-241] Moreover, endurance training normalizes the decrement in mitochondria-to-myofibril volume ratio, seen with pressure-overload hypertrophy.[244]

In mice, endurance training induced a stable cardiac hypertrophy (by 6 to 7%), but not changes in the activities of myocardial actomyosin ATPase, citrate synthase, succinate dehydrogenase, cytochrome c oxidase, malate dehydrogenase, and adenylate kinase. β-Gluceronidase activity increased by 20–25%.[245]

The myocardial lactate dehydrogenase activity may increase with endurance training.[246] However, it is not a common result.[247] Training does not affect the activities of phosphofructokinase,[223] glyceraldehyde-3-phosphate dehydrogenase, adenylate kinase, or creatine kinase[238] in the heart.

No significant difference was found in the mechanical efficiency of isolated hearts obtained from trained and untrained rats.[196] Training did not change the ATP/O ratio of mitochondria obtained from the myocardium.[239] Calculations made on the basis of recording the blood pressure contour in the axillary artery (diastolic pressure time index, tension time index) during a progressive multi-stage treadmill test, led to the conclusion that in humans, jogging training reduces myocardial O_2 demands, increases potential O_2 supply, and improves the supply/demand balance at any submaximal workload together with the increase of the whole body working capacity.[248]

At the same time endurance training suppresses the free radical oxidation of lipids. A prolonged swimming training program that caused a significant increase in cardiac weight, decreased activities of catalase in the right ventricle and in the subendo- and subepimyocardium. The activity of thioredoxin reductase decreased in each part of the myocardium and that of glutathione reductase in the right ventricle and in the subepimyocardium. The activity of glucose-6-phosphate dehydrogenase increased and the activity of glutathione peroxidase as well as the tissue content of carnosine and anserine and tissue sulphydryl groups remained unchanged. Only minor changes were found in the regional distribution of antioxidants.[249]

Coronary vasodilation during exercise can produce a three- to fivefold increase in coronary flow.[250,251] Even in strenuous exercise the myocardial oxygen delivery appears to be adequate and the existing flow reserve seems capable of handling the increased oxygen demand.[252] Correspondingly, the coronary flow reserve is not changed by chronic endurance exercise.[253,254] However, experiments on dogs indicated that endurance training significantly increases the coronary transport capacity. A 26 and 82% increase in maximal blood flow and capillary diffusion capacity, respectively, were detected.[255] There is also a difference between the effects of endurance and high-resistance training. Endurance-trained rats exhibited a higher left and total coronary cast weight when compared to either control or resistance-trained rats. In resistance-trained rats, a higher right coronary cast weight was observed in comparison with their sedentary counterparts.[145] It seems correct to conclude that exercises that substantially increase the cardiac output and coronary blood flow, stimulate a neovascular response, at least at the capillary level.[256,257]

Endurance training increases the glycogen store in the myocardium,[258,259] but no changes were found in the contents of phosphocreatine, ATP, ADP, and AMP.[259] Myocardial triglycerides[260] as well as phospholipids and cholesterol[259,260] did not alter with training.

ADDITIONAL ADAPTIVE CHANGES IN THE OXYGEN TRANSPORT SYSTEM

The adaptation to endurance exercises is also connected with an increased capillarization of the lung alveolus,[261] as well as changes in the respiratory muscles. In the diaphragm, activities of oxidation enzymes increase.[262,263] Increased glycogen content was found in type I and type IIb fibers of the diaphragm but not in type IIa.[263] Increased capillarization per area of muscle fiber was found in type IIb fibers of the diaphragm.[263] No changes in the oxidation enzymes were found in the intercostal muscles.[262] The activity of glycolytic enzymes remained without change.[262]

Endurance training stimulates erythropoietic processes in the bone marrow. This may be opposed by the 'sports anemia' related to plasma expansion, intensified hemolysis, iron deficiency, etc.[189]

REFERENCES

1. **Brooks, G.A.**, Anaerobic threshold: review of the concept and direction for further research, *Med. Sci. Sports Exerc.*, 17, 22, 1985.
2. **Heck, H., Mader, A., Hess, G., Mucke, S., Muller, R. and Hollmann, W.**, Justification of the 4 mmol/l lactate threshold, *Int. J. Sports Med.*, 6, 117, 1985.
3. **Sjøgaard, G.**, Muscle morphology and metabolic potential in elite road cyclists during a season, *Int. J. Sports Med.*, 5, 250, 1984.
4. **Hendriksson, J., and Reitman, J.S.**, Time course of changes in human skeletal muscle succinate dehydrogenase and cytochrome oxidase activity and maximal oxygen uptake with physical activity and inactivity, *Acta Physiol. Scand.*, 99, 91, 1977.
5. **Saltin, B., and Rowell, L.B.**, Functional adaptation to physical activity and inactivity, *Fed. Proc.*, 39, 1506, 1980.
6. **Londree, B.R., and Ames, S.A.**, Maximal steady state versus state of conditioning, *Eur. J. Appl. Physiol.*, 34, 269, 1975.
7. **MacDoughall, J.D.**, The anaerobic threshold: its significance for the endurance athlete, *Can. J. Appl. Sports Sci.*, 2, 130, 1977.
8. **Weltman, A., Natch, V., Sady, S., and Freeson, P.**, Onset of metabolic acidosis (anaerobic threshold) as a criterion measure of submaximum fitness, *Res. Q.*, 49, 117, 1978.
9. **Farrell, P.A., Wilmore, J.H., Coyle, E.F., Billing, J.E., and Costill, D.L.**, Plasma lactate accumulation and distance running performance, *Med. Sci. Sports*, 11, 338, 1979.
10. **LaFontaine, T.P., Londeree, B.R., and Spath, W.K.**, The maximal steady state versus selected running events, *Med. Sci. Sports Exerc.*, 13, 190, 1981.
11. **Sjödin, B., and Jacobs, I.**, Onset of blood lactate accumulation and marathon running performance, *Int. J. Sports Med.*, 2, 23, 1981.
12. **Kumagai, S., Tanaka, K., Matsuura, Y., Matsuzaka, A., Hirakoba, K., and Asano, K.**, Relationships of the anaerobic threshold with the 5 km, 10 km and 10 miles races, *Eur. J. Appl. Physiol.*, 49, 13, 1982.
13. **Tanaka, K., Matsuura, Y., Kumagai, S., Matsuzaka, A., Hironaba, K., and Asno, K.**, Relationships of anaerobic threshold and onset of blood lactate accumulation with endurance performance, *Eur. J. Appl. Physiol.*, 52, 51, 1983.
14. **Tanaka, K., and Matsuura, Y.**, Marathon performance, anaerobic threshold and onset of blood lactate accumulation, *J. Appl. Physiol.*, 57, 640, 1984.
15. **Rhodes, E., and McKenzie, D.**, Predicting marathon time from anaerobic threshold measurements, *Physician Sportmed.*, 19, 95, 1984.
16. **Sjödin, B., and Svedenhag, J.**, Applied physiology of marathon running, *Sports Med.*, 2, 83, 1985.
17. **Jacobs, I.**, Blood lactate: implication for training and sports performance, *Sports Med.*, 3, 10, 1986.
18. **Londeree, B.R.**, The use of laboratory test results with long distance runners, *Sports Med.*, 3, 201, 1986.
19. **Noakes, T.D.**, *Lore of Running*, Oxford University Press, Cape Town, 1986.
20. **Yoshida, T., Chida, M., Ichioka, M., and Sud, Y.**, Blood lactate parameters related to aerobic capacity and endurance performance, *Eur. J. Appl. Physiol.*, 56, 7, 1987.
21. **Aunola, S., Alanen, E., Marniemi, J., and Rusko, H.**, The relation between cycling time to exhaustion and anaerobic threshold, *Ergonomics*, 33, 1027, 1990.

22. **Heck, H.**, *Laktat in der Leistungsdiagnostik,* K. Hofmann Verlag, Schorndorf, 1990.

23. **Mader, A.**, Evaluation of the endurance performance of marathon runners and theoretical analysis of test results, *J. Sports Med. Phys. Fitness,* 31, 1, 1991.

24. **Föhrenbach, R., Mader, A., and Hollmann, W.**, Determination of endurance capacity and prediction of exercise intensity for training and competition in marathon runners, *Int. J. Sports Med.,* 8, 11, 1987.

25. **Magberg, J.M., and Coyle, E.F.**, Physiological determinants of endurance performance as studied in competitive race walkers, *Med. Sci. Sports Exerc.,* 15, 287, 1983.

26. **Farrell, P.A., Wilmore, J.H., Coyle, E.F., Billing,. J.L., and Costill, D.L.**, Plasma lactate accumulation and distance running performance, *Med. Sci. Sports Exerc.,* 11, 338, 1979.

27. **Sjödin, B.**, Anaerobic function, *Sport Sci. Rev.,* 1, 13, 1992.

28. **Mickelson, T.C., and Hagerman, F.C.**, Anaerobic threshold measurements of elite oarsmen, *Med. Sci. Sports Exerc.,* 14, 440, 1982.

29. **Kantola, H., and Rusko, H.**, *Sykettä Ladulle,* Valmennuskirjat Oy, Jyväskylä, 1985.

30. **Komi, P.V., Ito, A., Sjödin, B., Wallensstein, R., and Karlsson, J.**, Muscle metabolism, lactate breaking point, and biomechanical features of endurance running, *Int. J. Sports Med.,* 2, 148, 1981.

31. **Yoshida, T., Suda, Y., and Tunaichi, N.**, Endurance training regimes based upon arterial blood lactate: effects on anaerobic threshold, *Eur. J. Appl. Physiol.,* 49, 223, 1982.

32. **Kindermann, W., Simon, G., and Keul, J.**, The significance of the aerobic-anaerobic transition for the determination of work load intensities during endurance training, *Eur. J. Appl. Physiol.,* 42, 25, 1979.

33. **Verstappen, F.T.J., Janssen, G.M.E., and Does, R.J.M.M.**, Effects of endurance training and competition on exercise rest in relatively untrained people, *Int. J. Sports Med.,* 10 (Suppl. 3), S126, 1989.

34. **Henritze, J., Weltman, A., Schurrer, R., and Barlow, K.**, Effects of training at and above the lactate threshold on the lactate threshold and maximal oxygen uptake, *Eur. J. Appl. Physiol.,* 54, 84, 1985.

35. **Sjödin, B., Jacobs, I., and Svedenhag, J.**, Changes in onset of blood lactate accumulation (OBLA) and muscle enzymes after training at OBLA, *Eur. J. Appl. Physiol.,* 49, 45, 1989.

36. **Denis, C., Fouquet, R., Poty, P., Geyssant, A., and Lacour, J.R.**, Effect of 40 weeks of endurance training on the anaerobic threshold, *Int. J. Sports Med.,* 3, 208, 1982.

37. **Smith, B.W., McMurray R.G., and Symanski, J.D.**, A comparison of the anaerobic threshold of sprint and endurance trained swimmers, *J. Sports Med. Phys. Fitness,* 24, 94, 1984.

38. **Withers, R., Sherman, W., Miller, J., and Costill, D.**, Specificity of the anaerobic threshold in endurance trained cyclists and runners, *Eur. J. Appl. Physiol.,* 47, 93, 1981.

39. **Pierce, E.F., Weltman, A., Seip, R.L., and Snead, D.**, Effects of training specificity on the lactate threshold and VO_2 peak, *Int. J. Sports Med.,* 11, 267, 1990.

40. **Costill, D.L., Thomason, H., and Roberts, B.**, Fractional utilization of the aerobic capacity during distance running, *Med. Sci. Sports,* 5, 248, 1973.

41. **Costill, D.L., and Fox, E.L.**, Energetics of marathon running, *Med. Sci. Sports,* 1, 81, 1969.

42. **Costill, D.L.**, Physiology of marathon running, *JAMA,* 221, 1024, 1972.

43. **Brandsford, D.R., and Howley, E.T.**, Oxygen cost of running in trained and untrained men and women, *Med. Sci. Sports,* 9, 41, 1977.

44. **Daniels, J.T., Krahenbuhl, G., Foster, G., Gilbert, J., and Daniels, S.**, Aerobic responses of female distance runners to submaximal and maximal exercise, *Ann. N.Y. Acad. Sci.,* 301, 726,, 1977.

45. **Pollock, M.L.**, Submaximal and maximal working capacity of elite distance runners. Part 1. Cardiorespiratory aspects, *Ann. N.Y. Acad. Sci.,* 301, 310, 1977.

46. **Fox, E.L., and Costill, D.L.**, Estimated cardiorespiratory responses during marathon running, *Arch. Environ. Health,* 24, 316, 1978.

47. **Pollock, M., Jakcson, A.S., and Pate, R.R.**, Discriminary analysis of physiological differences between good and elite distance runners, *Res. Q. Exerc. Sport,* 51, 521, 1980.

48. **Conley, D.L., and Kranhenbuhl, G.S.**, Running economy and distance running performance, *Med. Sci. Sports Exerc.,* 12, 357, 1980.

49. **Conley, D.L.**, Percentage of maximal heart rate and distance running performance of highly trained athletes, *J. Sports Med. Phys. Fitness,* 21, 233, 1981.

50. **Daniels, J.T.A.**, A physiologist's view of running economy, *Med. Sci. Sports Exerc.,* 17, 332, 1985.

51. **Davies, C.T.M., and Thompson, M.W.**, Aerobic performance of female marathon and male ultramarathon athletes, *Eur. J. Appl. Physiol.,* 41, 233, 1979.

52. **Fay, L., Londree, B.R., LaFontaine, T.P., and Volek, M.R.**, Physiological parameters related to distance running performance in female athletes, *Med. Sci. Sports Exerc.,* 21, 319, 1989.

53. **Blomqvist, C.C., and Saltin, B.**, Cardiovascular adaptation to physical training, *Annu. Rev. Physiol.,* 45, 169, 1983.

54. **Anderson, P., and Saltin, B.**, Maximal perfusion of skeletal muscle in man, *J. Physiol.,* 336, 233, 1985.

55. **Nadel, E.R.**, Physiolgical adaptation to aerobic exercise, *Am. Sci.,* 73, 334, 1985.

56. **Ekblom, B.**, Factors determining maximal aerobic power, *Acta. Physiol. Scand.,* 128 (Suppl. 556), 15, 1986.

57. **Saltin, B.,** Maximal oxygen uptake: limitation and malleability, in *International Perspectives in Exercise Physiology*, Nazar, K., Terjung, R.L., and Budohoski, L., Eds., Human Kinetics Books, Champaign, 1990, 26.

58. **Saltin, B., and Strange, S.,** Maximal oxygen uptake: 'old and new' arguments for a cardiovascular limitation, *Med. Sci. Sports Exerc.*, 24, 30, 1992.

59. **Costill, D.L.,** The relationship between selected physiological variables and distance running performance, *J. Sports Med. Phys. Fitness*, 7, 61, 1967.

60. **Saltin, B., and Åstrand, P.O.,** Maximal oxygen uptake in athletes, *J. Appl. Physiol.*, 23, 353, 1967.

61. **Costill, D.L. and Winrow, E.,** Maximum oxygen intake among marathon runners, *Arch. Phys. Med. Rehab.*, 51, 317, 1970.

62. **Pärnat, J., Viru, A., Savi, T., and Nurmekivi, A.,** Indices of aerobic work capacity and cardio-vascular response during exercise in athletes specializing in different events, *J. Sports Med. Phys. Fitness*, 15, 100, 1975.

63. **Foster, C., Daniels, J.T., and Yarbrough, R.A.,** Physiological and training correlates of marathon running performance, *Aust. J. Sports Med.*, 9, 58, 1977.

64. **Rusko, H., Havu, M., and Karvinen, E.,** Aerobic performance capacity in athletes, *Eur. J. Appl. Physiol.*, 38, 151, 1978.

65. **Niinimaa, V., Dyon, M, and Shephard, R.J.,** Performance and efficiency of intercollegiate cross-country skiers, *Med. Sci. Sports*, 10, 91, 1978.

66. **Boileau, R.A., Mayhew, J.L., Reiner, W.F., and Lussier, L.,** Physiological characteristics of elite middle and long distance runners, *Can. J. Appl. Sports Sci.*, 7, 167, 1982.

67. **Svedenhag, J., and Sjödin, B.,** Maximal and submaximal oxygen uptakes and blood lactate levels in elite male middle- and long-distance runners, *Int. J. Sports Med.*, 5, 255, 1984.

68. **Pate, R.R., Sparling, P.B., Wilson, G.E., Cureton, K.J., and Miller, B.J.,** Cardiorespiratory and metabolic responses to submaximal and maximal exercise in elite women distance runners, *Int. J. Sports Med.,* 8 (Suppl. 2), 91, 1987.

69. **Daniels, J.T., Yarbrough, R.A., and Foster, C.,** Changes in VO_2max and running performance with training, *Eur. J. Appl. Physiol.*, 39, 249, 1978.

70. **Herbst, R.,** Der Gasstoffwechsel as Mass der Körperlichen Leistungsfähigkeit, *Dtsch. Arch. Klin. Med.*, 162, 33, 1928.

71. **Robinson, S., Edwards, H.T., and Dill, D.B.,** New records in human power, *Science*, 85, 409, 1937.

72. **Åstrand, P.-O.,** *Experimental Studies of Physical Work Capacity in Relation to Sex and Age,* Munkgaard, Copenhagen, 1952.

73. **Wyndham, C.N., Strydom, N.B., Rensburg van A.J., and Senade, A.J.S.,** Physiological requirements for world-class performances in endurance runners, *S. Afr. Med. J.*, 43, 996, 1989.

74. **Foster, C., Costill, D.L., Daniels, J.T., and Fink, W.J.,** Skeletal muscle enzyme activity, fiber composition and VO_2max in relation to distance running performance, *Eur. J. Appl. Physiol.*, 39, 73, 1978.

75. **Hagan, R.D., Smith, M.G., and Gettman, L.R.,** Marathon performance in relation to maximal aerobic power and training indices, *Med. Sci. Sports Exerc.*, 13, 185, 1981.

76. **Noakes, T.D.,** Implications of exercise testing for prediction of athletic performance: a contemporary perspective, *Med. Sci. Sports Exerc.*, 20, 319, 1988.

77. **Costill, D.L., and Winrow, E.,** A comparison of two middle-aged ultramarathon runners, *Res. Q. Exerc, Sport*, 41, 135, 1970.

78. **Scrimgeour, A.G., Noakes, T.D., Adams, B., and Myburgh, K.,** The influence of weekly training distance on fractional utilization of maximum aerobic capacity in marathon and ultramarathon runners, *Eur. J. Appl. Physiol.*, 55, 202, 1986.

79. **Sharp, R.L., Troup, J.F., and Costill, D.L.,** Relationship between power and sprint freestyle swimming, *Med. Sci. Sports Exerc.*, 14, 53, 1982.

80. **Jones, N.L., and McCartney, N.,** Influence of muscle power on aerobic performance and the effects of training, *Acta Med. Scand.*, 711, 115, 1986.

81. **Weltman, A., Janney, C., Rians, C.B., Strand, K., Berg, B., Tippitt, S., Wise, J., Cahill, B.R., and Katch, F.I.,** The effects of hydraulic resistance strength training in pre-pubertal males, *Med. Sci. Sports Exerc.*, 18, 629, 1986.

82. **Davies, K.J.A., Packer, L., and Brooks, G.A.,** Exercise bioenergetics following sprint training, *Arch. Biochem. Biophys.*, 215, 260, 1982.

83. **Strøme, S.B., Ingjer, F., and Meen, N.D.,** Assessment of maximal aerobic power in specifically trained athletes, *J. Appl. Physiol.*, 42, 833, 1977.

84. **Magel, J., Foglia, G., McArdle, W., Gutin, B., Pechar, G., and Katch, F.,** Specificity of swim training on maximum oxygen uptake, *J. Appl. Physiol.*, 38, 151, 1974.

85. **McArdle, W.D., Magel, J.R., Dello, D.J., Toner, M., and Chase, J.M.,** Specificity of run training on VO_2max and heart rate changes during running and swimming, *Med. Sci. Sports,* 10, 16, 1978.

86. **Pechar, G., McArdle, W., Katch, F., Magel, J., and DeLuca, J.,** Specificity of cardiorespiratory adaptation to bicycle treadmill training, *J. Appl. Physiol.*, 36, 753, 1974.

87. **Roberts, J., and Alspough, J.**, Specificity of training effects resulting from programs of treadmill running and bicycle ergometer riding, *Med. Sci. Sports*, 4, 6, 1972.
88. **Brouha, L.**, Training, in *Science and Medicine of Exercise and Sports,* Johnson, W., Ed., Harper & Row, New York, 1960.
89. **Ridge, B., Pyke, F., and Roberts, J.**, Responses to kayak ergometer performance after kayak and bicycle ergometer training, *Med. Sci. Sports*, 8, 18, 1976.
90. **Clausen, J., Lauson, K., Rasmussen, B., and Trap-Jensen, J.**, Central and peripheral circulatory changes after training of the arms or legs, *Am. J. Physiol.*, 225, 675, 1973.
91. **Gergley, T.J., McArdle, W.D., DeJesus, P., Toner, M.M., Jacobowitz, S., and Spino, R.J.**, Specificity of arm training on aerobic power during swimming and running, *Med. Sci. Sports Exerc.*, 16, 349, 1984.
92. **Lortie, G., Simoneuau, J.A., Hamel,. P., Boulay, M.R., Landry, F., and Bouchard, C.**, Responses of maximal aerobic power and capacity to aerobic training, *Int. J. Sports Med.*, 5, 232, 1984.
93. **Gaesser, G.A., and Rich, R.G.**, Effects of high- and low-intensity exercise training on aerobic capacity and blood lipids, *Med. Sci. Sports Exerc.*, 16, 269, 1974.
94. **Jürimäe, T., Viru, A., and Pedaste, J.**, Running training, physical working capacity and lipid and lipoprotein relationships in man, *Finn. Sports Exerc. Med.*, 3, 104, 1984.
95. **Jürimäe, T., Viru, A., Viru, E., and Peterson, T.**, Running training, physical working capacity and lipid and lipoprotein relationship in women, *Finn. Sports Exerc. Med.*, 3, 134, 1984.
96. **Jürimäe, T., Neissaar, I., and Viru, A.**, The effect of similar aerobic gymnastics and running programs on physical working capacity and blood lipids and lipoproteins in female university students, *Hung. Rev. Sports Med.*, 26, 251, 1985.
97. **Jürimäe, T., Viru, A., Pedaste, J., and Toode, K.**, Changes in physical working capacity and serum lipids and lipoproteins during running training program in female university students, *Biol. Sport*, 2, 243, 1985.
98. **Fox, E.L., Bastles, R.L., Billing, C.E., Mathews, D.K., Bason, R., and Webb, V.M.**, Intensity and distance of interval training programs and changes in aerobic power, *Med. Sci. Sports*, 5, 18, 1973.
99. **Fox, E.L., Bartles, R.L., Klinzing, J., and Ragg, K.**, Metabolic responses to interval training program of high and low power output, *Med. Sci. Sports*, 9, 191, 1977.
100. **Fox, E.L., Bartles, R.L., Billing, C.E., O'Brien, R., Bason, R., and Mathews, D.K.**, Frequency and duration of interval training programs and changes in aerobic power, *J. Appl. Physiol.*, 38, 481, 1975.
101. **Lesmes, G.R., Fox, E.L., Stevens, C., and Otto, R.**, Metabolic responses of females to high intensity interval training of different frequencies, *Med. Sci. Sports*, 10, 229, 1978.
102. **Knuttgen, H.G., Nordesjö, L.-O., Ollander, E., and Saltin, B.**, Physical conditioning through interval training with young male athlete, *Med. Sci. Sports*, 5, 220, 1973.
103. **Fox, E.L.**, Differences in metabolic alterations with sprint versus endurance interval training programs, in *Metabolic Adaptation to Prolonged Physical Exercise,* Howald, H. and Poortmans, J.R., Eds., Birkhäuser, Basel, 1975, 119.
104. **Viru, A., Jürgenstein, J., and Pisuke, A.**, Influence of training methods on endurance, *Track Tech.*, 47, 1495, 1972.
105. **Viru, A., Pisuke, A., and Jürgenstein, J.**, On exercise doses in using the interval method in middle-distance runners, *Teor. Prakt. Fiz. Kult.*, 32(12), 11, 1969 (in Russian).
106. **Volkov, N.I.**, Action of various rest intervals on training effect in repeated exercises, *Teor. Prakt. Fiz. Kult.*, 25, 32, 1962 (in Russian).
107. **Kindermann, W., and Keul, J.**, *Anaerobe Energiebereitstellung im Hochleistungssport,* Hofmann Verlag, Schorndorf, 1977.
108. **Saltin, B., Essén, B., and Pedersen, P.K.**, Intermittent exercise: its physiology and some practical applications, in *Advances in Exercise Physiology,* Karger, Basel, 1976, 23.
109. **Nurmekivi, A.**, *Use of Continuous and Up-Hill Running in Training of Middle- and Long-Distance Runners during the Preparative Period,* Thesis of acad. diss., Tartu University, Tartu, 1974.
110. **Bedford, T.G., Tipton, C.M., Wilson, N.C., Oppliger, R.A., and Gisolfi, C.V.**, Maximum oxygen consumption of rats and its changes with various experimental procedures, *J. Appl. Physiol.*, 47, 1278, 1979.
111. **Hickson, R.C., Rosenkoetter, M.A., and Brown, M.M.**, Strength training effects on aerobic power and short term endurance, *Med. Sci Sports Exerc.*, 12, 336, 1980.
112. **Fahey, T.D., Akka, L., and Rolph, R.**, Body composition and VO_2max of exceptional weight-training athletes, *J. Appl. Physiol.*, 39, 559, 1975.
113. **Dudley, G.A., and Djamil, R.**, Incompatibility of endurance and strength-training modes of exercise, *J. Appl. Physiol.*, 59, 1446, 1985.
114. **Dudley, G.A. and Fleck, S.J.**, Strength and endurance training: are they mutually exclusive, *Sports Med.*, 4, 79, 1987.
115. **Hurley, B.F., Seals, D.R., and Ebsani, A.**, Effect of high-intensity strength training on cardiovascular function, *Med. Sci. Sports Exerc.*, 16, 483, 1984.
116. **Tesch, P.A., Colliander, E.B., and Kaiser, P.**, Muscle metabolism during intense, heavy-resistance exercise, *Eur. J. Appl. Physiol.*, 55, 362, 1986.

117. **Pärnat, J., Viru, A., Savi, T., Kudu, F., and Markusas, F.**, Untersuchungen der Aeroben and Anaeroben Leistungsfähigkeit von Zehnkämfern, *Med. Sport,* 13, 366, 1973.
118. **Green, H.J., and Houston, M.E.**, Effect of a season of ice hockey on energy capacities and associated functions, *Med. Sci. Sports,* 7, 299, 1975.
119. **Green, H.J., Thomson, W.D., Daub, W.D., Houston, M.E., and Ranney, D.A.**, Fiber composition, fiber size and enzyme activities in vastus lateralis of elite athletes involved in high intensity exercise, *Eur. J. Appl. Physiol.,* 41, 109, 1979.
120. **Daub, W.B., Green, H.J., Houston, M.E., Thomson, J.A., Fraser, I.G., and Ranney, D.A.**, Specificity of physiological adaptations resulting from ice-hockey training, *Med. Sci. Sports Exerc.,* 15, 290, 1983.
121. **Newsholme, E.A.**, Application of principles of metabolic control to the problem of metabolic limitations in sprinting, middle-distance, and marathon running, *Int. J. Sports Med.,* 7 (Suppl.), 66, 1986.
122. **Henschen, S.**, *Skilauf and Skiwettlauf,* Jena, 1899.
123. **Herxheimer, H.**, Die Herzgrösse bei Sportleuten and ihre Beurteilung, *Klin. Wschr.,* 49, 2225, 1924.
124. **Deutsch, F., and Kauf, E.**, *Herz and Sport,* Wien, 1924.
125. **Reindell, H.**, *Diagnostik der Kreuslauffführschäden,* F. Enke, Stuttgart, 1949.
126. **Cureton, T.K.**, *Physical Fitness of Champion Athletes,* The University of Illinois Press, Urbana, 1951.
127. **Reindell, H., Klepzig, H., and Steim, H.**, *Die sportärztliche Herz- and Kreislaufberatung,* A. Wander A./G., Bern, 1957.
128. **Reindell, H., Klepzig, H., Steim, H., Musshoff, K., Roskamm, H., and Schildge, F.**, *Herz- and Kreislaufkranheiten and Sport,* J.A. Barth, München, 1960.
129. **Hollmann, W.**, *Arbeits- und Trainingseinfluss auf Kreislauf and Atmung,* Steinkopf-Verlag, Darmstadt, 1959.
130. **Karpman, V.L., Khruschov, S.V., and Borisova, Y.A.**, *Heart and Working Capacity of Sportsman,* FiS, Moscow, 1978.
131. **Reindell, H., Schildge, E., Klepzig, H., and Kirchhoff, H.W.**, *Kreislaufregulation,* Georg Thieme Verlag, Stuttgart, 1955.
132. **Linzbach, A.J.**, Herzhypertrophie and kritischer Herzgewicht, *Klin. Wschr.,* 26, 459, 1948.
133. **Harrison, F.R.**, *Failure of the Circulation,* Baltimore, 1935.
134. **Beickert, A.**, Tierexperimentelle Untersuchungen über die Leistungsfähigkeit der arbeitshypertropische Herzen, *Klin. Wschr.,* 32, 527, 1954.
135. **Komadel, L., Barth, E., and Kokavec, M.**, *Physiological Enlargement of the Heart,* Slovak. Acad. Sci., Bratislava, 1968 (in Russian).
136. **Bloor, C.M., Leon, A.S., and Pasyk, S.**, The effects of exercise of organ and cellular development in rats, *Lab. Invest.,* 19, 675, 1968.
137. **Thomas, M.-J., Bandiera, S., and Tibbits, G.T.**, Training-induced alteration in cardiomyocyte and sarcolemmal characteristics, *8th Int. Biochem. Exerc. Conf.,* Nagoya, 1991, 108.
138. **Petrén, T., Sjöstrand, T., and Sylven, B.**, Der Einfluss des Trainings auf die Häufigkeit der Capillaren in Herz- and Skeletmuskulatur, *Arbeitsphysiologie,* 9, 376, 1936.
139. **Thörner, W.**, Trainingsversuche an Hunder. III. Histologische Beobachtungen am Herz- and Skeletmuskeln, *Arbeitsphysiologie,* 8, 359, 1935.
140. **Poupa, O., and Rakusin, K.**, The terminal microcirculatory bed in the heart of athletic and nonathletic animals, in *Physical Activity in Health and Disease,* Evang, K. and Andersen, K.L., Eds., Universitetsforlaget, Oslo, 1966, 18.
141. **Leon, A.S., and Bloor, C.M.**, Effects of exercise and its cessation on the heart and its blood supply, *J. Appl. Physiol.,* 24, 485, 1968.
142. **Tomanek, R.J.**, Effect of age and exercise on the extent of the myocardial capillary bed, *Anat. Rec.,* 167, 55, 1970.
143. **Tharp, G.D., and Wagner, C.T.**, Chronic exercise and cardiac vascularization, *Eur. J. Appl. Physiol.,* 48, 97, 1982.
144. **Laughlin, M.H., and Tomanek, R.J.**, Myocardial capillarity and maximal capillary diffusions in exercise-trained dogs, *J. Appl. Physiol.,* 63, 1481, 1987.
145. **Ho, K.W., Roy, R.R., Taylor, J.F., Heksner, W.M., and Huss van W.D.**, Differential effects of running and weight-lifting on the rat coronary arterial tree, *Med. Sci. Sports Exerc.,* 15, 472, 1983.
146. **Tepperman, J., and Pearlman, D.**, Effects of exercise and anemia on coronary arteries of small animals as revealed by the corrosion-cast technique, *Circ. Res.,* 9, 576, 1961.
147. **Stevenson, J.A.F., Feleki, V., Rechnitzer, P., and Beaton, J.R.**, Effect of exercise on coronary tree size in the rat, *Circ. Res.,* 15, 265, 1964.
148. **Bloor, C.M., and Leon, A.S.**, Interaction of age and exercise on the heart and its blood supply, *Lab. Invest.,* 22, 160, 1970.
149. **Koerner, J.E., and Terjung, R.L.**, Effect of physical training on coronary collateral circulation of the rat, *J. Appl. Physiol.,* 52, 376, 1982.
150. **Penpargkul, S., and Scheuer, J.**, The effect of physical training upon the mechanical and metabolic performance of the rat heart, *J. Clin. Invest.,* 49, 4859, 1970.

151. **Roeske, W.R., O'Rourke, R.A., Klein, A., Leopold, G., and Karliner, J.S.,** Noninvasive evaluation of ventricular hypertrophy in professional athletes, *Circulation*, 53, 286, 1976.

152. **Underwood, R.H., and Schwade, J.D.,** Noninvasive analysis of cardiac function of elite distance runners — echocardiography, vectorcardiography, and cardiac intervals, *Ann. N.Y. Acad. Sci.*, 301, 297, 1977.

153. **Allen, H.D., Goldberg, S.J., Sahn, D.J., Schy, N., and Wojcik, R.,** A quantitative echocardiographic study of champion childhood runners, *Circulation*, 55, 142, 1977.

154. **Morganroth, J., Maron, B.J., Henry, W.L., and Epstein, S.E.,** Comparative left ventricular dimensions in trained athletes, *Ann. Intern. Med.*, 82, 521, 1975.

155. **Ikaheimo, M.J., Palatsi, I.J., and Takkunen, J.T.,** Noninvasive evaluation of the athletic heart: sprinters versus endurance runners, *Am. J. Cardiol.*, 44, 24, 1979.

156. **Longhurst, J.C., Kelly, A.R., Conyea, W.J., and Mitchell, J.H.,** Echocardiographic left ventricular masses in distance runners and weight lifters, *J. Appl. Physiol.*, 48, 154, 1980.

157. **Gilbert, C.A., Nutter, D.O., Felner, J.M., Perkins, J.V., Heysfield, S.B., and Schlant, R.C.,** Echocardiographic study of cardiac dimensions and function in the endurance-trained athletes, *Am. J. Cardiol.*, 40, 528, 1977.

158. **Paulson, W., Boughner, D.R., Ko, P., Cunningsham, D.D., and Persaud, J.A.,** Left ventricular function in marathon runners: echocardiographic assessment, *J. Appl. Physiol.*, 51, 881, 1981.

159. **Cohen, J.L., and Segal, K.R.,** Left ventricular hypertrophy in athletes: an exercise-echocardiographic study, *Med. Sci. Sports Exerc.*, 17, 695, 1985.

160. **Dickhuth, H.H., Simon, G., Kindermann, W., Wildberg, A., and Keed, J.,** Echocardiographic studies on athletes of various sport-types and non-athletic persons, *Z. Kardiol.*, 68, 449, 1979.

161. **Brown, S., Byrd, R., Jayringhe, M.D., and Jones, D.,** Echocardiographic characteristics of competitive and recreational weight lifters, *J. Cardiovasc. Ultrason.*, 2, 163, 1983.

162. **Monapace, F.J., Hammer, W.J., Ritzer, T.R., Kessler, K.M., Warner, H.F., Spann, J.F., and Bove, A.A.,** Left ventricular size in competitive weight lifters: an echocardiographic study, *Med. Sci. Sports Exerc.*, 14, 72, 1982.

163. **Fleck, S.J.,** Cardiovascular adaptations to resistance training, *Med. Sci. Sports Exerc.*, 20, S146, 1988.

164. **Stone, M.H., Wioson, G.D., Blessing, D., and Rozenek, R.,** Cardiovacular responses to short-term olympic style weight-training in young men, *Can. J. Appl. Sport Sci.*, 8, 134, 1983.

165. **Pearson, A.C., Schiff, M., Mrosek, D., Labovitz, A.J., and Williams, G.A.,** Left ventricular diastolic function in weight lifters, *Am. J. Cardiol.*, 58, 1254, 1986.

166. **Fleck, S.J., and Dean, L.S.,** Resistance training experience and the pressor response during resistance exercise, *J. Appl. Physiol.*, 63, 116, 1987.

167. **Colan, S.D., Sanders, S.P., McPherson, D., and Borrow, K.M.,** Left ventricular diastolic function in elite athletes with physiological cardiac hypertrophy, *J. Am. Coll. Cardiol.*, 6, 545, 1985.

168. **Snoecx, L.H.E.H., Abeling, H.F.M., Lambrechts, J.A.C., Schmitz, J.J.F., Verstappen, F.T.J., and Reneman, R.S.,** Echocardiographic dimensions in athletes in relation to their training programs, *Med. Sci. Sports Exerc.*, 14, 428, 1982.

169. **Cox, M.L., Benett, J.B., and Dudley, G.A.,** Exercise training-induced alterations of cardiac morphology, *J. Appl. Physiol.*, 61, 926, 1986.

170. **Fomin, N.A., Gorokhov, N.M., Vlassov, A.V., and Beshetov, A.V.,** Direction of adaptive transformations of heart in young sportsmen, *Teor. Prakt. Fiz. Kult.*, 5, 18, 1991 (in Russian).

171. **Ricci, G., Lajoie, D., Petitclerc, R., Peronnet, F., Ferguson, R.J., Fournier, M., and Taylor, A.W.,** Left ventricular size following endurance, sprint, and strength training, *Med. Sci. Sports Exerc.*, 14, 344, 1982.

172. **Rubal, B.J., Al-Muhailani, A.-R., and Rosentswieg, J.,** Effects of physical conditioning on the heart size and wall thickness of college women, *Med. Sci. Sports Exerc.*, 19, 423, 1987.

173. **Rost, R.,** The frontiers between physiology and pathology in the athlete's heart: to what limits can it enlarge and beat slowly, in *Sports Cardiology*, Lubich, T., Venerando, A., and Zeppilli, P., Eds., Aulo Gaggi, Bologna, 1989, 187.

174. **Pust, B., and Pevc, J.,** The influence of endurance training on left ventricular function, *J. Sports Med. Phys. Fitness*, 20, 359, 1980.

175. **Keul, J., Dickhuth, H.-H., Lehmann, M., and Staiger, J.,** The athlete's heart — haemodynamics and structure, *Int. J. Sports Med.*, 3 (Suppl. 1), 33, 1982.

176. **Loftin, M., Boileau, R.A., Massey, B.H., and Lohman, T.G.,** Effect of arm training on central and peripheral circulatory function, *Med. Sci. Sports Exerc.*, 20, 136, 1988.

177. **Dickhuth, H., Jakob, E., Wink, K., Bonzel, T., Keul, J., and Just, H.,** Lässt sich aus der maximalen Herzhypertrophill ein absolutes kritisches Herzgewicht albeiten? in *Training and Sport zur Prävention and Rehabilitation in der technischen Umwelt*, Franz, J., Mellerowicz, H., and Noack, W., Eds., Springer, Berlin, 1985, 722.

178. **Spataro, A., Pelliccia, A., Amici, E., Caselli, G., and Eiffi, A.,** Ipertrofia cardiaca estrema in athleti: Studio ecocardiografico morfologica e funzionale, *G. Ital. Cardiol.*, 18, 171, 1988.

179. **Peronnet, F., Perrault, H., Cleroux, J., Cousineau, D., Nadeau, R., Pham-Huy, H.G., Tremblay, G., and Lebau, R.**, Electro- and echocardiographic study of the left ventricle in man after training, *Eur. J. Appl. Physiol.*, 45, 125, 1980.

180. **Åstrand, P.-O., Cuddy, T.E., Saltin, B., and Stenberg, J.**, Cardiac output during submaximal and maximal work, *J. Appl. Physiol.*, 19, 268, 1964.

181. **Ekblom, B., and Hermansen, L.**, Cardiac output in athletes, *J. Appl. Physiol.*, 25, 619, 1968.

182. **Clausen, J.P.**, Effect of physical training on cardiovascular adjustments to exercise in man, *Physiol. Rev.*, 57, 779, 1977.

183. **Rowell, L.B.**, *Human Circulation Regulation during Physical Stress*, Oxford University Press, Oxford, 1986.

184. **Barnard, R.J.**, Long-term effects of exercise on cardiac function, *Exerc. Sport Sci. Rev.*, 3, 113, 1975.

185. **Riedhammer, H.N., Rufflenbeul, W., Weihe, H., and Krayenbuhl, H.P.**, Left ventricular contractile function in trained dogs with cardiac hypertrophy, *Basic Res. Cardiol.*, 71, 297, 1976.

186. **Scheuer, J., and Tipton, C.M.**, Cardiovacular adaptations to physical training, *Ann. Rev. Physiol.*, 39, 221, 1977.

187. **Ritzer, T.F., Bove, A.A., and Carey, R.A.**, Left ventricular performance characteristics in trained and sedentary dogs, *J. Appl. Physiol.*, 48, 130, 1980.

188. **Oscai, L.B., Williams, B.T., and Hertig, B.A.**, Effect of exercise on blood volume, *J. Appl. Physiol.*, 24, 624, 1968.

189. **Szygula, Z.**, Erythrocytic system under the influence of physical exercise and training, *Sports Med.*, 10, 181, 1990.

190. **Hopper, M.K., Coggan. A.R., and Coyle, E.F.**, Exercise stroke volume relative to plasma-volume expansion, *J. Appl. Physiol.*, 64, 404, 1988.

191. **Frick, M.H., Konttinen, A., and Sarajas, H.S.S.**, Effects of physical training on circulation at rest and during exercise, *Am. J. Cardiol.*, 12, 142, 1963.

192. **Ekblom, B.**, Effect of training on oxygen transport system in man, *Acta Physiol. Scand. Suppl.*, 328, 1969.

193. **Whitehorn, W.V. and Grimmengo, A.S.**, Effect of exercise on properties of the myocardium, *J. Lab. Clin. Med.*, 48, 959, 1956.

194. **Molé, P.A., and Rabb, C.**, Force-velocity relations in exercise-induced hypertrophied rat heart muscle, *Med. Sci. Sports*, 5, 69, 1973.

195. **Molé, P.A.**, Increased contractile potential of papillary muscles from exercise trained rat hearts, *Am. J. Physiol.*, 234, H431, 1978.

196. **Penpargkul, S., and Scheuer, J.**, The effect of physical training upon the mechanical and metabolic performance of the rat heart, *J. Clin. Invest.*, 49, 1859, 1970.

197. **Scheuer, J., and Stezoski, S.W.**, Effect of physical training on the mechanical and metabolic responses of the heart to hypoxia, *Circ. Res.*, 30, 418, 1972.

198. **Meerson, F.Z., Kapelko, V.J., and Shaginova, S.I.**, Contractile function of heart muscle in adaptation to physical exercise, *Kardiologia*, 13(4), 5, 1973 (in Russian).

199. **Schaible, T.F., and Scheuer, J.**, Cardiac function in hypertrophied hearts from chronically exercised female rats, *J. Appl. Physiol.*, 50, 1140, 1981.

200. **Schaible, T.F., and Sheuer, J.**, Effects of physical training by running or swimming on ventricular performance of rat hearts, *J. Appl. Physiol.*, 46, 854, 1979.

201. **Schaible, T.F., Pénpargkul, S., and Scheuer, J.**, Cardiac response to exercise training in male and female rats, *J. Appl. Physiol.*, 50, 112, 1981.

202. **Nutter, D.O., Preist, R.E., and Fuller, E.O.**, Endurance training in the rat. I. Myocardial mechanics and biochemistry, *J. Appl. Physiol.*, 51, 934, 1981.

203. **Dowell, R.T., Cutilletta, A.F., Rudnik, M.A., and Sodt, P.C.**, Heart functional response to pressure overload in exercised and sedentary rat, *J. Appl. Physiol.*, 230, 199, 1976.

204. **Baldwin, K.M., Ernst, S.B., Herrick, R.E., and MacIntosch, A.M.**, Effects of physical training and thyroxine on rodent cardiac functional and biochemical properties, *Pflügers Arch. ges. Physiol.*, 391, 190, 1981.

205. **Fuller, E.O., and Nutter, D.O.**, Endurance training in the rat. II. Performance of isolated and intact heart, *J. Appl. Physiol.*, 51, 941, 1981.

206. **Mullin, W.J., Herrick, R.E., Valdez, V., and Baldwin, K.M.**, Adaptive responses of rats trained with reductions in exercise heart rate, *J. Appl. Physiol.*, 54, 1378, 1984.

207. **Crews, J., and Aldinger, E.E.**, Effect of chronic exercise on myocardial function, *Am. Heart J.*, 74, 536, 1967.

208. **Dowell, R.T., Stone, H.L., Sordahl, L.A., and Asimakis, G.**, Contractile function and myofibrillar ATPase in the exercise-trained dog heart, *J. Appl. Physiol.*, 43, 977, 1977.

209. **Sordahl, L.A., Asinakis, G.K., Dowell, R.T., and Stone, H.L.**, Functions of selected biochemical systems from exercise-trained dog heart, *J. Appl. Physiol.*, 42, 426, 1977.

210. **Barnard, R.J., Duncan, H.W., Baldwin, K.M., Grimditch, G., and Buckberg, G.D.**, Effects of intensive training on myocardial performance and coronary blood flow, *J. Appl. Physiol.*, 49, 444, 1980.

211. **Gleeson, T.T., Mullin, W.J., and Baldwin, K.M.,** Cardiovascular response to treadmill exercise in rats: effects of training, *J. Appl. Physiol.*, 54, 789, 1983.

212. **Scheuier, J., Penpargkul, S., and Bhan, A.K.,** Experimental observation in the effect of physical training upon intrinsic cardiac physiology and biochemistry, *Am. J. Cardiol.*, 33, 744, 1974.

213. **Bhan, A.K., and Scheuer, J.,** Effects of physical training on cardiac myosin ATPase activity, *Am. J. Physiol.*, 228, 1178, 1975.

214. **Pagani, E.D., and Solaro, J.J.,** Swimming exercise, thyroid state and the distribution of myosin isoenzyme in rat heart, *Am. J. Physiol.*, 245, H713, 1983.

215. **Baldwin, K.M.,** Effects of chronic exercise on biochemical and functional properties of the heart, *Med. Sci. Sports Exerc.*, 17, 522, 1985.

216. **Rupp, H.,** The adaptive changes in the isoenzyme pattern of myosin from hypertrophied rat myocardium as a result of pressure overload and physical training, *Basic Res. Cardiol.*, 76, 79, 1981.

217. **Malhorta, A., Penpargkul, S., Schaible, T., and Scheuer, J.,** Contractile proteins and sarcoplasmic reticulum in physiologic cardiac hypertrophy, *Am. J. Physiol.*, 241, H263, 1981.

218. **Bhan, A.K., Malhorta, A., and Scheuer, J.,** Biochemical adaptation in cardiac muscle: effects of physical training on sulfhydryl groups of myosin, *J. Mol. Cell. Cardiol.*, 7, 435, 1975.

219. **Medugorac, I., Kämmereit, A., and Jacob, R.,** Einfluss einer chronischen Schwimmtrainings auf Struktur und Enzymaktivität von Myosin beim Rattenmyokard, *Z. Physiol. Chem.*, 356, 1161, 1975.

220. **Penpargkul, S., Malhorta, A., Schaible, T., and Scheuer, J.,** Cardiac contractile proteins and sarcoplasmic reticulum in heart of rats trained by running, *J. Appl. Physiol.*, 48, 409, 1980.

221. **Resink, T.J., Evers, W.G., Noakes, T.P., and Opie, L.H.,** Increased cardiac myosin ATPase activity as a biochemical adaptation to running training: enhanced response to catecholamines and a role for myosin phosphorylation, *J. Mol. Cell. Cardiol.*, 13, 679, 1981.

222. **Baldwin, K.M., Winder, W.W., and Holloszy, J.O.,** Adaptation of actomyosin ATPase in different types of muscle to endurance exercise, *Am. J. Physiol.*, 229, 422, 1973.

223. **Baldwin, K.M., Cooke, D.A., and Cheadle, W.G.,** Time course adaptations in cardiac and skeletal muscle to different running programs, *J. Appl. Physiol.*, 42, 267, 1977.

224. **Penpargkul, S., Repke, D.I., Katz, A.M., and Scheuer, J.,** Effect of physical training on calcium transport by rat cardiac sarcoplasmic reticulum, *Circ. Res.*, 40, 134, 1977.

225. **Carey, R.A., Ritzer, T.T., and Bove, A.A.,** Effect of endurance training on skeletal and cardiac muscle myosin ATPase activity in the dog, *Med. Sci. Sports Exerc.*, 11, 308, 1979.

226. **MacIntosh, A.M., Baldwin, K.M., Herrick, R.E., and Mullin, W.M.,** Effect of training on biochemical and functional properties of neonatal heart, *J. Appl. Physiol.*, 59, 1440, 1985.

227. **Baldwin, K.M., Fitzsimons, D.P., and Morris, G.S.,** Effects of acute and chronic exercise on the biochemical properties of the heart, in *Sports Cardiology,* Vol. 2, Lubich,. T., Venerando, A., and Zeppilli, P., Eds., Aulo Gaggi, Bologna, 1989, 17.

228. **MacIntosh, A.M., Wullin, W.M., Fitzsimons, D.P., Herrick, R.E., and Baldwin, K.M.,** Cardiac biochemical and functional adaptation to exercise in sympathectomized neonatal rats, *J. Appl. Physiol.*, 60, 991, 1986.

229. **Franks, K., Cooke, R., and Stull, J.T.,** Myosin phosphorylation decreases ATPase activity of cardiac myofibrils, *J. Mol. Cell. Cardiol.*, 16, 597, 1984.

230. **Pemrick, M.J.,** The phosphorylated L_2 light chain of skeletal myosin is a modifier of actomyosin ATPase, *J. Biol. Chem.*, 255, 8836, 1980.

231. **Tibbits, G.F., Barnard, R.J., Baldwin, K.M., Cugalj, N., and Roberts, N.K.,** Influence of exercise on excitation-contraction coupling in rat myocardium, *Am. J. Physiol.*, 240, H472, 1981.

232. **Tibbits, G.F., Nagatomo, T., Sasaki, M.B., and Bernard, R.J.,** Cardiac sarcolemma: compositional adaptation to exercise, *Science,* 213, 1271, 1981.

233. **Tibbits, G., Koziol, B.J., Roberts, N.K., Baldwin, K.M., and Barnard, R.J.,** Adaptation of the rat myocardium to endurance training, *J. Appl. Physiol.*, 44, 85, 1978.

234. **Barnard, R.J., Corre, K., and Cho, H.,** Effect of training on the resting heart rate of rats, *Eur. J. Appl. Physiol.*, 35, 285, 1976.

235. **Acros, J.C., Schal, R.S., Sun, S., Argus, M.F., and Burch, G.H.,** Changes in ultrastructure and respiratory control in mitochondria of rat heart hypertrophied by exercise, *Exp. Mol. Pathol.*, 8, 49, 1968.

236. **Kraus, H., and Kirsten, R.,** Die Wirkung vor körperlichen Training auf die mitochondriale Energieproduktion im Herzmuskel and in der Leber, *Pflügers Arch. ges. Physiol.*, 320, 334, 1970.

237. **Hearn, G.R., and Wainio, W.W.,** Succinic dehydrogenase activity of the heart and skeletal muscle of exercised rats, *Am. J. Physiol.*, 155, 348, 1956.

238. **Walpurger, G., and Anger, H.,** Enzymatic organization of energy metabolism in rat heart after training in swimming and running, *Z. Kreislaufforsch.*, 59, 438, 1970.

239. **Oscai, L.B., Molé, P.A., and Holloszy, J.O.,** Effects of exercise on cardiac weights and mitochondria in male and female rats, *Am. J. Physiol.*, 220, 1944, 1971.

240. **Oscai, L.B., Molé, P.A., Brei, B., and Holloszy, J.O.,** Cardiac growth and respiratory enzyme levels in male rats subjected to a running program, *Am. J. Physiol.,* 220, 1238, 1971.
241. **Dohm, G.L., Huston, R.L., Askew, E., and Weiser, P.C.,** Effects of exercise on activity of heart and muscle mitochondria, *Am. J. Physiol.,* 223, 783, 1972.
242. **Gollnick, P.D., and Ianuzzo, C.D.,** Hormonal deficiencies and the metabolic adaptations of rats to training, *Am. J. Physiol.,* 223, 278, 1972.
243. **Hooker, A.M., and Baldwin, K.M.,** Substrate oxidation specificity in different types of mammalian skeletal muscle, *Am. J. Physiol.,* 236, C66, 1979.
244. **Crisman, R.P., and Tomanek, R.J.,** Exercise training modifies myocardial mitochondria and myofibril growth in spontaneously hypertensive rats, *Am. J. Physiol.,* 248, H8, 1985.
245. **Kainulainen, H., Ahomäki, E., and Vihko, V.,** Selected enzyme activities in mouse cardiac muscle during training and terminated training, *Basic Res. Cardiol.,* 79, 710, 1984.
246. **Gollnick, P.D., and Hearn, G.R.,** Lactic dehydrogenase activities of heart and skeletal muscle of exercised rats, *Am. J. Physiol.,* 201, 694, 1961.
247. **Gollnick, P.D., Struck, P.J., and Bogyo, T.P.,** Lactic dehydrogenase activities of rat heart and skeletal muscle after exercise and training, *J. Appl. Physiol.,* 22, 623, 1967.
248. **Barnard, R.J., MacAlpin, R., Kattus, A.A., and Buckberg, G.D.,** Effect of training on myocardial oxygen supply/demand balance, *Circulation,* 56, 289, 1977.
249. **Kihlström, M., Ojala, J., and Sahkinen, A.,** Decreased level of cardiac antioxidants in endurance trained rats, *Acta Physiol. Scand.,* 135, 549, 1989.
250. **Bache, R.J., and Vrobel, T.R.,** Effects of exercise on blood flow in the hypertrophied heart, *Am. J. Cardiol.,* 44, 1029, 1979.
251. **Hultgren, P.B., and Bove, A.A.,** Myocardial blood flow and mechanics in volume overload-induced left ventricular hypertrophy in dogs, *Cardiovasc. Res.,* 15, 522, 1981.
252. **Bove, A.A.,** Effects of strenuous exercise on myocardial blood flow, *Med. Sci. Sports Exerc.,* 17, 517, 1985.
253. **Carey, R.A., Santamore, W.P., Michele, J.J., and Bove, A.A.,** Effects of endurance training on coronary resistance in dogs, *Med. Sci. Sports Exerc.,* 11, 355, 1983.
254. **Liang, I.Y.S., Hamra, M., and Stone, H.L.,** Maximum coronary blood flow and minimum coronary resistance in exercise-trained dogs, *J. Appl. Physiol.,* 56, 641, 1984.
255. **Laughlin, M.H.,** Effects of training on coronary transport capacity, *J. Appl. Physiol.,* 58, 468, 1985.
256. **Scheuer, J.,** Effects of physical training on myocardial vascularity and perfusion, *Circulation,* 66, 491, 1982.
257. **Thomas, D.P.,** Effects of acute and chronic exercise on myocardial ultrastructure, *Med. Sci. Sports Exerc.,* 17, 546, 1985.
258. **Poland, J.L., and Blount, D.H.,** The effects of training on myocardial metabolism, *Proc. Soc. Exp. Biol. Med.,* 129, 171, 1968.
259. **Scheuer, J., Kapner, L., Stringfellow, C.A., Armstrong, C.L., and Penpargkul, S.,** Glycogen, lipid and high energy phosphate stores in hearts from conditioned rats, *J. Lab. Clin. Med.,* 75, 924, 1970.
260. **Watt, E.W., Foss, M.L., and Block, W.D.,** Effects of training and detraining on the distribution of cholesterol, triglycerides and nitrogen in tissues of albino rats, *Circ. Res.,* 31, 908, 1972.
261. **Minarovjech, V.,** Changements de la structure des poumons causès par l'entrainement, *1st Congr. Eur. Méd. Sportive,* Praha, 1963, 17.
262. **Moore, R.L., and Gollnick, P.D.,** Response of ventilatory muscles of the rat to endurance training, *Pflügers Arch. ges. Physiol.,* 392, 268, 1982.
263. **Green, H.J., Plyley, M.J., Smith, D.M., and Kile, J.B.,** Extreme endurance training and fiber type adaptation in rat diaphragm, *J. Appl. Physiol.,* 66, 1914, 1989.

Chapter 7

SPECIFICITY OF TRAINING EFFECTS ON CONTROL FUNCTIONS AND THE CONNECTIVE TISSUE

ENDOCRINE FUNCTIONS

Three specific variants of training effects on endocrine functions may be discriminated. When training is directed to the improvement of sports performance in sprint or highly intensive anaerobic exercises (e.g., the 400- or 1500-m race), the development of an opportunity for rapid and intensive adrenaline output is expected. The development of possibilities for enhanced adrenaline secretion in training,[1,2] as well as the correlation between high catecholamine levels in the blood and high levels in supramaximal exercise performance[3,4] is demonstrated. However, the specific relation between corresponding training exercises and the development of these qualities awaits striking argumentation. Still, it was observed that 30 s of running at maximum speed caused after sprint training a higher rise in the blood noradrenaline level.[5] Neither sprint[5] nor endurance[6] training changed the catecholamine level in the blood after 2 min of running at 110% VO_2max.

The second variant is common for endurance training. In a number of studies endurance-training effects on the functional stability of the sympatho-adrenal and pituitary-adrenocortical systems have been shown. A certain relation was found between this quality and endurance capacities.[1,7-10] However, as these facts were established by the time of maintaining a stable high level of hormone excretion with urine, these results have to be re-examined against more precise methodological backgrounds.

In rats an actual morphofunctional improvement of adrenocorticocytes was found as a result of running or swimming training for 5 or 11 weeks.[11] An increased number of mitochondria, their vesicular cristae, elements of endoplasmic reticulum, and polysomes were found in the fascicular zone as well as an elevated content of cytochrome a-a_3 in the whole adrenal cortex. Morphometric analysis, together with the other obtained data, showed four variants of alterations in the adrenals, depending on the training regime: (1) an adrenal hypertrophy due to enlargement of the medulla and the glomerular zone; this variant was characteristic of adaptation to short-term sprint exercises during the first week of training; (2) a pronounced adrenal hypertrophy due to enlargement of the fascicular and reticular zones and the medulla without any pronounced changes in the adrenal corticosterone content; this was characteristic of adaptation to prolonged continuous exercise; (3) a slight adrenal hypertrophy due to the fascicular and reticular zones, accompanied by an augmented adrenal corticosterone content; this was connected with adaptation to anaerobic exercises; (4) a slight adrenal hypertrophy accompanied by a decrease in the adrenal corticosterone content; this was specific for prolonged adaptation to short-term sprint exercises.

The third variant of the specificity of training effects on the endocrine function may be the strength-training influence on possibilities to produce testosterone, stimulating muscular hypertrophy. Almost nothing is known about whether training changes the possibility for testosterone secretion and whether such an effect is specifically related to training for improved strength. But promising results have been obtained. It was found that in rats, training increased the Leydig cell capacity to produce testosterone and cAMP during gonadotropin stimulation.[12] However, it was the result of endurance, not strength training. Nevertheless, data were obtained suggesting that resistance training also stimulates testosterone production. A two-year study showed that even in elite athletes a prolonged intensive strength training leads to increased serum levels of testosterone. The correlation of change in maximal force with changes both in testosterone/cortisol and testosterone/sex hormone-binding globulin ratios indicates that the increase in the serum testosterone level creates more optimal conditions for strength improvement.[13]

In addition, the training specificity may be related to changes on the level of cellular receptors (see Chapter 3). Human experiments with insulin euglycemic clamp techniques demonstrated that glucose metabolism was significantly higher both in long-distance runners and weight-lifters in comparison with control persons. The results obtained by using various insulin doses suggested that the enhancement of insulin action by training is due to the increase in insulin sensitivity rather than insulin responsiveness. Endurance training appeared to be more effective than strength training for the improvement of insulin sensitivity.[14]

NEURAL ADAPTATION

Neural adaptation takes place at the level of spinal motoneurons as well as at higher levels of the central nervous system. The existence of neural adaptation explains why (1) the changes in cross-sectional area of muscle fibers are much smaller than the changes in maximal force production,[15-18] (2) training-induced increases in voluntary strength may occur without increases in twitch and tetanic tension evoked by electrical stimulation,[19] (3) training of one limb causes increases in strength of the contralateral limb (see p. 189–190), and (4) a specificity of training effects exists; increases in voluntary strength are specific to the movement pattern,[20,21] joint position,[22] contraction type,[23,24] and movement velocity[20,25,26] used in training.

Neural adaptation is suggested to be related to improved coordination or learning,[21] increased activation of prime mover muscles,[27] and changes in the recruitment pattern of motor units.[28] One of the expressions is a better synchronization of the activity of motor units.[29] Correlations were found between the increases in voluntary strength and the increases in integrated electromyogram[27,30] (Figure 7-1), indicating that strength-trained subjects can more fully activate prime mover muscles for maximal voluntary contractions.[31]

In each sport event the muscular activity is founded on specific motor programming. In some events the programs have to be acquired for a long time before competitions in order to reserve possibilities for a careful improvement of motor skill to ensure the perfection and beauty of the performance (e.g., gymnastics). In some other events an accomplished motor program is essential for maximal utilization of physical abilities (e.g., track and field events). However, there is also a group of events founded on quick motor programming during the competition performance (e.g., sports games). In this case the arsenal of necessary skill has to be acquired in previous training. During performance the necessary skills will be chosen and used according to rapid alterations in the situation.

The motor programming takes place in the premotor cortex, the supplementary motor areas, and other association areas of the brain cortex. Inputs from these areas, from the cerebellum, and, to some extent, from the basal ganglia converge to the primary motor cortex and finally excite or inhibit the corticobulbar and corticospinal neurons of the motor cortex. These output neurons of the motor cortex have a powerful influence on interneurons and motoneurons of the brain stem and of the spinal cord. Accordingly, the primary motor cortex can influence spinal motoneurons directly via the pyramidal tract and indirectly by modulating the activity of the descending brain stem system (the vestibulospinal and reticulospinal tracts). The final point is the spinal α-motoneuron. The net membrane current of the motoneuron determines the firing pattern of the motor unit and, thus, the muscular activity.[32]

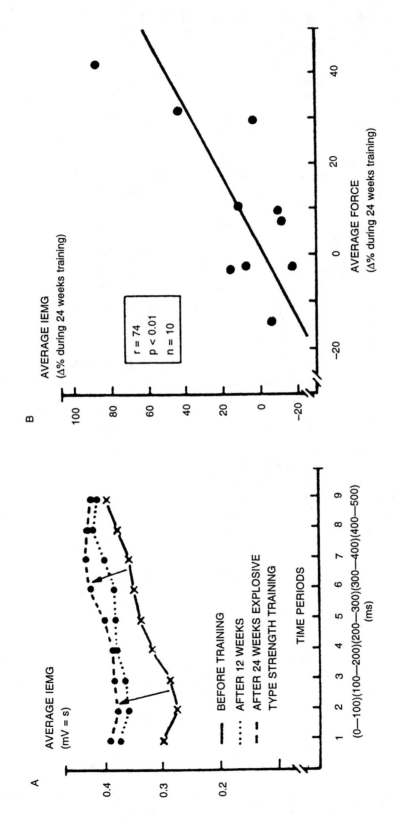

FIGURE 7-1. Average IEMG-time curves calculated from averaged IEMGs of the vastus lateralis (VL), vastus medalis (VM), and rectus femoris (RF) muscles produced during the early 500 ms in rapid maximal isometric bilateral leg extension in the subjects accustomed to strength training before and after the 12- and 24-week explosive (power) type strength training (A) and the relationship between the relative changes in average 'early' IEMG and the relative changes in average 'early' force (B) after the corresponding 24-week training. (From Häkkinen, K., *J. Sports Med. Phys. Fitness*, 29, 9, 1989. With permission.)

D.G. Sale[33] considers as possible mechanisms of neural adaptation in training:

1. Increased activation of agonists
2. Selective recruitment of motor units within agonists
3. Selective activation of agonists within a muscle group
4. Co-contraction of antagonists

In addition, the training effects on motoneurons' excitability and lability have to be taken into consideration. Strength training with weight-lifting or isometric exercises causes an increase in the reflex potentiation of EMG responses.[34,35] Reflex potentiation is enhanced in weight-lifters[36,37] and elite sprinters.[38] The potentiation of reflex responses by voluntary effort is probably related to elevated motoneuron excitability.[34,35] Training increased the time that the highest threshold motor units could be kept active in sustained maximal contractions.[39] Training allows both low- and high-threshold motor units to maintain regular firing intervals at lower rates than before training.[40]

Naturally, a marked specificity exists in the response to strength training, including its action on motoneuron excitability.[41,42] Isometric strength training resulted in an elevated ability of subjects to discharge motor units at regular firing intervals, whereas high repetition dynamic training resulted in a trend towards reduced ability to maintain regular firing intervals.[43] A comparison of various training methods for improved strength showed that the force improvement was the highest in maximal voluntary isometric contraction as well as in maximal electrically evoked tetanic contraction when isometric training was used. The lowest improvement was found with isokinetic training at the movement velocity of $160°·s^{-1}$. Isokinetic training with the movement velocity of $40°·s^{-1}$ gave medium effects. The training effect on the torque at various velocities of movement was the highest when the movement velocity corresponded to the movement velocity of training exercises.[44] This result is in accordance with others indicating that at least in isokinetic training the training velocity contributes in improving peak torque.[45] It was calculated that in a 60-day training with the aid of maximal isokinetic knee extensions at an angular velocity of 2.09 rad·s^{-1}, hypertrophy accounted for 40% of the increase in force while the remaining 60% was attributable to an increased neural drive and, possibly, to changes in muscle architecture.[46]

A training program that included various types of jumping exercises resulted in an earlier preactivation of leg extensor muscles before impact in the performance of test exercises. This was associated with a more powerful eccentric working phase. Higher preactivation of muscle, higher flexion of knee, and increased dorsioflection of ankle joints in the beginning of contact caused an increased tendomuscular stiffness, possibly through more powerful reflex activation.[47]

Six weeks of daily electrostimulation sets augmented the muscle force by changing peripheral processes associated with intracellular events, without modifying the nervous command of the contraction. Comparison of the peripheral changes recorded during submaximal training by electrostimulation and voluntary contractions suggest that electrostimulation is less efficient, but complementary to voluntary training because the number and the type of trained motor units are different in the two procedures.[48]

It was noted earlier that there are certain differences between the effects of training for improved strength and for improved power (Figure 7-2). The main difference between exercises applied in heavy resistance and power training is founded on the time of development of peak force during movements. In heavy resistance exercises the aim is to apply the highest possible force or one close to it. The time for force development is not the main condition of these exercises. In power exercises the aim is to achieve the highest possible power output by the movement. Therefore, the time of force development becomes a main determinant. Correspondingly, there are substantial differences in the results of systematical use of heavy resistance or power exercises. These differences have to be related to adaptive changes on muscle level (hypertrophy vs. improvement of the excitation-coupling system,

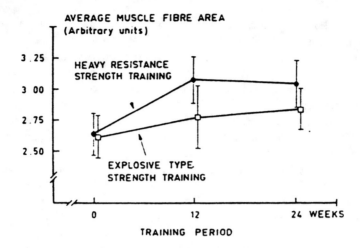

FIGURE 7-2. Average (arbitary units ± SE) total fiber area of the fast- and slow-twitch fiber types of the vastus lateralis during the 24-week heavy resistance strength training and during 24-week explosive type strength training in subjects accustomed to strength training. (From Häkkinen, K., *J. Sports Med. Phys. Fitness*, 29, 9, 1989. With permission.)

sarcoplasmic reticulum function, and cross-bridge formation rate) or on the level of central nervous control. Usually, both groups of adaptive changes are revealed together. Only the ratio between them is different depending on the training exersies. There also seems to be a certain time sequence in development of various adaptive changes in training for improved strength. Early changes in voluntary strength can usually be accounted for largely by neural factors with a gradually increasing contribution of hypertrophy factors as the training proceeds.[28] During prolonged heavy resistance training the capacity of the neuromuscular system for fast force production may even decrease after the initial slight improvement.[49]

CHANGES IN THE CENTRAL NERVOUS SYSTEM

In a number of studies, training-induced structural, biochemical, and functional changes were found in the nervous system. Mice subjected to physical activity during late post-natal development show significantly higher brain weight than inactive controls. Histological examination of the cerebellum revealed significantly greater dendritic field, branch length, synaptic density of dendritic spikes, and total number of spikes per unit length per cell.[50] The training effect on spinal neuron size was recorded in rats.[51] A histochemical study indicated increased oxidative potential of motoneurons.[52] A high significance belongs also to the increased activity of cholinesterase in motor end-plate[53] and changes in axonal conduction velocity.[54] Most of these adaptations appear to be specific to motor unit types and cannot be generalized beyond motor unit population.[55] The responsiveness of the monosynaptic component of the spinal stretch reflex to training has been demonstrated in limb muscles of monkeys.[56]

In conclusion, the mechanism of neural adaptation includes increased activation of prime movers in a specific movement, and appropriate changes in the activation of synergists and antagonists.[21] All these manifestations are essential not only for improved muscular strength and power, but also for improved speed of movement and endurance. The neural adaptation mechanism is decisive for improved skill and coordination.

CROSS-EFFECTS OF TRAINING ON UNTRAINED MUSCLES

There are very old evidences that resistive training with muscles of one limb increases the strength of the muscles of the contralateral limb.[57,58] During the last half-century it has been confirmed by physiological experiments.[59-62] More recently, it was demonstrated that the strength increase in the contralateral untrained arm was associated with an increase in integral electromyogram[63] but not in muscle size.[63,64] Consequently, the cross-training effect was considered to be the result of neural adaptation.[37]

In an experiment of one-legged exercise a positive cross-effect on the contralateral leg was confirmed in regard to peak torque of both quadriceps and hamstring muscles. Also, an increased endurance of these muscles of the untrained leg was found after 8 weeks of training of the contralateral leg.[65]

The cross-training effect is revealed also in regard to the velocity of movement. However, the training effect on the muscle strength as well as on the velocity of movement is more pronounced in the trained than in the untrained leg.[44]

The one-leg training experiments are rather conclusive that endurance exercises affect only muscles directly involved in mechanical energy production.[66-68] This is the case in regard to enzyme adaptation as well as energy stores. The glycogen concentration of the trained leg was from 6 to 60 mmol·kg^{-1} wet wt. higher. In bicyclists and swimmers the muscle glycogen content is higher in the trained than in the other muscles with differences varying from 20 to 101 mmol·kg^{-1} wet wt.[69] One-leg training experiments indicated the increase of glycogenetic enzymes (glycogen synthase and hexokinase) only in trained muscles.[66]

In triathlonists the mean percentage of type I fibers was 58, 63, and 60% in the gastrocnemius, vastus lateralis, and deltoid muscles, respectively. However, the respiratory capacity as well as the activity of citrate synthase were lower in the deltoid muscle compared with leg muscles.[70] In another study, 8 weeks of cycling increased the peak VO_2 by 13%, capillary density by 15%, and volume of mitochondria by 40% in the vastus lateralis muscle. In the unexercised deltoid muscle the peak VO_2 increased by 9%, but the volume of mitochondria decreased by 17%. Capillary density did not change.[71]

The dependence of adaptive changes within muscular fibers on their actual use indicates that the inductors of these modifications are local in nature and depend on the internal conditions within the muscle fibers. The cross-effects of unilateral training are not actualized through any possible influence acting generally on muscle tissue.

TRAINING EFFECTS ON THE CONNECTIVE TISSUE

The main types of connective tissue (ligaments, tendons, collagenous structures within muscles, bone, and cartilage) contain collagen, which is extracellularly located and which constitutes 25 to 30% of the total body protein. To continue discussion on the specific nature of training effects in regard to the connective tissue, the main questions are (1) does training influence the synthesis and turnover of collagen and other proteins of the connective tissue? (2) how are these effects related to the training specificity? and (3) do the training-induced changes in the connective tissue improve the strength of the structures of the tissue?

Most of the animal studies indicate that endurance training can increase the maximum strength of tendons[72-76] and ligaments.[75-80] Accordingly, the breaking load of ligaments and tendons increases. These changes were accompanied by an increased mass of studied tendons and ligaments.[72,75,76,80,81] However, these results were not obtained in all studies. There seems to exist a number of factors determining the action of training on connective structures. Among these the significance of age, sex, and localization of the structure is demonstrated.

As a result of endurance training, an increased number of nuclei and an increased tendon mass were found in young mice,[72] but this was not found in elder animals.[73] Endurance training programs increased the maximal load that the attachment of the medical collateral ligament to tibia could sustain in growing male rats[80] and male dogs.[79] This effect was not observed in female rats.[73,81,82] However, in a paper a training-induced increase in the load necessary to disrupt the medical collateral ligament in female rats was reported.[83] In contrast to the positive training effect on the maximal tensile strength of various tendons,[73,84] this effect was not observed using a Calcaneus-Achilles tendon-gastrocnemius-femur preparation.[84]

Hypophysectomy,[85] adrenalectomy,[86] and diabetes,[87] but not thyroidectomy[88] or ovariectomy,[82] excluded the training effect on ligamentous strength. Treatment of hypophysectomized rats with thyrotropin restored the training effect.[85] Treatment of hypophysectomized rats with somatotropin[77,85] or corticotropin[85] was ineffective in regard to restoring the training effect.

Collagen can be measured determining the hydroxyproline content. As expected, training increased both hydroxyproline concentration and the breaking strengths of tendons[74] or ligaments.[81,89] However, a possibility was also indicated that the breaking strength increases without any change in the hydroxyproline content.[80] It is likely that this discrepancy may be related to the increase in collagen degradation, found in the Achilles tendon of trained animals.

The water content of ligaments and tendons does not change with training.[81] The activity of aerobic enzymes increases in tendons.[89-91] Sprint training has been seen to enhance ligament weight and the weight/length ratio.[92] The same is assumed as a result of resistive training.[93-95] The maximum voluntary contraction represents approximately 30% of the maximum tensile strength of tendons.[96] This leaves a great safety margin.

Exercises for improved flexibility are connected with stretching ligaments and tendons. It was shown that an experimental stretching of a tendon to 108% of its original length altered the tendon's qualities. The tendon remained at 104% of its original length when unloaded. In the second trial the tendon was stretched more. Nevertheless, there were no changes observed in the maximal load at breaking.[97]

Systematic physical activity also increases bone density and mass.[98-103] First of all, the bone mass of the main active limbs increases.[99,104,105] In regard to changes in the bone tissue, the major factors are training intensity and load-bearing.[95] However, there are differences in stimulation of bone density and of bone length growth. Low-intensity training may stimulate the growth in bone length and in bone girth in growing animals. Relatively high-intensity training inhibits these processes, but results in increased bone density. Lower-intensity training does not change bone density.[75,106-108]

Increased bone density with high-intensity training or increased load-bearing is founded on increases in calcium[74,100,109] and hydroxyproline concentration[74] in bones. Bone enlargement together with increased bone density, collagen concentration, and mineral content warrant a rise in breaking strength.[74,75]

The thickness of cartilage in all joints was greater in trained than in nontrained rabbits.[110]

Training also induces changes in the endomyseal connective tissue. In rats a compensatory hypertrophy of the soleus muscle after severing the attachment of the gastrocnemius and plantaris muscles to the Achilles tendon, doubled the number of fibroplasts in the soleus.[111] After severing the gastrocnemius from the Achilles tendon the collagen content increased in the plantaris muscle.[112] Endurance exercises did not increase the total collagen of the endomyseal connective tissue sheaths.[113,114] On the other hand, life-long endurance training maintains a higher level of biosynthesis[115] as well as hydroxyproline concentration in the soleus muscle.[116] Swimming training, which lacks weight-bearing and eccentric components, caused an increase in prolyl 4-hydroxylase and galactorylhydroxylysyl glucoryltransferase activities in the soleus, suggesting that muscle contractile activity per se is a positive regulator of collagen biosynthesis.[117] In the rectus femoris muscle the training effect on hydroxyproline concentration was not observed. In slow muscles the basement membrane is more collagenous than in the fast muscle. Aging and training further distinguish the composition of the basement membrane in slow and fast muscles.[118]

In young men, strength training stimulated the endomyseal connective tissue growth.[74,119] In body-builders the collagen amount was increased in the biceps muscle, but the proportion of collagen in the total amount of noncontractile proteins was similar in untrained persons, elite, and novice body-builders.[120]

In the rat heart, endurance training decreased the hydroxyproline concentration.[121] However, this result was not confirmed in the mouse heart. In young mice no changes in myocardial hydroxyproline concentration were found with daily running.[122] Myocardial collagen content increased with endurance training (running) in 4-month-old rats but not in 8.5-month-old rats.[123] During training the hydroxyproline concentration increased in the skin of mice.[124] At the same time, training may improve the skin elasticity in older men and women.[125]

REFERENCES

1. **Viru, A.**, *Hormones in Muscular Activity.* Vol. II, Adaptive Effects of Hormones in Exercise, CRC Press, Boca Raton, FL, 1985.
2. **Kjaer, M.**, Epinephrine and some other hormonal responses to exercise in man. With special reference to physical training, *Int. J. Sports Med.,* 10, 1, 1989.
3. **Vendsalu, A.**, Studies on adrenaline and noradrenaline in human plasma, *Acta Physiol. Scand.,* 49 (Suppl. 173), 1960.
4. **Häggendal, J., Hartley, L.H., and Saltin, B.**, Arterial noradrenaline concentration during exercise in relation to the relative work levels, *Scand. J. Clin. Lab. Invest.,* 26, 337, 1970.
5. **Brooks, S., Cheetham, M.E., and Williams, C.**, Sprint training and the catecholamine response to brief maximal exercise in man, *J. Physiol.,* 369, P71, 1988.
6. **Brooks, S., Cheetham, M., and Williams, C.**, Endurance training and the catecholamine response to brief maximum exercise in man, *J. Physiol.,* 361, P81, 1985.
7. **Matlina, E.S., and Kassil, G.N.**, Metabolism of catehcolamines during physical exercise in man and animals, *Usp. Fiz. Nauk,* 2, 13, 1976 (in Russian).
8. **Viru, A.**, *Functions of the Adrenal Cortex in Muscular Activity,* Medizina, Moscow, 1977 (in Russian).
9. **Kassil, G.N., Vaisfeldt, I.L., Matlina, E.S., and Schreiberg, G.L.**, *Humoral-Hormonal Mechanisms of Regulation of Functions in Sports Activities,* Nauka, Moscow, 1978 (in Russian).
10. **Viru, A., and Matsin, T.**, Functional stability of adrenocortical activity during bicycle ergometer and running exercise, *Biol. Sports,* 5, 305, 1988.
11. **Viru, A., and Seene, T.**, Peculiarities of adjustments in the adrenal cortex to various training regimes, *Biol. Sports,* 2, 91, 1985.
12. **Näveri, H., Kuoppasalmi, K., Karvonen, S.-L., Huhtaniemi, I., and Härkönen, M.**, Androgens and physical exercise in the male rats, *Int. J. Sports Med.,* Suppl. (22nd World Congr. Sports Med.), 62, 1982.
13. **Häkkinen, K., Pakarinen, A., Alen, M., Kauhanen, H., and Komi, P.V.**, Neuromuscular and hormonal adaptations in athletes to strength training in two years, *J. Appl. Physiol.,* 65, 2406, 1988.
14. **Sato, J., Osawa, I., Oshida, Y., Sato, Y., Kikura, Y., Higuchi, M., and Kobayashi, S.**, Effects of different types of physical training on insulin action in human peripheral tissues — use of the euglycemic clamp technique, *8th Int. Biochem. Exerc. Conf.,* Nagoya, 1991, 133.
15. **Ikai, M., and Fukunaga, T.**, A study on training effect on strength per unit cross-sectional area of muscle by means of ultrasonic measurement, *Eur. J. Appl. Physiol.,* 28, 173, 1970.
16. **Thorstensson, A.**, Observations on strength training and detraining, *Acta Physiol. Scand.,* 100, 491, 1977.
17. **Komi, P.V., Viitasalo, J., Rauramaa, R., and Vihko, V.**, Effect of isometric strength training on mechanical electrical and metabolic aspects of muscle function, *Eur. J. Appl. Physiol.,* 40, 45, 1978.
18. **Costill, D.L., Coyle, E.F., Fink, W.F., Lesmes, G.R., and Witzman, F.A.**, Adaptation in skeletal muscle following strength training, *J. Appl. Physiol.,* 46, 96, 1979.
19. **McDonagh, M.J.N., Hayward, C.M., and Davies, C.T.M.**, Isometric training in human elbow flexor muscles, *J. Bone Joint Surg.,* 65., 355, 1983.
20. **Häkkinen, K., and Komi, P.V.**, Training-induced changes in neuromuscular performance under voluntary and reflex conditions, *Eur. J. Appl. Physiol.,* 55, 147, 1986.
21. **Rutherford, O.M., and Jones, D.A.**, The role of learning and coordination in strength training, *Eur. J. Appl. Physiol.,* 55, 100, 1986.
22. **Lindh, M.**, Increase of muscle strength from isometric quadriceps exercise at different knee angles, *Scand. J. Rehab. Med.,* 11, 33, 1979.
23. **Komi, P.V., and Buskirk, E.R.**, Effect of eccentric and concentric muscle conditioning on tension and electrical activity of human muscle, *Ergonomics,* 15, 417, 1972.
24. **Kanahisa, H., and Miyashita, M.**, Effect of isometric and isokinetic muscle training on static strength and dynamic power, *Eur. J. Appl. Physiol.,* 50, 365, 1983.

25. **Coyle, E., Feiring, C., and Rotkins, T.**, Specificity of power improvements through slow and fast isokinetic training, *J. Appl. Physiol.*, 51, 1437, 1981.
26. **Kanahisa, H., and Miyashita, M.**, Specificity of velocity in strength training, *Eur. J. Appl. Physiol.*, 52, 104, 1983.
27. **Häkkinen, K., and Komi, P.V.**, Electromyographic changes during strength training and detraining, *Med. Sci. Sports*, 15, 455, 1983.
28. **Sale, D.G.**, Neural adaptation in strength and power training, in *Human Muscle Power*, Jones, N.L., McGartnes, N., and McComas, A.J., Eds., Human Kinetics, Champaign, 1986, 281.
29. **Milner-Brown, H.S., Stein, R.B., and Lee, R.G.**, Synchronization of human motor units: possible roles of exercise and supraspinal reflexes, *EEG Clin. Neurophysiol.*, 38, 245, 1975.
30. **Komi, P.V.**, Training of muscle strength and power: interaction of neuromotoric, hypertrophic and mechanical factors, *Int. J. Sports Med.*, 7 (Suppl. 1), 10, 1986.
31. **Häkkinen, K., and Komi, P.V.**, Changes in electrical and mechanical behaviour of leg extensor muscles during heavy resistance strength training, *Scand. J. Sports Sci.*, 7, 55, 1985.
32. **Noth, J.**, Cortical and peripheral control, in *Strength and Power in Sport*, Komi, P.V., Ed., Blackwell Scientific, Oxford, 1992, 9.
33. **Sale, D. G.**, Neural adaptation to strength training, in *Strength and Power in Sport*, Komi, P.V., Ed., Blackwell Scientific, Oxford, 1992, 249.
34. **Sale, D.G., MacDougall, J.D., Upton, A.R.M., and McComas, A.J.**, Effect of strength training upon motoneuron excitability in man, *Med. Sci. Sports Exerc.*, 15, 57, 1983.
35. **Häkkinen, K., and Komi, P.V.**, Changes in neuromuscular performance in voluntary and reflex contraction during strength training in man, *Int. J. Sports Med.*, 4, 282, 1983.
36. **Sale, D.G., Upton, A.R.M., McComas, A.J., and MacDoughall, J.D.**, Neuromuscular function in weight-training, *Exp. Neurol.*, 82, 521, 1983.
37. **Sale, D.G.**, Neural adaptation to resistance training, *Med. Sci. Sports Exerc.*, 20, S135, 1988.
38. **Upton, A.R.M., and Radford, P.F.**, Motoneuron excitability in elite sprinters, in *Biomechanics VA*, Komi, P.V., Ed., University Park Press, Baltimore, 1975, 82.
39. **Grimby, L., Hannerz, J., and Hedman, B.**, The fatigue and voluntary discharge properties of single motor units in man, *J. Physiol.*, 316, 545, 1981.
40. **Kawakami, M.**, Training effect and electromyogram. I. Spatial distribution of spike potentials, *Jpn. J. Physiol.*, 51, 1, 1955.
41. **Sale, D.G., and MacDoughall, D.**, Specificity in strength training: a review for the coach and athlete, *Can. J. Appl. Sports Sci.*, 6, 87, 1981.
42. **Sale, D.G., McComas, A.J., MacDoughall, J.D., and Upton, A.R.M.**, Neuromuscular adaptation in human thenar muscles following strength training and immobilization, *J. Appl. Physiol.*, 53, 419, 1982.
43. **Cracraft, J.D., and Petajan, J.H.**, Effect of muscle training on the pattern of firing of single motor units, *Am. J. Phys. Med.*, 56, 183, 1977.
44. **Bravaya, D.Y.**, Comparative analysis of the effect of static (isometric) and dynamic (isokinetic) force training, *Sports Training Med. Rehab.*, 1, 71, 1988.
45. **Lesmes, G.R., Costill, D.L., Coyle, E.F., and Fink, W.J.**, Muscle strength and power changes during maximal isokinetic training, *Med. Sci. Sports*, 10, 266, 1978.
46. **Narici, M.V., Roi, G.S., Landoni, L., Minetti, A.E., and Ceretelli, P.**, Changes in force, cross-sectional area and neural activation during strength training and detraining of the human quadriceps, *Eur. J. Appl. Physiol.*, 59, 310, 1989.
47. **Kyröläinen, H., Komi, P.V., and Kim, D.H.**, Effects of power training on neuromuscular performance and mechanical efficiency, *Scand. J. Med. Sci. Sports*, 1, 78, 1991.
48. **Duchateau, J., and Hainut, K.**, Training effects of submaximal electrostimulation in a human muscle, *Med. Sci. Sports Exerc.*, 20, 99, 1988.
49. **Häkkinen, K.**, Lihasvoiman lisääntymisen mekanismi ja voimaharjoitelun keskeisel periaatteet, *Finn. Sports Exerc. Med.*, 2, 147, 1983.
50. **Pysh, J.J., and Weiss, G.M.**, Exercise during development induces an increase in Purkinje cell dendritic tree size, *Science*, 206, 230, 1979.
51. **Gilliam, T.B., Roy, R.R., Taylor, J.F., Heusner, W.W., and Van Huss, W.D.**, Ventral motor neuron alteration in rat spinal cord after chronic exercise, *Experimentia*, 15, 665, 1977.
52. **Gerchman, L.B., Edgerton, V.R., and Carrow, R.E.**, Effect of physical training on the histochemistry and morphology of central motor neurons, *Exp. Neurol.*, 49, 790, 1975.
53. **Crockett, J.L., Edgerton, V.R., Max, S.R., and Barnard, R.J.**, The neuromuscular junction response to endurance training, *Exp. Neurol.*, 51, 207, 1976.
54. **Dirks, S.J., and Hutton, R.S.**, Endurance training and short latency reflexes in man, *Scand. J. Sports Sci.*, 6, 21, 1984.
55. **Hutton, R.S.**, The central nervous system, in *The Olympic Book of Sports Medicine*, Dirix, A., Knuttgen, H.G., and Tittel, K., Eds., Blackwell Scientific, Oxford, 1988, 69.

56. **Wolpaw, J.R.**, Adaptive plasticity in the spinal strength reflex: an accessible substrate of memory, *Cell. Mol. Neurobiol.*, 5, 147, 1985.

57. **Fechner, G.T.**, Berichte, die zu beweisen schneinen daß durch die Übung der Geieder der einen Seite die der anderen Seite mitgeübt werden, *Ber. Sächweiz. Ges. Wiss. Math. Phys. Kl.*, 10, 70, 1858.

58. **Scriptue, E.W., Smith, T.L., and Brown, E.M.**, On the education of muscular control and power, *Stud. Yale Psych. Lab.*, 2, 114, 1894.

59. **Hellebrandt, F.A., Parrish, A.M., and Houtz, S.J.**, Cross education. The influence of unilateral exercise on the contralateral limb, *Arch. Phys. Med.*, 28, 76, 1947.

60. **Hellebrandt, F.A.**, Cross education: ipsilateral and contralateral effects of unimanual training, *J. Appl. Physiol.*, 4, 136, 1951.

61. **Zimkin, N.V.**, *Physiological Characteristics of Strength, Speed and Endurance*, FiS, Moscow, 1956 (in Russian).

62. **Hollmann, W., and Hettinger, T.**, *Sportmedizin — Arbeits and Trainingsgrundlagen*, Schattauer, Stuttgart, 1976.

63. **Moritani, T., and deVries, H.A.**, Neural factors vs. hypertrophy in time course of muscle strength gain, *Am. J. Phys. Med. Rehabil.*, 58, 115, 1979.

64. **Landin, S., Hagenfeldt, L., Saltin, B., and Wahren, J.**, Muscle metabolism during exercise in patients with Parkinson's disease, *Clin. Sci. Mol. Med.*, 47, 493, 1974.

65. **Kannus, P., Alosa, D., Cook, L., Johnson, R.J., Runström, P., Pope, M., Beynnon, B., Yasuda, K., Nichols, C., and Kaplan, M.**, Effect of one-legged exercise on the strength, power and endurance of the contralateral leg, *Eur. J. Appl. Physiol.*, 64, 117, 1992.

66. **Piehl, K., Adolfsson, S., and Nazar, K.**, Glycogen storage and glycogen synthase activity in trained and untrained muscle of man, *Acta Physiol. Scand.*, 90, 779, 1974.

67. **Saltin, B., Nazar, K., Costill, D.L., Stein, E., Jansson, E., Essen. B., and Gollnick, P.D.**, The nature of training response, peripheral and central adaptations to one-legged exercise, *Acta Physiol. Scand.*, 96, 289, 1976.

68. **Henriksson, J.**, Training-induced adaptation of skeletal muscle and metabolism during submaximal exercise, *J. Physiol.*, 270, 677, 1977.

69. **Saltin, B., and Gollnick, P.D.**, Skeletal muscle adaptability: significance for metabolism and performance, in *Handbook of Physiology*. Section 10: Skeletal Muscle, Peachy, L.D., Adrian, R.H., and Geiger, S.R., Eds., Williams and Wilkins, Baltimore, 1983, 555.

70. **Flynn, M.G., Costill, D.L., Kirwan, J.P., Fink, W.J., and Dengel, D.R.**, Muscle fiber composition and respiratory capacity in triathletes, *Int. J. Sports Med.*, 8, 383, 1987.

71. **Rösler, K., Hoppeler, H., Conley, K.E., Claassen, H., Gehr, P., and Howell, H.**, Transfer effects in endurance exercise. Adaptation in trained and untrained muscles, *Eur. J. Appl. Physiol.*, 54, 355, 1985.

72. **Ingelmark, B.E.**, Der Bau der Sehnen wahrend verschieder altersperioden und unter Wechselenlendes funktionellen Bedingungen. I. Fine qualitative morphologische Untersuchungen an den Achillessehnen wasser Ratten, *Acta Anat.* (Basel), 6, 113, 1948.

73. **Viidik, A.**, The effort of training on the tensile strength of isolated rabbit tendons, *Scand. J. Plast. Recontr. Surg.*, 1, 141, 1967.

74. **Kiiskinen, A., and Heikkinen, E.**, Effect of prolonged physical training on the development of connective tissues in growing mice, in *Metabolic Adaptation to Prolonged Physical Exercise*, Howald, H. and Poortmans, J.R., Eds., Birkhäuser, Basel, 1975, 253.

75. **Booth, F.W., and Gould, E.W.**, Effects of training and disuse on connective tissue, *Exerc. Sport Sci. Rev.*, 3, 83, 1975.

76. **Viidik, A.**, Adaptability of connective tissues, in *Biochemistry of Exercise VI*, Saltin, B., Ed., Human Kinetics, Champaign, 1986, 545.

77. **Tipton, C.M., Schild, R.J., and Tomarek, R.J.**, Influence of physical activity on the strength of knee ligaments in rats, *Am. J. Physiol.*, 212, 783, 1967.

78. **Viidik, A.**, Elasticity and tensile strength of the anterior cruciate ligament in rabbits as influenced by training, *Acta Physiol. Scand.*, 74, 372, 1968.

79. **Tipton, C.M., James, S.L., Merger, W., and Tchang, T.K.**, Influence of exercise on strength of medial collateral knee ligaments of dogs, *Am. J. Physiol.*, 218, 894, 1970.

80. **Tipton, C.M., Mathes, R.D., and Sandage, D.S.**, In situ measurements of junction strength and ligament elongation in rats, *J. Appl. Physiol.*, 37, 758, 1974.

81. **Tipton, C.M., Martin, R.K., Matthews, R.D., and Carey, R.D.**, Hydroxyproline concentrations in ligaments from trained and nontrained dogs, in *Metabolic Adaptation to Prolonged Physical Exercise*, Howald, H. and Poortmans, J.R., Eds., Birkhäuser, Basel, 1975, 262.

82. **Booth, F.W., and Tipton, C.M.**, Effects of training and 17-estradiol upon heart rates, organ weights, and ligamentous strength of female rats, *Int. Z. angew. Physiol.*, 27, 187, 1969.

83. **Adams, A.**, Effect of exercise upon ligament strength, *Res. Q.*, 37, 163, 1966.

84. **Viidik, A.**, Tensile strength properties of Achilles tendon systems in trained and untrained rabbits, *Acta Orthop. Scand.*, 40, 261, 1969.
85. **Tipton, C.M., Tchang, T.-K., and Mergner, W.**, Ligamentous strength measurements from hypophysectomized rats, *Am. J. Physiol.*, 221, 1144, 1971.
86. **Tipton, C.M., Struck, P.-J., Baldwin, K.M., Matthes, R.D., and Dowell, R.T.**, Response of adrenalectomized rats to chronic exercise, *Endocrinology*, 91, 573, 1972.
87. **Vailas, A.C., Tipton, C.M., Matthes, R.D., and Beaford, T.G.**, The influence of physical activity on the strength of junctions and ligaments of diabetic rats, *Med. Sci. Sports*, 10, 57, 1978.
88. **Tipton, C.M., Terjung, R.L., and Barnard, R.J.**, Response of thyroidectomized rats to training, *Am. J. Physiol.*, 215, 1137, 1968.
89. **Heikkinen, E., and Vuori, I.**, Effect of physical activity on the metabolism of collagen in aged mice, *Acta Physiol. Scand.*, 84, 543, 1972.
90. **Heikkinen, E., Suominen, H., Vihersaari, T., Vuori, I., and Kiiskinen, A.**, Effect of physical training on enzyme activities of bones, tendons and skeletal muscle in mice, in *Metabolic Adaptation to Prolonged Exercise*, Howald, H. and Poortmans, J.R., Eds., Birkhäuser, Basel, 1975, 448.
91. **Vailas, A.C., Tipton, C.M., and Mergner, W.**, Ligamentous strength measurements from hypophysectomy on the aerobic capacity of ligaments and tendons, *J. Appl. Physiol.*, 44, 542, 1978.
92. **Tipton, C.M., Matthes, R.D., Maynard, J.A., and Carey, R.A.**, The influence of physical activity on ligaments and tendons, *Med. Sci. Sports*, 7, 165, 1975.
93. **Woo, S.L.Y., Gomex, M.A., Woo, Y.-K., and Aneson, W.H.**, Mechanical properties of tendons and ligaments. II. The relationship between immobilization and exercise on tissue remodeling, *Biorheology*, 19, 397, 1982.
94. **Fleck, S.J., and Falkel, J.E.**, Value of resistive training for the reduction of sports injuries, *Sports Med.*, 3, 61, 1986.
95. **Stone, M.H.**, Implications for connective tissue and bone alterations resulting from resistance exercise training, *Med. Sci. Sports*, 20 (Suppl.), S.162, 1988.
96. **Hirch, G.**, Tensile properties during tendon healing, *Acta Orthop. Scand. Suppl.*, 153, 145, 1974.
97. **Viidik, A.**, Simultaneous mechanical and light microscopic studies of collagen fibers, *Z. Anat. Entwicklungsgesch.*, 136, 204, 1972.
98. **Heleta, T.**, Variations in thickness of cortical density of bone in two populations, *Ann. Clin, Res.*, 1, 227, 1969.
99. **Nilsson, B.E., and Westlin, N.E.**, Bone density in athletes, *Clin. Orthop.*, 77, 179, 1971.
100. **Dalen, N., and Olson, K.E.**, Bone mineral content and physical activity, *Acta Orthop. Scand.*, 45, 170, 1974.
101. **Block, J.E., Friedlander, A.L., Brocks, G.A., Steiger, P., Stubbs, H.A., and Genat, H.K.**, Determinants of bone density among athletes engaged in weightbearing and nonweightbearing activity, *J. Appl. Physiol.*, 67, 1100, 1989.
102. **Snow-Horter, C., and Marcus, R.**, Exercise bone mineral density and osteoporosis, *Exerc. Sport Sci. Rev.*, 19, 351, 1991.
103. **Eisman, J.A., Kelly, P.J., Sambrock, P.N., Pocock, N.A., Ward, J.J., Eberl, S., and Yeates, M.J.**, in *Osteoporosis: Physiological Basis, Assessment and Treatment*, DeLuca, H.F. and Maress, R., Eds., Elsevier, New York, 1990, 227.
104. **Jones, H.H., Priest, J.D., Hayes, W.C., Tichnor, C.C., and Nagel, D.A.**, Humeral hypertrophy in response to exercise, *J. Bone Joint Surg.*, 59A, 204, 1977.
105. **Montoye, H.J., Smith, E.L., Fardon, D.F., and Howley, E.T.**, Bone mineral in senior tennis players, *Scand. J. Sports Sci.*, 2, 26, 1980.
106. **Saville, P.D., and Whyte, M.P.**, Muscle and bone hypertrophy, *Clin. Orthop.*, 65, 81, 1969.
107. **Kiiskinen, A., and Heikkinen, E.**, Effects of physical training on development and strength of tendons and bones in growing mice, *Scand. J. Clin. Lab. Invest.*, 29 (Suppl. 123), 20, 1973.
108. **King, D.W., and Pengelly, R.G.**, Effect of running on the density of rat tibias, *Med. Sci. Sports*, 5, 68, 1973.
109. **Heaney, R.P.**, Radiocalcium metabolism in disuse osteoporosis in man, *Am. J. Med.*, 33, 188, 1962.
110. **Holmdahl, D.E., and Ingelmark, B.E.**, Der Bau des Gelenkkuorpels under verschiedenen funktionellen Verhaltnissen, *Acta Anat.*, 6, 309, 1948.
111. **Jeblecki, C.K., Neuser, J.E., and Kaufman, S.**, Autoradiographic localization of new RNA synthesis in hypertrophying skeletal muscle, *J. Cell. Biol.*, 57, 743, 1973.
112. **Turto, H., Lindy, S., and Halme, J.**, Precollagen proline hydroxylase activity in work-induced hypertrophy of rat muscle, *Am. J. Physiol.*, 226, 63, 1974.
113. **Kovanen, V., Suominen, H., and Heikkinen, E.**, Connective tissue of fast and slow skeletal muscle in rats — effects of endurance training, *Acta Physiol. Scand.*, 108, 173, 1980.
114. **Kovanen, V., Suominen, H., and Heikkinen, E.**, Collagen of slow twitch and fast twitch muscle fibers in different types of rat skeletal muscle, *Eur. J. Appl. Physiol.*, 52, 235, 1984.
115. **Kovanen, V., and Suominen, H.**, Age- and training-related changes in the collagen metabolism of rat skeletal muscle, *Eur. J. Appl. Physiol.*, 58, 765, 1989.

116. **Kovanen, V., Suominen, H., and Peltonen, L.**, Effects of aging and life-long physical training on collagen in slow and fast skeletal muscle in rats, *Cell Tissue Res.,* 248, 247, 1987.

117. **Karpakka, J., Väänänen, K., Orava, S., and Takala, T.E.S.**, The effects of preimmobilization training and immobilization on collagen synthesis in skeletal muscle, *Int. J. Sports Med.,* 11, 484, 1990.

118. **Kovanen, V., Suominen, H., Risteli, J., and Risteli, L.**, Type IV collagen and laminin in slow and fast skeletal muscle in rats. Effects of age and life-time endurance training, *Collagen Rel. Res.,* 8, 145, 1988.

119. **Brzank, K.D., and Pieper, K.S.**, Effect of intensive, strength building exercise training on the fine structure of human skeletal muscle capillaries, *Anat. Anz.,* 161, 243, 1986.

120. **MacDoughall, J.D., Sale, D.G., Alway, S.E., and Sutton, J.R.**, Muscle fiber number in biceps brachii in body builders and control subjects, *J. Appl. Physiol.,* 57, 1399, 1984.

121. **Tomanek, R.J., Taunton, C.A., and Liskop. K.S.**, Relationship between age, chronic exercise and collagen tissue of the heart, *J. Gerontol.,* 27, 33, 1972.

122. **Kiiskinen, A., and Heikkinen, E.**, Physical training and connective tissues in young mice-heart, *Eur. J. Appl. Physiol.,* 35, 167, 1976.

123. **Bartosová, D., Chvapil, M., Korecky, B., Poupa, O., Rakusan, K., Turek, Z., and Visek, M.**, The growth of the muscular and collagenous parts of the rat heart in various forms of cardiomegaly, *J. Physiol.,* 200, 285, 1969.

124. **Kiiskinen, A., and Heikkinen, E.**, Physical training and connective tissue in young mice, *Br. J. Dermatol.,* 95, 525, 1976.

125. **Suominen, H., Heikkinen, E., Moisio, H., and Viljama, K.**, Physical and chemical properties of skin in habitual trained and sedentary 31 to 70 years old men, *Br. J. Dermatol.,* 99, 147, 1978.

Chapter 8

MOLECULAR MECHANISMS
OF TRAINING EFFECTS

In the previous chapter it was shown that systematically repeated exercises induce a great variety of changes in the body. These include morphological changes, up to the subcellular structures, metabolic and functional changes, and improved coordination of the body's activities regarding nervous, hormonal, and cellular autonomic regulations. They are specifically related to the training exercises used. Improvements in performance and various body faculties are founded on these changes.

There was never any doubt that changes induced by training express adaptation to conditions of increased muscular activity. Thus, various concepts related to these adaptive processes were used to explain the mechanism of training effects:

1. J.-B. Lamarck's[1] statement that function creates organ
2. W. Roux's[2] postulation that any functional change induces a trophic stimulation and thereby specific action on the organic form
3. W. Weigert's law[3] of supercompensation for energy expenditure
4. W.A. Engelhardt's[4] rule that the degradation process is always a specific stimulus for the synthetic process
5. I. P. Pavlov's[5] theory of conditioned reflexes

These concepts cannot be considered alternatives. Partly, they are additive, contributing mechanisms for different changes (changes in organic form vs. supercompensation for energy stores, improvement of the body's resources and cellular structures vs. coordination of functions). At the same time there exists a possibility for regarding some of these concepts as expressions of the process of development in understanding the same manifestation. J.B. Lamarck's idea was based on analysis of the process of evolution. It was speculative to use this idea for understanding processes going on within the ontogenesis of an individual organism. Therefore, an additional postulation like that of W. Roux's was necessary. But what does trophic stimulation mean, and what is the mechanism by which it acts? These questions have remained without answers. A number of biochemical results enabled W.A. Engelhardt to establish a close relationship between synthetic and degradation processes in the organism. Soon evidence was obtained that this relationship is founded on cellular autoregulation of enzyme activities as well as on various mechanisms of neurohormonal regulation. What was important in Engelhardt's rule was the affirmation that a stimulus for the synthetic process is born in the degradation process. Consequently, this rule made it possible to recognize the trophic stimulus as a result of previous degradation. In the same way the stimulus for repletion of energy stores and their supercompensation can be understood. However, the trophic stimulus must not only warrant restoration of the previous stores and abilities, but also induce improvement of the organism's faculties. Therefore, the changes constituting the background for improvement of the organism's faculties have to transfer various qualities to a new, more or less stable level. Only if this is the case, can the training effects be understood.

Analysis of recovery processes after various exercises (Chapter 4) showed that restitution of the body's abilities is followed by a period of intensive adaptive protein synthesis and supercompensation for energy stores. However, this period is only transitory. Consequently, the effect of a single exercise bout is not enough for achieving any training effects. Accordingly, the experience of sports practice is very striking: only systematically repeated exercises can lead to training effects.

The concept of symmorphosis postulates that the quantity of structural elements is regulated to satisfy but not to exceed the requirements of the functional system.[6] Chronically maintained high demands are necessary for a stable improvement.

Sportsmen's experience also shows that progress in sports results is possible only by using exercises requiring extensive mobilization of the body's abilities. Animal experiments performed in N.N. Yakovlev's laboratory likewise led to the conclusion that systematically repeated exercises promote the improvement of fitness only if they cause substantial changes in the biochemical content of the internal milieu, i.e., alterations in the 'biochemical homeostasis'.[7]

Therefore, training effects can be achieved: (1) if the exercises are repeated, and (2) if they demand an extensive mobilization of the adaptation abilities of the organism.

The classical studies by W.B. Cannon[8] and H. Selye[9] laid the basis necessary for intimate understanding of adaptation processes. Subsequent progress in the theory of adaptation helped to draw a more complete picture about the training mechanism. In this context, understanding of the connection between a high functional activity and the activation of the cellular genetic apparatus is the most important item. In 1965 it was suggested by F.Z. Meerson[10] that an intracellular mechanism exists that interrelates the physiological function and the genetic apparatus of cells. Through this mechanism, the intensity of the functional activity of cellular structures determines the activity of the genetic apparatus. Thereby, a specific stimulation of protein synthesis follows. The significance of adaptive protein synthesis in the development of fitness has been assumed by various authors.[11-18] It has been hypothesized[15] that the mobilization of bodily resources and their utilization during training exercise causes accumulation of metabolites that will specifically induce adaptive synthesis of structure and enzyme proteins related to the most active cellular structures and biochemical reactions, respectively. The accompanying activation of the mechanism of general adaptation warrants hormonal changes necessary for amplification of the inductor effect of metabolites as well as for the supply of protein synthesis by 'building materials'. As a result, an effective renewal of protein structures, their enlargement, and increase in the number of molecules of the most responsible enzymes will be created (Figure 8-1).

In order to evaluate this hypothesis it is necessary (1) to demonstrate the specific relation between training exercises and induction of adaptive protein synthesis, (2) to establish what the metabolic inductors in various kinds of training exercises are, (3) to obtain evidence for the essential role of hormones in amplifying the action of metabolic inductors, (4) to confirm the necessity for repeated series of training exercises in order to achieve any training effects, and (5) to clarify interrelations between series of repeated exercises.

PROTEIN SYNTHESIS IN TRAINING

The above-presented data are collectively rather conclusive that (a) training exercises stimulate an enlargement of cellular structures and correspondingly increase the contents of various proteins, and (b) these processes are specifically related to the training exercises used. Differences in training effects suggest that in the training process the adaptive protein synthesis is utilized in many ways. The main locus of the adaptive protein synthesis varies between tissues and organs. In striated muscle tissue different distribution of the adaptive protein synthesis exists between muscles, and within a muscle between motor units (types of muscle fiber). Within a cell, the adaptive protein synthesis is differently distributed between cellular structures and between individual proteins. In all cases there exist two main determinants of the distribution of the adaptive protein synthesis:

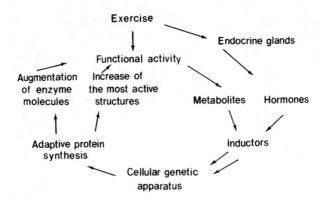

FIGURE 8-1. Induction of the adaptive protein synthesis and its results.

1. The rate of functional activities during exercise performance or in the first stage of the recovery period
2. The significance of the organ, muscle, motor unit, cellular structure, and metabolic pathway in acute adaptation to the performed exercise and in the realization of the concrete motor task

Undoubtedly, the proteins in which synthesis is stimulated, are different in training for improved endurance and in training for improved strength. Strength training mainly increases the content of myofibrillar proteins in the first place in fast-twitch glycolytic fibers, but rather significantly also in fibers of other types. However, these changes are almost exclusively located in the muscles bearing the most strain during exercise. The increased activity of oxidative enzymes and elevated content of mitochondrial proteins indicate that the effect of endurance training is located in the first place in mitochondria. This effect has been found in various types of muscle fibers. It has been demonstrated that in the recovery period after an endurance exercise the protein synthesis rate increased in fast-twitch oxidative-glycolytic fibers but not in fast-twitch glycolytic fibers (see Chapter 4, Figure 4-12). Within oxidative-glycolytic fibers the synthesis rate of mitochondrial proteins increased more than that of myofibrillar proteins.

EVIDENCES OF AUGMENTED PROTEIN SYNTHESIS IN TRAINING

A number of results have confirmed the increased rate of protein synthesis in muscles during their hypertrophy.[11,18-20] Simultaneously, an increase in the RNA content takes place.[21,22] The increased activity of genome of the skeletal muscle fibers was indicated by elevated activities of DNA-dependent RNA polymerase[22-26] and amino-acyl-RNA-synthase.[23,27] This result was obtained both with endurance and strength training. An increased synthesis of RNA *in vivo* was detected within 24 h after initiating the compensatory hypertrophy of muscles.[22]

The increased physical working capacity resulting from endurance training was found to be influenced by actions on the induction of adaptive protein synthesis. Actinomycin D, a blocker of DNA-dependent synthesis of RNA, decreased the working capacity. At the same time, exercise decreased the resistance of animals to actinomycin. Administration of a combination of cofactors and precursors of nucleic acids (folic acid, vitamin B_{12}, and orotic acid) promoted the increase in working capacity during training.[28] Actinomycin D administration prevented the compensatory hypertrophy of muscles.[29]

A program of chronic treadmill running induced an increase in citrate synthase activity of 30 to 41% together with a similar rise (27 to 57%) in mRNA for cytochrome c in the rat soleus, plantaris, red quadriceps, and gastrocnemius muscles. An increase was also found in mRNA for α-actin but only in fast-twitch fibers.[30]

The results are in a good accord with data obtained in experiments with chronic indirect electrical stimulation of the extensor digitorum longus or tibialis anterior muscles. In these experiments the muscle contractions were moderate in force output, but the period of daily stimulation was up to 24 h. A pronounced elevation in the activities of citrate synthase and cytochrome oxidase accompanied with an increase in mRNA for citrate synthase,[31] β-subunit of F_1ATPase, VIC subunit of cytochrome oxidase, and cytochrome b.[32,33] In a study of the muscle-disuse effect, parallel changes of cytochrome c protein synthesis and cytochrome c mRNA were confirmed.[34] It was concluded that in muscular activity similar to endurance type exercises, the chronic adaptation is founded on a pre-translational control mechanism.[18]

To imitate human resistance training, a model was employed in rats. Calf muscles were electrically stimulated to contract against a heavy resistance, resulting in plantar flexion. Both ankle extensors and flexors in the same limb were induced to contract; the gastrocnemius muscle (ankle extensor) shortened while the antagonist tibialis anterior muscle (ankle flexor) lengthened during active cross-bridge formation. Using a vigorous program of such heavy resistance training, the concentrically trained gastrocnemius muscle did not reveal hypertrophy. A significant hypertrophy was established in eccentrically trained tibialis anterior muscle. A milder resistance training program caused similar hypertrophy in the eccentric and concentric contracted muscle.[35] After a single bout of either 192 concentric or eccentric contractions, both mixed and myofibrillar protein synthesis rate increased 50 to 60% in the post-exercise recovery period (between 12 to 41 h after the exercise bout). However, skeletal α-actin mRNA and cytochrome c mRNA did not change.[36,37] While mitochondrial adaptation is not expected in heavy resistance training, the lack of change in α-actin mRNA suggests that the myofibrillar protein synthesis might be stimulated through an increase in protein translation.[18] The increased protein synthesis after concentric contractions was not associated with muscle hypertrophy when this kind of activity was used in training.[35] Obviously, the increased protein synthesis rate, caused by a protein translation control mechanism, was balanced by a comparable increase in protein degradation. Against this background, a post-translational control mechanism was suggested in concentric resistance training.[18]

The eccentrically trained tibialis anterior muscle enlarged, however, in relation with daily contraction. After a 10-week heavy resistance training program, increases of 41% in α-actin mRNA, of 38% in total RNA, and of 28% in protein were recorded in the tibialis anterior muscle.[36] Consequently, multiple control sites (pre-translational, translational, and post-translational) can be elicited by training.[18]

When a weight is chronically attached to the wing of a chicken, a 140% increase in the protein content occurs in the slow-twitch anterior latissimus dorsi muscle.[38] It was calculated that only 20% of the increase in the protein synthesis rate accounts for net muscle growth, while 80% of the increase contributes to an increased turnover of proteins. In fast-twitch muscle hypertrophy, even a larger proportion of increase in protein synthesis contributes to the normal replacement and wastage of protein structures (up to 91%). The actual muscle growth was warranted only by 9% of the increase in protein synthesis.[39]

In regard to the action of increased muscular activity on protein turnover, there is no full agreement between the results of various authors. First, it was observed that the compensatory hypertrophy is founded on both increased protein synthesis and decreased protein breakdown in muscles bearing the highest load.[40,41] Later, a 73% increase in the fractional rate of protein degradation was detected in fast-twitch muscle during the third to seventh day of its compensatory hypertrophy. Most of the increase in the degradation rate was blocked by administration of a prostaglandin inhibitor.[42]

In rats a study of the action of exercises causing muscular hypertrophy indicated the existence of significant differences depending on the fiber type. In brachialis muscle, containing mainly fast-twitch fibers, the protein content increased due to the elevated rate of protein synthesis while the breakdown rate did not change. In slow-twitch soleus muscle the protein synthesis rate remained stable but the degradation rate diminished.[43]

Six weeks of running exercises resulted in a 50% increase in cytochrome c concentration in the quadriceps muscle of rats. This change was associated with a 50% increase in the half-life of cytochrome c from 32 days in sedentaries to 48 days in runners. The increase in the synthesis rate was comparatively small and amounted to about 20%. Thus, the decrease in the degradation rate appeared to play the main role in the response of this mitochondrial protein to training.[44] Later this result was not confirmed. A more pronounced increase of mitochondrial protein synthesis was found in comparison with a decrease in their breakdown or the increased synthesis appeared with a lack of changes in the degradation rate.[45,46] In a study, a pronounced decrease in the cytochrome c half-life (from 30 to 8 days) was established after endurance training.[47] The main reason of the discrepancy in results seems to be related to differences in the involvement of muscle fibers of various types.[46]

The differences in training effects related to the intensity and duration of exercises can be expected by the results of a study in the uptake of ^{3}H-leucine into different fractions of the rat skeletal muscle following acute endurance and sprint exercises. The changes appeared to be different after prolonged moderate running vs. short-term intensive dashes. Endurance exercises caused a post-exercise increase of labeled amino acid incorporation into the protein of the mitochondrial fraction both in the red and white vastus muscle. Sprint exercise caused the same only in the white muscle. During post-exercise recovery, episodes of increased label incorporation into the soluble fractions of proteins were found only in the red vastus after endurance exercise, but in both types of muscles after sprint exercise.[48]

While endurance training induces an elevated rate of myosin heavy chain turnover in all types of skeletal muscle fibers, sprint training causes the same change in fast-twitch glycolytic and fast-twitch oxidative-glycolytic, but not in slow-twitch oxidative fibers. The actin turnover rate becomes more rapid in both training regimes in all fiber types as compared to sedentary rats.[49]

In regard to the specific adaptation to sprint training it is worth remembering that the velocity of contraction is proportionally related to the myosin content.[50] Besides that, a great significance may belong to the ratio between myosin isozymes. A 2-week endurance training increased the content of slow myosin isozyme in the vastus lateralis muscle. The same was the result of 2-week sprint training. In the soleus muscle, neither training program changed the ratio between myosin isozymes.[51]

A model of strength training consisting of repeated fast clambering with an additional load (100 to 400 g) induced an increased rate of synthesis of actomyosin proteins in fast-twitch glycolytic fibers.[52] While in endurance training the enhanced turnover rate was founded on approximately equal increase in the synthesis and degradation of contractile proteins, in strength training a consistent prevalence in the increase of synthesis persisted.

For a study of myosin isozyme induction, two models were used. One of them was compensatory hypertrophy of the fast plantaris and the slow soleus induced by surgical removal of the gastrocnemius muscle. The other model was spontaneous running of rats living in an exercise wheel, in which they ran voluntarily as much as 18 km daily.[53,54] After 11 weeks of development of compensatory hypertrophy there was three times as much slow myosin and twice the amount of intermediate myosin as in the control plantaris muscle. These increases were balanced by losses of fast myosin, particularly of fast myosin I, which was greatly reduced in 4 weeks and had completely disappeared by 11 weeks. A different situation appeared after a running period. There was no increase in the size of the plantaris muscle, and the fast myosin I isozyme was still present at levels of control animals. When both stimuli were present in the same muscle (a combination of synergist removal and running exercise), the stimulus to hypertrophy overrode that of exercise. The fast myosin I disappeared and intermediate myosin content doubled. A nearly sixfold increase in the proportion of slow myosin was found. This rise was equal to the sum of increases found with each treatment alone. The changes in specific myosin heavy chain messenger RNAs indicated the relation of the mentioned changes to gene expressions. There were increases in slow myosin heavy chain mRNA as well as in fast IIa myosin heavy chain mRNA, while the fast IIb myosin heavy chain mRNA decreased. Therefore, the increase in slow myosin with hypertrophy was due to an increase in the slow myosin heavy chain mRNA, and the increase in intermediate myosin was associated with an increase in the fast IIa myosin heavy chain mRNA. For comparison the results of Riede et al.[55] may be mentioned. Hypertrophy of the soleus and plantaris muscles was induced by extripation of the gastrocnemius muscle. The following 13 weeks of endurance training caused similar increase in succinate dehydrogenase activity in hypertrophied and control muscles.

In the soleus muscle the compensatory hypertrophy was accompanied by a loss of intermediate and fast myosin in association with a corresponding decrease in the mRNA for fast IIa myosin heavy chain. The slow myosin heavy chain mRNA increased as in the plantaris muscle. Thus, the fast IIa myosin heavy chain gene was regulated in opposite directions in fast and slow muscles, whereas the slow myosin heavy chain was up-regulated in both muscle types. Therefore, the individual muscles responded differently to a common signal.[54] It is noteworthy that the tissue-specific regulation of the myosin heavy chain gene family was also induced by thyroid hormone.[56]

With hypertrophy there was a slight decrease in the fast myosin light chains LC1f, LC2f, and LC3f as well as in LC2f mRNA in the plantaris muscle. These changes were balanced by increases in the slow light chain LC1s and LC2s. Little or no changes appeared in the soleus.[54]

The compensatory hypertrophy of skeletal muscles is associated with an increased incorporation of ^{3}H-inositol into phosphatidyl-inositol. After unilateral tendectomy of the gastrocnemius muscle, during growth the soleus muscle and the plantaris muscle incorporated ^{3}H-inositol more rapidly than the contralateral muscles of the control limb. After the growth ceased, the incorporation into phosphatidyl-inositol gradually returned toward control levels.[57] These results indicate an increased formation of membrane phospholipids. By contrast, in rats that had been forced to swim (for 30 min during the first 4 days and for 1 h during the next 16 days), there was no increase in ^{3}H-inositol incorporation.[57] Therefore, in the cellular membrane levels there also may be differences in the training effects.

An increase in muscle collagen synthesis during increased muscular activity was demonstrated on isolated rabbit muscles incubated in a medium containing radioactive proline. The muscles, incubated under a constant tension, synthesized proteins at 22% of the rate observed *in vivo*. Intermittent mechanical stretching resulted in an increase of 73% in the rate of total protein synthesis up to 38% of that found *in vivo*. Collagen synthesis was affected in the same way as total protein synthesis in both types of incubation. The relative rates of collagen and total proteins synthesis were unchanged.[58]

It can be suggested that training-induced adaptive protein synthesis extends to many structures, tissues, and organs, following the above-discussed training effects. An increase in the protein synthesis rate was detected in hearts from endurance-trained rats.[59] In a study a reduced phenylalanine incorporation into myocardial proteins was observed in perfused hearts isolated from rats trained in running for 10 weeks.[60] Because the rats were sacrificed 1 day after the last training bout, the question remains whether the result reflects the training effect or the recovery period after the last training sessions.

METABOLIC CONTROL OF PROTEIN SYNTHESIS IN TRAINING

CONTROL OF TRANSCRIPTION

Studies performed in the laboratory of N.N. Yakovlev indicated that an accumulation of nonprotein nitrogen and a decrease of protein nitrogen in skeletal muscles during their activity is followed by increased protein nitrogen during the recovery period.[61-62] A certain quantitative relation was observed: a more pronounced decrease during exercise was followed by a more rapid increase in the protein content after the exercise.[62] These results suggest that a link exists between the protein degradation during exercise and the post-exercise protein synthesis. In agreement with this suggestion, exercises for improved strength caused a more pronounced accumulation of protein metabolites than other exercises;[63] hypertrophy of the muscles is caused only by such types of exercise. Prolonged exercises of moderate intensity did not result in any substantial changes in protein nitrogen during and after exercise.[64] In sportsmen the accumulation of protein metabolites was compared after weight exercises with bars corresponding to 25, 50 and 75% of the athlete's maximal strength. The 75% exercise caused a larger accumulation of nonprotein nitrogen in the blood than exercises with bars corresponding to 25 or 50%. Further longitudinal study showed that training was most effective in improving strength when the bar corresponded to 75% of the athlete's ability.[65]

Recently the suggestion about the link between exercise-induced protein degradation and the following protein synthesis was supported by the results of a study performed on the molecular level. Experiments with attachment of a weight to the chicken wing indicated that those muscles that had lost the greatest amount of slow myosin I protein within 48 h had the highest slow myosin I synthesis rate. Obviously, a feedback stimulation of slow myosin I synthesis occurred in response to the slow myosin I degradation.[54,66]

The link between protein degradation and the subsequent protein synthesis may be specific or unspecific. The specific link means that inductors for adaptive protein synthesis are produced as a result of protein degradation. This would suggest that balanced protein turnover is achieved by the influence of protein metabolites on the genes whose expression is the synthesis of degraded proteins. If the same mechanism provides the adaptive increase in protein content, the training-induced development of both protein structures and enzyme systems must be related to the inductor-action of some products of protein breakdown. The unspecific links may be founded on the production of inductors in other metabolic processes that take place simultaneously with but independently of protein degradation.

Protein Degradation Products

It was suggested that low molecular weight products of protein degradation may have significance in the control of protein synthesis by their direct action on the transcriptional process, causing its depression or activation.[24] However, the response specifically related to the performed exercise can only be brought about by specific adjustment of transcriptional activity, mainly of the 'housekeeping' genes, to meet the cell's protein demands. Specific activation of the genetic apparatus will be achieved if the related low molecular weight compounds are protein-specific fragments (specific fragments of protein subunits) produced by protein degradation.[16] This view is supported by evidence that cytoplasmic proteins or their subunits are needed to activate the transcription.[67,68] If protein-specific fragments act as an apoinducer at the gene or operon enhancer region, formation and dissociation of the protein-specific fragments enhancer complex (affecting the fragments concentration) determine the gene or operon transcription activity.[16]

The products of intracellular proteolysis may influence protein synthesis through autoimmune processes.[69] This suggestion is still not experimentally confirmed.

Creatine

Among protein metabolites, creatine[24,70-74] and some amino acids, particularly leucine,[75-77] are known to induce protein synthesis in skeletal muscles. Creatine was found to stimulate myosin synthesis.[70,71] In experiments on the rat myocardium, stimulation of the synthesis of myosin heavy chain was detected.[74] In the myocardium, creatine specifically increased the activity of phosphocreatine kinase as well.[74] Incubation of the growing myoblast culture of the chicken embryo with creatine resulted in 1.5-fold increase in ^{14}C-orotic acid incorporation into RNA, 1.9-fold increase in the activity of nuclear RNA-polymerase, and 29% increase in the incorporation of ^{14}C-leucine into myosin.[73] However, a study of muscle tissue culture failed to confirm the creatine effect on myosin synthesis.[78] Creatine administration *in vivo* did not increase the synthesis rate of sarcoplasmic or myofibrillar proteins in muscle fibers of various types.[79]

Until the muscle cells retain their integrity, the main source of intracellular release of free creatine is the ATP-phosphocreatine system. Besides the role of this system in energy transport from mitochondria to myofibrils, it is decisive in energy attaining in short-term very intensive sprint or strength exercises. It is logical that liberated creatine may induce myosin synthesis while both the force of power output by muscle contraction and ATP breakdown depend on the amount of myosin in myofibrils. In this connection it is possible to explain the increased effect of power exercises for improvement of sprinters' specific performance by supplement of a mixture of creatine and amino acids to the diet.[80] Oral creatine supplementation also increased the possibility to maintain muscle peak torque during repeated contractions[81] and the specific endurance of runners of 400 to 1500 m.[82]

The rapid reutilization of free creatine for phosphocreatine resynthesis at the beginning of the post-exercise recovery period makes doubtful the accumulation of this substrate and, thereby, its main role in the stimulation of muscle protein synthesis. However, administration of exogenous creatine induces increases both in creatine[79,83] and phosphocreatine[83] contents in skeletal muscles of humans[83] and rats.[79] Besides stimulation of the synthesis of some muscle proteins responsible for performance, the positive effect of performance might be related to promotion of phosphocreatine resynthesis at myofibrils as well as in mitochondria due to the increased intracellular creatine content. As a result, a rapid energy supply for myofibrils was ensured both by the increased local phosphocreatine store and the favored transport of oxidation energy from mitochondria to myofibrils.

Amino Acids

The leucine effect on protein synthesis was blocked by inhibition of RNA synthesis.[75] Consequently, the leucine action consists in stimulation of transcription. Within physiological limits, comparatively high doses of leucine inhibited protein degradation in the rat diaphragm. Moderate doses did not exhibit this effect. Stimulation of protein synthesis was observed in both cases. However, the leucine effect on proteolysis ceased after a blockade of leucine transamination. A product of the latter, α-ketoisocapronic acid, was effective in acting on proteolysis but not on protein synthesis. Also the blockade of leucine transamination did not change the leucine effect on protein synthesis.[84] Thus, the inductor effect of leucine is separated from its action on protein breakdown.

Administration of leucine *in vivo* failed to convincingly confirm its stimulatory action on the muscle protein synthesis.[85-86]

Addition of valine, glutamine, metionine, phenylalanine or tyrosine to the incubation medium *in vitro* did not change the rate of protein synthesis in striated muscle tissue. Isoleucine inhibited the rate.[75] In skeletal muscle, raised intracellular glutamine concentrations increase protein synthesis and inhibit overall but not myofibrillar protein degradation *in vitro*.[86] When isoleucine and valine were added in combination, the labeled amino acid incorporation was augmented, but to a smaller extent than in administration of leucine alone.[76] Branched-chain amino acids (leucine, valine, and isoleucine) stimulated protein synthesis also when they were administered *in vivo*. This effect was pronounced in the myocardium, diaphragm, and soleus muscle,[77] i.e., in muscles possessing a high oxidation potential. An increased perfusate concentration of branched-chain amino acids increased protein synthesis rate in the skeletal muscles of young rats, but not in fasted adult rats.[87]

A question arises about the physiological role of 3-methylhistidine. This amino acid is synthesized by adding the methyl group to the histidine molecule after it is included into the peptide chain for formation of myosin or actin. In degradation of contractile proteins,

3-methylhistidine is released and without any changes or reutilization will be excreted with urine. Does this particular amino acid contribute to the link between degradation and synthesis of contractile proteins? This possibility was supported by the results collected in a study of the dynamics of 3-methylhistidine excretion during an 8-week period of resistive training. The training sessions were followed by an increased 3-methylhistidine excretion with peak values on the next night. Training with 70% one-repetition maximum (1RM) exercises was more effective than 50% 1RM exercises in improvement of muscular strength, as well as in development of muscle hypertrophy. The 3-methylhistidine excretion increased during the training period to a higher level in 70% 1RM exercises.[88] These results do not prove the contribution of 3-methylhistidine in induction of the synthesis of contractile proteins. More likely, the higher 3-methylhistidine release corresponded to the more intensive turnover of contractile proteins in case of more effective training.

According to the results of N. N. Yakovlev,[89] muscular activity causes subsequent activation of arginase, ornithine-decarboxylase, and ornithine-α-ketoglytarate transaminase in active muscles. The final result is an augmented formation of polyamines spermidine and spermine. They are inductors of the protein synthesis.[90] In resistance exercises the formation of spermidine and spermine was more pronounced than in endurance exercises. However, this metabolic pathway itself depends on protein synthesis. After administration of cyclohexamide the accumulation of putrescine, spermidine, and spermine was less pronounced, and the activation of ornithine-decarboxylase failed.[91]

Specific tRNA

Besides direct inductor action, leucine and other free amino acids may stimulate protein synthesis through loading the specific tRNA molecules. The unloaded tRNAs consistently inhibit the initiation of translation of the majority of the mRNA in polysomes. Decreased charging of $tRNA^{His}$ or $tRNA^{Leu}$ by inhibition of amino acid activation also suppressed translational initiation rate of mRNA in polysomes. Therefore, the amino acid inflow to the cellular protein synthesis system as well as their activation are important factors in releasing the translational system from such inhibition.[92] By this mechanism the free amino acid accumulation due to intracellular proteolysis may have significance at least in creation of favorable conditions for translation of the formed mRNA.

The Km for leucine of the leucyl-tRNA synthetase was measured to be below the intracellular concentration of leucine. The charging of muscle leucyl- and phenylalanyl-tRNA showed similar behavior, although only leucine affected the protein synthesis. These results suggest that the stimulation of protein synthesis by additional leucine inflow is probably not related to an increased level of leucyl-tRNA.[84]

Energy Balance

A number of metabolites other than products of protein degradation were tested in order to establish their contribution to the control of protein metabolism in muscular activity. It has been suggested that the main stimulus for the adaptive protein synthesis may arise from an increase in the phosphorylation potential

$$\frac{|ADP| \cdot |P_1|}{|ATP|}$$

at least in the myocardium.[93] The intensity of contractile activity must be rather high to decrease the pool of high-energy phosphates in order to cause a decrease in the rate of protein synthesis.[94] No evidence is available on the stimulation of protein synthesis by increased phosphorylation potential or decreased ATP content.

The changes in ATP concentration may contribute in the control of protein synthesis via energy-dependent activation of amino acids. The background for the amino acid activation is the formation of diadenosine $5 \cdot 5^{III}$-P^1, P^4-tetraphosphate. It was suggested that this compound serves as a metabolic 'signal nucleotide' that is formed at the onset of protein synthesis and is a positive pleiotypic activator. It correlates the rate of protein synthesis to other cellular functions that determine the rate of cell division. However, this compound is rapidly depleted after decreases in the ATP/ADP ratio.[95] All these data and suggestions support the view that decreases in the ATP/ADP ratio may inhibit the protein synthesis. Evidence of the opposite action of decreased ATP/ADP ratio is lacking.

Addition of glucose increased the incorporation of ^{14}C-tyrosine into the myocardial proteins. Glucose was effective in the diaphragm and, to a smaller extent, in the soleus muscle, but only when it was administered in combination with branched-chain amino acids.[77] Lactate, pyruvate, malate, and ketones failed to stimulate labeled amino acid incorporation into muscle proteins.[78,84]

The intracellular reduction/oxidation state influences the inhibition of proteolysis caused by leucine or its transamination product α-ketoisokapronic acid in the atrium or diaphragm.[96] Changes in the reduction-oxidation ratio may have significance in the regulation of protein synthesis by influence on the eukaryotic initiation factor 2. When this factor is oxidized, its ability to form a ternary complex with initiator methionyl-tRNA and GTP is promoted. The contribution of this change in regulation of protein synthesis during muscular activity is rather doubtful.[97]

Muscle Stretch

Stretch is capable of inducing increased protein synthesis in either cultured or whole muscle or muscle cells.[54,98-101] The gastrocnemius muscle atrophies less when it is fixed in a stretched rather than a shortened position in an immobilized limb.[102] It has been hypothesized that a stimulation of muscle growth may arise from mechanical stretch of muscle.[103,104] According to this hypothesis the initiating role in adaptive protein synthesis may belong to the sarcolemma. Three possibilities are suggested: protein synthesis may be influenced through the function of Na,K-pump, Ca shifts, or prostaglandin synthesis.

The suggestion of the Na,K-pump involvement in the stretch-induced cell growth of cultured cells is founded on two facts: (1) cultured skeletal myotubes respond to passive stretch by increased activity of the Na,K-pump, and (2) ouabain, a blocker of the Na,K-pump, prevents the stretch-induced increase in protein synthesis.[105] The possible contribution of the Na,K-pump to adaptive synthesis after exercise has not been evaluated.

Calcium

Ca^{2+} as a universal cellular regulator is necessary both for protein degradation and synthesis. Deprivation of extracellular calcium by changing the incubation medium decreased muscle protein degradation by 22% after 2 h. Increase in intracellular calcium by Ca ionophore A23187 increased proteolysis by 40 to 60%. This change was similar to that observed in isometric or isotonic work of muscles. Increase in free calcium, obtained with the aid of potassium depolarization, increased proteolysis by 55% in muscles.[106] Increased uptake of external Ca^{2+} into rat soleus muscle by divalent cation ionophore also increased protein synthesis, but the magnitude of this change (+44%) was lower than the increase in protein breakdown (+114%). The stretch effect on protein synthesis was much more pronounced when stretch was tested in combination with calcium ionophore.[107] Some experiments have not confirmed that calcium ionophore stimulates the synthesis rate of total muscle protein.[108,109]

In the sarcoplasma the concentration of free Ca^{2+} is highest at the onset of each contraction. It must be clarified whether these short-term changes influence the protein synthesis in the post-exercise recovery period and how this action is carried out.

Prostaglandins

The post-exercise adaptive protein synthesis may be causally related to various intracellular or tissue compounds, known by their regulatory influences. Among them the contribution of prostaglandins seems to be rather convincing. An experiment on cultured avian skeletal muscle showed that mechanical stimulation of muscle increases the lipid-related second messengers arachidonic acid, diacylglycerol, and prostaglandins through the activation of specific phospholipases.[110-112] Accordingly, stretch-stimulated increase in protein synthesis also may be caused by activation of sarcolemmal phospholipases, release of arachidonic acid, and a consequent increase in prostaglandin synthesis. Thereby, arachidonic acid is considered to be a signal for protein synthesis.[109] Arachidonic acid itself fails to stimulate protein synthesis despite its stimulatory action on protein degradation. Only in the soleus muscle was a slight stimulatory effect of arachidonic acid on protein synthesis found. Of the metabolites of arachidonic acid, effective in the stimulation of protein synthesis is prostaglandin $F_{2\alpha}$.[108] In a study the increase in protein synthesis was obtained also by prostaglandin A_1 in addition to the effect of $F_{2\alpha}$.[109] Addition of prostaglandin $F_{2\alpha}$ increased the effect of muscle stretch on protein synthesis.[111] When the enzyme cyclo-oxygenase, which converts free arachidonic acid into prostaglandins, was inhibited by indomethicin or methofuramic acid, protein synthesis did not change in muscle incubated under constant tension. In this situation protein synthesis decreased in isolated intermittently stretched muscles.[109]

Prostaglandin failed to stimulate the synthesis of proteins in calcium-deprived muscle preparations.[112] On the other hand, stimulation of protein degradation in muscle by Ca^{2+} is mediated by prostaglandin F_2 and does not require the calcium-activated protease.[113]

A prostaglandin inhibitor, fenbufen, did not prevent compensatory hypertrophy in rats but reduced the increase in protein synthesis rate on the seventh day of hypertrophy.[114]

There is a possibility that cAMP may contribute in the stimulation of protein synthesis.[115] The related evidence concerns mainly the mitochondrial proteins (see below) or influence on the myocardium.[116]

Tissue Growth Factors

Almost nothing is known about the contribution of various tissue growth factors in training-induced adaptive protein synthesis. However, there is no background to exclude their possible significance. In related studies, attention has to be paid also to nuclear regulating factors. The muscle-specific proteins have a common DNA sequence of a CC (A + T rich)$_6$GG nucleotide base motif (CArG-box).[117] It has been suggested that the CArG motif appears to be the main component for muscle-specific transcriptional stimulation of the contractile protein genes.[118] Physiological signals may induce adaptive response through gene expression by interaction of nuclear factors (trans-acting factors) with DNA sequences that regulate the transcription of specific genes.[17] The presence of a trans factor in the skeletal muscle is reported.[119] In cases where sets of genes have been found to be coordinated by the same trans factor, a consensus sequence in the genes' 5'-flanking region, which binds this regulatory protein, have been found. It remains to be determined whether the coordinate expression of a subset of muscle genes, which respond to exercise training, may occur by means of recognition of a consensus DNA sequence by an 'exercise signal' consisting of a single protein or single oligonucleotide.[17]

Specialized cells must contain an array of positive and negative regulators that modify the actions of transcriptional activators.[120] Recently, the family of myogenic factors (myogenesis-controlling genes) was discovered. This family includes myoD, myogens, MRF-1, and Myf-5, which are expressed in skeletal muscle cells. They activate the myogenic program in fibroblasts. All these proteins activate their own transcription in transfected cells. They influence also the transcription of other proteins. The muscle-specific enhancer regions contain binding-sites for regulatory proteins as well as MyoD.[121]

R. Eftimie et al.[122] found that in denervated muscle of the adult calf, myogenin and MyoD mRNAs reach levels that are approximately 40- and 15-fold higher than those found in innervated muscle. Myogenin mRNAs began to accumulate rapidly between 8 and 16 h after denervation, and MyoD transcripts levels began to increase sharply between 16 h and 1 day after denervation. Direct electrical stimulation of the soleus muscle with extracellular electrodes repressed the increase of myogenesis and MyoD transcripts after denervation by 4- to 3-fold, respectively. The authors have suggested that myogenin and/or MyoD may regulate a repertoire of skeletal muscle genes that are down-regulated by 'electrical activity'.

The protein Id has been shown to interact with myogenic transcription factors (MyoD, myogenin, MRF4, and Myf-5) by forming complexes that will not bind to DNA. Id is a negative regulator of transcription.[123] Experiments on the rat and mouse muscle showed that Id is increased under conditions that lead to atrophy, such as denervation or nerve impulse block. When Id is overexpressed in a fiber type-specific fashion, the fibers with the highest levels of Id-expression show atrophy. Therefore, the Id might play a role in regulation of muscle fiber size at the transcriptional level.[124]

In turn, the myogenic factors are regulated by three families of growth factors, which have major effects on the differentiation of skeletal muscle cells. Fibroblast growth factors (FGF) and transforming growth factors-β (TGF-β) are potent inhibitors. The insulin growth factor (IGF, somatomedin) exhibits a biphasic stimulatory action.[125] Thereby, the IGFs exert pleiotypic anabolic action on skeletal muscle cells.[125] All three growth factors affect the expression of myogenin, and FGF and TGF-β have shown to inhibit the expression of MyoD.[126]

In regard to exercise training the significance of myogenic factors as well as of growth factors still awaits evaluation. Such an approach is indicated by the increase in IGF in result of strength exercises.[127]

MUSCLE SATELLITE CELLS

The proliferation capacity of skeletal muscle tissue is documented for muscle regeneration.[128] It is based on the existence of satellite cells as the stem cells of muscle fibers.[129] Hypertrophy as well as hyperplasia might be induced by the activation of satellite cells.[130] Hyperplasia in the cat muscle undergoing strength training was associated with the appearance of satellite-like cells.[131] Satellite cell proliferation is described to be far more than necessary for repair of fiber damage.[132]

After 6 weeks of treadmill running at 35 m·min^{-1} the number of satellite cells in trained rats was increased more than 2.5-fold in comparison with sedentary control rats.[133] Accordingly, in men, 6 weeks of aerobic cycling caused activation of satellite cells in the vastus lateralis muscle. Very small myofibers with central muscles were found. At the ultrastructural level it was observed that these fibers turned out to be myotubes.[134] The participation of satellite cells in muscular hypertrophy as well as activation of myosin synthesis seems rather plausible. However, the extent of their role in muscular hypertrophy as well as their relation to other mechanisms are yet to be established.

CONTROL OF SYNTHESIS OF MITOCHONDRIAL PROTEINS

There are principal differences between exercises and training regimes causing either muscular hypertrophy or an improvement on the mitochondrial level. Accordingly, there must be differences either in inductors of adaptive protein synthesis or in the mechanisms of recognition of inductors at the levels of genetic apparatus and gene expression. This problem has not been systematically studied. It may be assumed that since different qualitative amounts of gene expression occur, different levels of the repeated trans factors would exist in the nuclei from skeletal muscles that have undergone endurance training vs. muscles that have experienced weight training.[17]

By a hypothesis, elevated level of cAMP within skeletal muscle during its chronic continuous stimulation results in an increase in mRNAs transcribing the proteins of mitochondria.[135] The background for this suggestion is a correlation between the increase of cAMP and/or β-adrenergic receptor density on the one hand, and the increase of mRNAs for mitochondrial proteins on the other hand in response to chronic stimulation of a striated muscle.[135] Immediately after a single run for 5, 10, or 30 min cAMP concentration doubles in the red and white quadricep muscles.[136] Using 10- or 30-min runs as training exercises for 13 weeks, no change was found in training with the 10-min runs, but with the 30-min exercises increases of cytochrome c concentration (+31%) and of citrate synthase activity (+37%) were detected in the gastrocnemius muscle.[137] Obviously, either the exercise-induced cAMP accumulation is not the sole factor, or the post-exercise duration of the elevated cAMP is more important. In the heart, a single 60-min run resulted in cAMP being increased for 24 h after exercise.[138]

Experiments with β-adrenoreceptor blockade support the role of cAMP in training-induced mitochondrial proliferation. The normally observed increase in citrate synthase, cytochrome oxidase, β-hydroxyacyl-CoA dyhydrogenase, malate dehydrogenase, and alanine aminotransferase in aerobically trained skeletal muscles in rats was almost completely blocked by administration of propranol, but not by β_1-selective blocker atenolol.[139] In another study, β-blockade excluded training-induced rises in the activities of succinate dehydrogenase, malate dehydrogenase, and citrate synthase in the rat skeletal muscles.[140] In humans, chronic β-blockade significantly reduced the increase in succinate dehydrogenase, cytochrome-c oxidase, and β-hydroxyacyl-CoA dehydrogenase activities in the vastus lateralis muscle by cycling training for 8 weeks.[141] Endurance training induced an increase in β-adrenoreceptor density. This response is considered specific for skeletal muscles as well as for vascular and bronchiolar smooth muscles but not for the heart and adipose tissue.[142,143] The increased number of β-adrenoreceptor favors cAMP accumulation and, thereby, mitochondrial proliferation.

In a study, β-adrenergic blockade in rats failed to prevent enzymatic adaptation to exercise in skeletal muscles.[144] There may be individual differences in sensitivity to the blocker. However, the existence of other factors contributing to increased biogenesis of mitochondria in training have to be considered. In this way the mitochondrial enzyme adaptation in skeletal muscles in swimming training in adrenaldemedullated and/or sympathectomized rats may be explained. At least some of them have resulted from contractile activity of the same muscle fiber, because the mitochondrial adaptation is located only in the fibers participating in the performance of the training exercise.[18,145] Thus, the ineffectiveness of daily injections of adrenaline to sedentary rats during 6 weeks in the increase of skeletal muscle respiratory capacity (judging by the activities of citrate synthase and succinate dehydrogenase, and cytochrome c concentration)[146] is not contradictory to the cAMP role in the normal response of mitochondria to endurance training.

It is assumed that an 'exercise stimulus' interacts at a site distal to the β-adrenergic receptor. In such an event, catecholamines would be permissive in priming the pathway for the local autocrine signal from exercise that leads to mitochondrial proliferation.[17]

The 'exercise stimulus' may be related to the energy balance in mitochondria. The role of energy balance was indicated by results showing that a depletion of high-energy phosphates by feeding the creatine analog β-guanidinopropine stimulates mitochondrial protein synthesis even though the daily physical activity was reduced.[147]

It has been suggested that the key role in the increased activity of mitochondrial enzymes belongs to the induction of δ-aminolevulinic acid synthase by exercise.[145] The effect of thyroxine is analogous. The activity of this enzyme in the red portion of the vastus lateralis muscle was doubled 17 h after a 4000-m run in rats. A similar change was obtained 14 h after injections of thyroxine. Before that, no change in heme-containing cytochrome c concentration occurred.[148] δ-Aminolevulinic acid synthase is a rate-limiting enzyme in heme synthesis. This observation thus implies that up-regulation of heme synthesis is an early regulatory event mediated by muscle contraction and leading to an improvement of respiratory capacity.[18]

The role of hypoxic conditions for mitochondrial development has been discussed. There seems no convincing evidence that the endurance training-induced improvement in mitochondrial capacity is related to intracellular hypoxia.

TRANSLATION CONTROL

Multiple sites (pre-translational, translational, and post-translational) are inferred to be evoked as protein quantities adapt to new levels of muscular activity.[18] It was noted earlier that the charging of tRNA by specific amino acids is an important event in releasing the protein synthesizing system from tonic inhibition. The control of muscle protein synthesis could be modulated at the translational level by the cytoplasmic redox potential.[149] An increase in the sarcoplasmic $NAD^+/NADH$ ratio is accompanied by a decrease in protein synthesis.[77]

The translation process is related to the GTP:GTD ratio. This ratio may decrease because the adenylate energy change decreases in the contracting skeletal muscle. If this occurs, the translation rate would decrease. GTP is also required for peptide chain elongation.[97] Experimental data support the view that if during heavy exercise the energy change of muscle is affected, then the translation and elongation steps of protein synthesis are temporarily decreased.[94]

In conclusion, it is reasonable to suggest that in addition to specific influences on gene transcription, systematically performed muscular activity may induce alterations in mRNA stability, protein translation, protein assembly, and protein degradation.[18] The integral result of all these events is rather likely the specific response through the adaptive protein synthesis (Figure 8-2).

HORMONAL ACTION ON ADAPTIVE PROTEIN SYNTHESIS IN TRAINING

Various experiments have provided a lot of results on the inductor action of hormones as well as on the contribution of hormones in translation control. Plotting these results with the wide spectrum of exercise-induced changes in hormone levels (see Chapter 2), the role of hormones in the actualization of training effects becomes plausible. Adrenocortical, thyroid, insulin, or catecholamine deficiencies aggravate or eliminate the increase in working capacity (determined by endurance tests) in endurance training (Table 8-1). However, in regard to various training-induced changes in the organism, the influence exerted by hormone deficiencies is various and in a number of cases the training effects have remained without alteration (Table 8-2).

Hormones may participate in the regulation of training-induced adaptive protein synthesis in two ways. As has been suggested, hormones amplify the inductive action arisen from metabolic changes during or after training exercises.[14,15,173] There also exists a possibility that the contribution of hormones means a permissive action: a sufficient hormone level is necessary for the activity of other mechanisms of transcriptional, translational, and post-translational control. However, the lack of alterations in a number of training effects in various hormone deficiencies (Table 8-2) suggests that the permissive role of hormones in the control of adaptive protein synthesis is rather questionable. If any of the above-discussed mechanisms of the control of genome activity depends on the permissive action of hormones, the hormone deficiencies have to exclude the adaptive protein synthesis and its results. Therefore it is more likely to assume that there are two separate mechanisms for the regulation of the control of genome activity and gene expression: (1) by metabolic factors and (2) by hormonal influences.

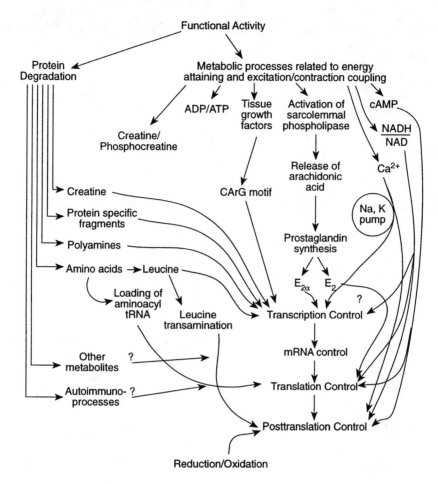

FIGURE 8-2. Stimulation of the adaptive protein synthesis by metabolites.

Table 8-1. Effects of Hormonal Deficiencies on the Improvement of Working Capacity during Training

Cause of hormone deficiency	Training effect	Ref.
Adrenalectomy	No increase in working capacity	150
	Restoration of ability to perform exercise used for training up to the level of untrained intact rats; no increase in other exercises	151,152
Blockade of adrenocortical response to training exercises by dexamethasone administration	No increase in working capacity	153
Thyroid-deficiency	No increase in working capacity	154
	Less pronounced increase	155
Diabetes	Less pronounced increase	156
Chemical sympathectomy	No increase in working capacity	157

These two mechanisms may be additive or integrative in their action. The control of metabolic changes has to be highly specific and determine the choice of proteins for their adaptive synthesis. The hormonal control mechanism may be less specific and more dependent on the overall influence of training sessions on the endocrine function. In terms of the above-described theory of the adaptation process (see Chapter 1), the training session has to

Table 8-2. Action of Hormone Deficiencies on Training-Induced Adaptive Changes

Training effect	Training	Cause of hormone deficiency	Change in the training effect	Ref.
Compensatory hypertrophy of soleus and plantaris muscles	Increased load due to tendotomy of gastrocnemius in rats	Hypophysectomy Diabetes	Without change Without change	158 159,160
Hypertrophy of gastrocnemius and plantaris muscles	Running with progressively increased incline in rats	Thyroidectomy	No effect	161
Increased content of mitochondrial proteins or increased activity of mitochondrial enzymes	Endurance training in rats	Hypophysectomy Thyroidectomy Diabetes Adrenalectomy Adrenalectomy Adrenaldemedullation + sympathectomy Propylthiouracil-induced hypothyroidism Methylthiouracil-induced hypothyroidism	Without change Without change Without change Without change Without change Diminished increase of cytochrome c content, SDH increase without change Without change No response Increase only to level lower than in normal sedentary rats	156 156,161 156,162 154 163 163 164 154 155
Content of myofibrillar and sarcoplasmic proteins in glycolytic and oxidative-glycolytic portion of quadriceps muscle	Running training in rats	Methylthiouracil-induced hypothyroidism	Increase only to levels lower than in normal sedentary rats	165
Increased activity of glycolytic enzymes	Endurance training in rats	Diabetes	Without change, only increase in hexokinase activity lower	162
Increase in muscle glycogen content	Endurance training in rats or rabbits	Sympathectomy Diabetes Adrenalectomy Castration in male rats	Less pronounced More pronounced change No change Less pronounced	166,167 168 150 169
Muscle phosphocreatine content	Endurance training in rats	Sympathectomy	No effect	167
Increase in liver glycogen content	Endurance training in rats	Adrenalectomy	No effect	151,152
Cardiac hypertrophy	Endurance training in rats	Hypophysectomy Thyroidectomy Adrenalectomy Ovariectomy	Less pronounced No effect More pronounced Without change	170 165,171 151,152 172
Increase in cardiac myosin or myofibrillar ATPase activity	Endurance training in rats	Hypothyroidism Thyroidectomy Adrenalectomy	No effect Decrease instead of increase Slightly increased effect	164,165 165 151,152

be sufficient in its intensity and duration to activate the general adaptation mechanism and thereby induce the changes in endocrine functions.

The role of various hormones in regulation of the protein synthesis was discussed in Chapter 4. This discussion led to the suggestion that the two main hormones participating in the induction of the adaptive protein synthesis in post-exercise periods are testosterone and thyroxine/triiodothyronine. Induction of myofibrillar proteins by testosterone makes it important in the actualization of strength training-induced hypertrophy. There is a number of papers indicating a further augmentation of protein synthesis in the muscles if training is accompanied by administration of androgen preparation of anabolic action.[26,174,175] The prohibited use of these preparations by sportsmen made their training more effective and improved their results in strength and power events. In the theoretical aspect, here we have a striking example of the amplifying action of a hormone on the metabolic effect of training.

Thyroid hormones are known to exert a stimulatory influence on the biogenesis of mitochondria. More than 20 years ago it was demonstrated that treatment with triiodothyronine enhanced the training-induced increase in the activities of glycerol-p-dehydrogenase and succinate dehydrogenase.[154] In order to support the role of thyroid hormones in adaptive synthesis of mitochondrial proteins in endurance training, rather suggestive are the results indicating that the specific increase in the synthesis of mitochondrial proteins in oxidative-glycolytic muscle fibers after an endurance exercise (30-min run at 35 m·s^{-1}) does not appear in hypothyroid rats (see p. 103). When the intensity of exercise was high (10 min of swimming with additional load of 40% b.w.), the thyroid hormone level increased after exercise even in rats made hypothyroid by methimazol administration. In this case, post-exercise increase in the synthesis of mitochondrial proteins took place.

In regard to studies on thyroid-deficient rats (Table 8-2), attention must be directed to the low initial level of the muscle oxidative capacity in those rodents. In all cases training only nearly replaced the influence of thyroid deficiency and restored the oxidative capacity. In no case was any increase beyond the levels of sedentary intact rats obtained. Therefore, the observed elevation in the mitochondrial function has only a relative meaning. Experiments indicated an increase in the cytochrome aa$_3$ content due to training both in the oxidative-glycolytic and glycolytic portions of the quadriceps muscle in rats treated with methylthiouracil. However, the post-training level of cytochrome aa$_3$ was substantially lower than in normal sedentary rats. A real increase in the mitochondrial marker content (cytochrome aa$_3$) beyond the level of sedentary rats was observed only in normal rats after training. In these experiments the activation of the thyroid function during training was evidenced by a gain in the thyroid weight (by 22% in normal rats). The gain in the thyroid weight was particularly pronounced in methylthiouracil-treated rats (by 7%). Obviously, the decreased feedback influences lead to a very pronounced pituitary thyrotropin response. The new thyroid tissue, developed under this influence, proved to be capable of synthesizing thyroxine. The blood level of thyroxine increased in the methylthiouracil-treated group from 1.95 ± 0.73 to 5.70 ± 0.43 µg·100 ml^{-1} after training. The hormone level in sedentary controls was 9.52 ± 0.63 µg·100 ml^{-1}.[155] These results are suggestive of the fact that the training-induced mitochonrial changes may also be thyroid dependent in hypothyroid rats.

Thyroid hormones and androgens seem to be important in separately amplifying the two main directions of training effects on muscle proteins (Figure 8-3). However, it does not mean that thyroid hormones do not contribute to the synthesis of myofibrillar proteins or testosterone to the synthesis of other proteins. Nevertheless, a certain specificity remains. For example, administration of synthetic androgens of anabolic action did not potentiate the effects of sprint training in young male rats.[176,177] On the other hand, by its anticatabolic action, testosterone also participates in post-translational control. Administration of retabolil diminished the decrease of myosin Mg^{2+}-ATPase activity in red muscles caused by forced training in rats.[178]

The main hormonal regulators of the translation process are insulin and somatotropin. In sports practice there is a tendency to use somatotropin as doping. However, there is no

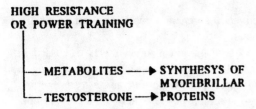

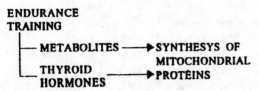

FIGURE 8-3.   Difference in induction of the adaptive protein synthesis in strength and endurance training.

convincing evidence of the actual increase of training effects by somatotropin injection.[179] Nevertheless, somatotropin has to be taken into consideration as a factor of translation control. In a muscle undergoing compensatory hypertrophy, somatotropin treatment caused proportional growth as it occurred in the contralateral control muscles. It was suggested that muscle size is determined by at least two independent factors: somatotropin, and muscular work. Somatotropin appears to act on a biochemical 'amplifying system' for the cells anabolic machinery and determines the absolute changes in muscle size, which result from changes in muscular work.[180]

The elevated output of spermine and spermidine during muscular exercises was mentioned above. These polyamines are known to stimulate proliferation and protein synthesis (see p. 205). Somatotropin stimulates the metabolic processes leading to the formation of spermidine and spermine.[90]

Table 8-1 indicates the lack of training-induced increase in endurance when during training exercises the normal adrenocortical response was blocked. This fact may be related to the two regulatory effects of glucocorticoids. First, the glucocorticoid catabolic effect is necessary for mobilization of precursors for protein synthesis. On the other hand, the same catabolic effect may be involved to warrant an intensive protein turnover and, thereby, an effective renewal of the most responsible protein structures. The latter suggests the contribution of glucocorticoids in post-translational control.

More pronounced cardiac hypertrophy in adrenalectomized rats than in normals (Table 8-2) suggests that glucocorticoids may contribute to the determination of the optimal magnitude of structural changes of the myocardial cells. However, apart from these results, in intact female rats glucocorticoid treatment increased the training-induced cardiac enlargement.[181]

High unphysiological doses of glucocorticoids induce muscle atrophy. Training is capable of avoiding or reducing this harmful result of glucocorticoid administration.[182-184] Using moderate doses of a glucocorticoid, the decrease of fast-twitch fibers weight never exceeded 12%. Training did not prevent the modest effect of muscle weight, but in this case enhanced muscle oxidative capacity and maximal oxygen uptake as well as delayed the appearance of exhaustion during a submaximal exercise bout were detected.[185] These results suggest that in training, glucocorticoid may change the main direction of protein synthesis by contributing to post-translational control.

For a complete interpretation of experimental results related to hormone administration, hormone deprivation, or changes in hormone levels, one must take into consideration that in all these cases the recorded results depend not only on the amount of hormone in body fluids, but also on the tissue sensitivity, determined by a number of factors, among which the most important are the number of specific hormone receptors and the affinity of the receptors to

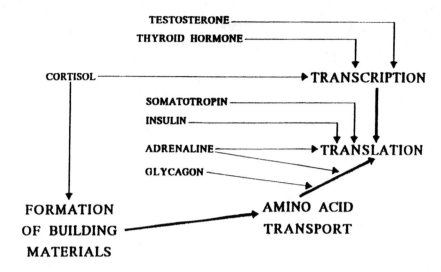

FIGURE 8-4. Participation of hormones in the control of the adaptive protein synthesis.

hormone. Because of the regulation of the hormonal signal at the receptor level the actual hormone action may not be described completely by the hormone concentration or administered doses. Hormonal control in adaptive protein synthesis may be understood as shown in Figure 8-4.

ADAPTIVE PROTEIN SYNTHESIS IN THE MYOCARDIUM

There is no serious background to suggest the existence of significant differences in the control of adaptive protein synthesis between skeletal and heart muscles. However, differences may exist in metabolic inductors and conditions that are responsible for the production of necessary inductors. It was suggested that the main determinants of the cardiac hypertrophy are ventricular systolic stretch due to increased afterload and ventricular diastolic stretch due to increased preload.[186] In the first case a parallel sarcomere replication occurs that leads to an increased ventricular wall size (Figure 8-5). The result is a concentric hypertrophy. In the case of ventricular diastolic stretch series, sarcomere replication takes place with the final result of increased ventricular chambers. The latter means eccentrical hypertrophy commonly observed in most athletes (see p. 169). However, eccentrical hypertrophy is also related to protein synthesis and its relation to protein degradation. The factors modulating these processes are the hormones catecholamine, somatotropin, thyroid hormones, insulin, and cortisol, the metabolites lactate, pyruvate, amino acids, and free fatty acids, as well as such factors as hemodynamic load and hypoxia (Figure 8-6).

OTHER THEORIES OF TRAINING MECHANISMS

In investigations on the supercompensation of energy stores after exercise an interesting fact was established. When the subsequent exercise set begins from the level of supercompensated stores, their decrease reaches levels of glycogen and phosphocreatine contents higher than after the first exercise (Figure 8-7). The following supercompensation leads the energy stores to a higher level now in comparison with supercompensation after the first exercise set.[187-189] On this background it was assumed that in training the augmentation of energy stores is founded on the performance of the subsequent exercise set from the level of supercompensation after the previous one (Figure 8-7).[7]

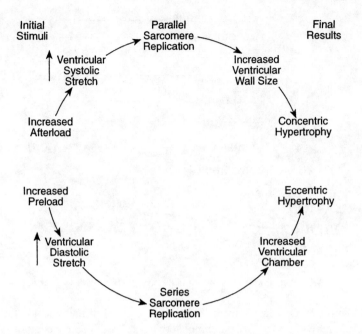

FIGURE 8-5. Induction of concentric and eccentric hypertrophy of the myocardium.[186] (From Minelli, R., and Riccardi, L., in *Sports Cardiology,* Vol. 2, Lubich, T., Venerando, A., and Zeppilli, P., Eds., Aulo Caggi, Bologna, 1983, 29. With permission.)

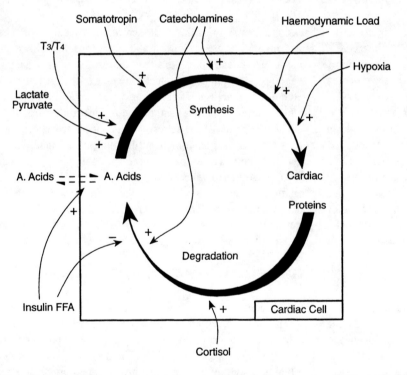

FIGURE 8-6. Factors stimulating protein synthesis or degradation in the myocardium.[186] (From Minelli, R., and Riccardi, L., in *Sports Cardiology,* Vol. 2, Lubich, T., Venerando, A., and Zeppilli, P., Eds., Aulo Caggi, Bologna, 1983, 29. With permission.)

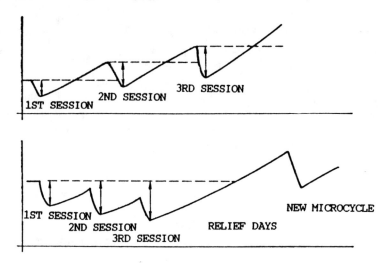

FIGURE 8-7. Training-induced increase in the organism's energy reserve, founded on the post-exercise supercompensation. Constructed according to N. Yakovlev.[7]

For further evaluation of this theory it is necessary to clarify the changes in enzyme/ substrate ratios when the next set of exercise follows the previous one from the supercompensation level, as well as the relation of augmentation of energy stores to adaptive synthesis of related enzymes. In any case, results were obtained indicating that glycogen replenishment depends on synthesis of regulatory protein(s), induced by glucocorticoids (see p. 101).

The essential significance of the formation of new conditioned reflexes and their systems (dynamics stereotypes) in training was postulated by A.N. Krestovnikov.[190] He followed the ideas of his teacher I.P. Pavlov on the leading role of brain cortex in functions of the organism as a whole and, particularly, in the adaptation to new conditions of life activities. He assumed that the formation of conditioned reflexes determines the acquisition of new forms of motor coordination, as well as the actual degree of utilization of motor potential of a sportsman. This view was propagated by various Soviet physiologists but not evaluated in carefully controlled experiments. In any event, it is worth paying attention to this idea in order to understand the improved coordination of motor and other functions in training.

CONCLUSION

Muscle fibers are capable of synthesis of various proteins, including any kind of myofibrillar proteins. The actualization of these possibilities depends on the inductive stimulus. Consequently, the different effects of endurance vs. strength training on the skeletal muscle proteins are rather indicative of the fact that the cellular genetic apparatus is influenced by different inductors formed during endurance or strength exercises. The inductors generated by endurance exercises do not influence the genes responsible for an increase in the overall amount of myofibrillar proteins. At the same time, the inductors generated by strength exercises do not stimulate the genes related to an increase in the synthesis rate of mitochondrial proteins.

The specific initiation of adaptive protein synthesis in muscular activity depends not only on the possible differences between metabolic inductors. There exist a number of mechanisms that may modulate the actual transcription. It is not excluded that the specificity of induction of the adaptive protein synthesis depends on the modulatory mechanisms or on the interrelation between the action of inductors and the activity of the modulatory mechanism. The gene expression is regulated on the translational and post-translational levels as well. All these processes may contribute to the specific results of the adaptive protein synthesis. Hormones intensively secreted during and after exercise add their influence as inductors or regulators of transcription and gene expression. The hormones' actions may have a permissive role. However, the influence of at least some hormones is additive, amplifying the exercise-induced initiation of adaptive protein synthesis and corresponding gene expression. There exists a rather strong plausibility that the amplifying action of hormones is necessary to increase the protein synthesis to higher rates than those necessary for the normal renewal of the protein content of active protein structures.

The integral result of all these regulatory events is the specific response of the adaptive protein synthesis. The latter ensures improvements of cellular capacities for the performance of functional tasks specifically related to training exercises.

There is a serious background for considering the general picture presented. Nevertheless, it must be pointed out that little is known about what the specific inductors ensuring links between performed training exercises and adaptive changes at the cellular level are. Further studies are also necessary for understanding the role of hormones in every concrete case.

REFERENCES

1. **Lamarck, J.-B.**, *Philosophie Zoologique*, Dentu Libraire, Paris, 1809.
2. **Roux, W.**, *Gesammelte Abhandlunger über Entwicklungsmechanik des Organismus, Bd. 1. Funktionelle Anpassung*, Leipzig, 1895.
3. **Weigart, K.**, *Neue Auffassung der Zellwucherung auf äussere Reize*, 1873.
4. **Englehardt, W.A.**, Die Beziehungen Zwischen Atmung and Pyrophosphatumsatz in Vogelerythrocyten, *Biochem. Z.*, 251, 343, 1932.
5. **Pavlov, I.P.**, *Lectures on Conditioned Reflexes*. Twenty-five years of objective study of the higher nervous activity (behaviour) of animals, International Publishers, New York, 1928.
6. **Taylor, C.R., and Weibel, E.R.**, Design of the Mammalian respiratory system. I. Problem and strategy, *Respir. Physiol.*, 44, 1, 1981.
7. **Yakovlev, N.N.**, *Sportbiochemie*, Barth, Leipzig, 1977.
8. **Cannon, W.B.**, *Bodily Changes in Pain, Hunger, Fear and Rage*, 2nd ed., D. Appleton & Co, New York, 1925.
9. **Selye, H.**, *The Physiology and Pathology of Exposure to Stress*, Medical Publishers, Montreal, 1950.
10. **Meerson, F.Z.**, Intensity of function of structures of the differentiated cell as a determinant of activity of its genetic apparatus, *Nature*, 206, 483, 1965.
11. **Poortmans, J.R.**, Effects of long lasting physical exercises and training on protein metabolism, in *Metabolic Adaptation to Prolonged Physical Exercise*, Howald, H. and Poortmans, J.R., Eds., Birkhäuser, Basel, 1975, 212.
12. **Yakovlev, N.N.**, Biochemical mechanisms of adaptation of skeletal muscles to muscular activity, *Ukr. Biokhim. Zh.*, 48, 388, 1976.
13. **Hollmann, W., and Hettinger, T.**, *Sportsmedizin — Arbeits and Trainingsgrundlagen*, Schattauer, Stuttgart, 1976.
14. **Viru, A.**, *Hormonal Mechanisms of Adaptation and Training*, Nauka, Leningrad, 1981 (in Russian).
15. **Viru, A.**, The mechanism of training effects: a hypothesis, *Int. J. Sports Med.*, 5, 219, 1984.
16. **Mader, A.**, A transcription-translation activation feedback circuit as a function of protein degradation, with the quality of protein mass adaptation related to the average functional load, *J. Theor. Biol.*, 134, 135, 1988.
17. **Booth, F.W.**, Perspectives on molecular and cellular exercise physiology, *J. Appl. Physiol.*, 65, 1461, 1988.
18. **Booth, F.W., and Thomason, D.B.**, Molecular and cellular adaptation of muscle in response to exercise: perspectives of various models, *Physiol. Rev.*, 71, 541, 1991.
19. **Hamosh, M., Lesch, M., Baron, J., and Kaufman, S.**, Enhanced protein synthesis in a cell-free system from hypertrophied skeletal muscle, *Science*, 157, 935, 1967.
20. **Poortmans, J.R.**, Protein turnover during exercise, in *3rd Int. Symp. Biochem. Exerc.*, Landrey, F. and Orban, W.A.R., Eds., Symposia Specialists, Miami, 1978, 159.
21. **Millward, D.J., Garlick, P.J., James, W.P.T., Nganyelugo, D.O., and Ryatt, J.S.**, Relationship between protein synthesis and RNA content in skeletal muscles, *Nature*, 241, 204, 1973.

22. **Sobel, B.E., and Kaufman, S.,** Enhanced RNA polymerase activity in skeletal muscle undergoing hypertrophy, *Arch. Biochem. Biophys.*, 137, 469, 1970.

23. **Silber, M.L., Pliskin, A.V., and Rogozkin, V.A.,** Action of physical exercise on synthesis of nuclear RNA in skeletal muscles, *Vopr. Med. Khim.*, 17, 280, 1972 (in Russian).

24. **Rogozkin, V.A.,** The role of low molecular weight compounds in the regulation of skeletal muscle genome activity during exercise, *Med. Sci. Sports*, 8, 74, 1976.

25. **Feldkoren, B.I., Silber, M.L., and Rogozkin, V.A.,** Synthesis of proteins of skeletal muscles and DNA depending RNA polymerase activity of nuclei during action of cyclohexamide, *Ukr. Biokhim. Zh.*, 50, 292, 1978 (in Russian).

26. **Rogozkin, V.A., and Feldkoren, B.I.,** The effect of retabolil and training on activity of RNA polymerase in skeletal muscle, *Med. Sci. Sports*, 11, 345, 1979.

27. **Rogozkin, V.A.,** Some aspects of skeletal muscle metabolism regulation during their functional activity, in *Metabolism and Biochemical Evaluation of Sportsmens Fitness*, Yakovlev, N.N., Ed., Leningrad Res. Inst. Phys. Cult., Leningrad, 1974, 79 (in Russian).

28. **Meerson, F.Z., and Rozanova, L.S.,** Action of actinomycin-2703 and a complex of stimulators of RNA synthesis on the development of fatigue and training state, *Dokl. Akad. Nauk. USSR*, 166, 496, 1966 (in Russian).

29. **Goldberg, A.L., and Goodman, H.M.,** Amino acid transport during work-induced growth of skeletal muscle, *Am. J. Physiol.*, 216, 1111, 1969.

30. **Morrison, P.B., Biggs, R.B., and Booth, F.W.,** Daily running for 2 wk and mRNA for cytochrome c and α-actin in rat skeletal muscle, *Am. J. Physiol.*, 257, C936, 1989.

31. **Seedorf, U., Leberer, E., Kirschbaum, B.J., and Pette, D.,** Neural control of gene expression in skeletal muscle. Effects of chronic stimulation on lactate dehydrogenase isoenzymes and citrate synthase, *Biochem. J.*, 239, 115, 1986.

32. **Williams, R.S., Garcia-Moll, M., Mellor, J., Salmons, S., and Harlan, W.,** Adaptation of skeletal muscle to increased contractility activity, *J. Biol. Chem.*, 262, 2764, 1987.

33. **Kraus, W.E., Bernard, T.S., and Williams, R.S.,** Interactions between sustained contractile activity and β-adrenergic receptors in regulation of gene expression in skeletal muscles, *Am. J. Physiol.*, 256, C506, 1989.

34. **Morrison, P.R., Montgomery, J.A., Wong, T.S., and Booth, F.W.,** Cytochrome c protein-synthesis rates and mRNA contents during atrophy and recovery in skeletal muscle, *Biochem. J.*, 241, 257, 1987.

35. **Wong, T.S., and Booth, F.W.,** Skeletal muscle enlargement with weight-lifting exercise by rats, *J. Appl. Physiol.*, 65, 950, 1988.

36. **Wong, T.S., and Booth, F.W.,** Protein metabolism in rat tibialis anterior muscle after stimulated chronic eccentric exercise, *J. Appl. Physiol.*, 69, 1709, 1990.

37. **Wong, T.S., and Booth, F.W.,** Protein metabolism in rat tibialis anterior muscle after stimulated chronic concentric exercise, *J. Appl. Physiol.*, 69, 1718, 1990.

38. **Laurent, G.J., Sparrow, M.P., Bates, P.C., and Millward, D.J.,** Turnover of muscle protein in the fowl. Changes in rates of protein synthesis and breakdown during hypertrophy of the anterior and posterior latissimus dorsi muscles, *Biochem. J.*, 176, 407, 1978.

39. **Millward, D.J.,** Protein turnover in cardiac and skeletal muscle during normal growth and hypertrophy, in *Degradative Processes in Heart and Skeletal Muscle*, Wildenthal, K., Ed., Elsevier/North-Holland, Amsterdam, 1980, 161.

40. **Goldberg, A.L.,** Protein turnover in skeletal muscle. I. Protein metabolism during work-induced hypertrophy and growth induced with growth hormone, *J. Biol. Chem.*, 244, 3217, 1969.

41. **Goldberg, A.L., Jabelecki, C., and Li, J.B.,** Effects of use and disuse on amino acid transport and protein turnover in muscle, *Ann. N.Y. Acad. Sci.*, 228, 190, 1974.

42. **McMillan, D.M., Reeds, P.J., Lobley, and Palmer, R.M.,** Changes in protein turnover in hypertrophying plantaris muscles of rats: effects of fenburen — an inhibitor of prostaglandin synthesis, *Prostaglandins*, 34, 841, 1987.

43. **Kelly, F.J., Watt, P.W., Goldspink, D.F., and Goldspink, G.,** Exercise-induced changes in skeletal muscle in the rat, *Biochem. Soc. Trans.*, 10, 174, 1982.

44. **Terjung, R.L., Winder, W.W., Baldwin, K.M., and Holloszy, J.O.,** Effect of exercise on the turnover of cytochrome c in skeletal muscle, *J. Biol. Chem.*, 248, 7404, 1973.

45. **Booth, E.W., and Holloszy, J.O.,** Cytochrome c turnover in rat skeletal muscles, *J. Biol. Chem.*, 252, 416, 1977.

46. **Terjung, R.L.,** The turnover of cytochrome c in different skeletal-muscle fibre types of the rat, *Biochem. J.*, 178, 569, 1979.

47. **Terjung, R.L.,** Cytochrome c turnover in skeletal muscle, *Biochem. Biophys. Res. Commun.*, 66, 173, 1975.

48. **Wenger, H., Wilkinson, J., Dallaire, J., and Nihei, T.,** Uptake of ^{3}H-leucine into different fractions of rat skeletal muscle following acute endurance and sprint exercise, *Eur. J. Appl. Physiol.*, 47, 83, 1981.

49. **Seene, T., and Alev, K.,** Effect of muscular activity on the turnover rate of actin and myosin heavy and light chains in different types of skeletal muscle, *Int. J. Sports Med.*, 12, 204, 1991.

50. **Barany, M.**, ATPase activity of myosin correlated with speed of muscle shortening, *J. Gen. Physiol.*, 50 (Suppl., Part 20), 197, 1967.

51. **Guezennec, C.Y., Gilson, E., and Serrarier, B.**, Comparative effects of hind limb suspension and exercise on skeletal muscle myosin isozymes in rats, *Eur. J. Appl. Physiol.*, 60, 430, 1990.

52. **Pehme, A., and Seene, T.**, Importance of the relation of power to total volume of work on the protein synthesis on different types of skeletal muscles during strength training on rats, *Acta Comment. Univ. Tartuensis*, 814, 15, 1988.

53. **Gregory, P., Low, R.B., and Stirewalt, W.S.**, Changes in skeletal muscle myosin isozymes with hypertrophy and exercise, *Biochem. J.*, 238, 55, 1986.

54. **Gregory, P., Prior, G., Periasamy, M., Gagnon, J., and Zak, R.**, Molecular basis of myosin heavy chain isozyme transitions in skeletal hypertrophy, in *Biochemistry of Exercise VII*, Taylor, A.W., Ed., Human Kinetics Books, Champaign, 1990, 133.

55. **Riede, M., Moore, R.L., and Gollnick, P.D.**, Adaptive response of hypertrophied skeletal muscle to endurance training, *J. Appl. Physiol.*, 59, 127, 1985.

56. **Izumo, S., Nadal-Ginard, B., and Mahdavi, A.**, All members of the MHC multigene family respond to thyroid hormone in a highly tissue-specific manner, *Science*, 231, 597, 1986.

57. **Jabelcki, C., Diantag, J., and Kaufman, S.**, ^{3}H inositol incorporation into phosphatidyl-inositol in work-induced growth of rat muscle, *Am. J. Physiol.*, 232, E324, 1977.

58. **Palmer, R.M., Reeds, P.J., Labley, G.E., and Smith, R.H.**, The effect of intermittent changes in tension on protein and collagen synthesis in isolated rabbit muscle, *Biochem. J.*, 198, 491, 1981.

59. **Amsterdam, E.A., Wickman-Coffelt, J., Choquet, Y., Kamiyama, T., Lenz, J., Zelis, R., and Mason, D.T.**, Response of the rat heart to strenuous exercise: physical, biochemical and functional correlates, *Clin. Res.*, 20, 361, 1972.

60. **Kainulainen, H., Komulainen, J., Takala, T., and Vihko, V.**, Regional glucose uptake and protein synthesis in isolated perfused rat hearts immediately after training and later, *Basic Res. Cardiol.*, 82, 9, 1987.

61. **Popova, N.K.**, Action of muscular activity on the uptake of nitrogen compounds by muscles, *Sechenov Physiol. J. USSR*, 37, 103, 1951 (in Russian).

62. **Chagovets, N.R.**, Biochemical changes in muscles in restitution period after physical work, *Ukr. Biokhim. Zh.*, 29, 450, 1957.

63. **Makarova, A.F.**, Biochemical changes in muscles of animals during experimental training of various kinds, *Ukr. Biokhim. Zh.*, 30, 903, 1958 (in Russian).

64. **Rogozkin, V.A.**, Nitrogen metabolism in muscular activity of various intensity, *Ukr. Biokhim. Zh.*, 31, 489, 1959 (in Russian).

65. **Makarova, A.F.**, Biochemical characteristics of strength exercises, *Ukr. Biokhim. Zh.*, 30, 366, 1958 (in Russian).

66. **Kennedy, J.M., Kamel, S., Tambone, W.W., Vrbova, G., and Zak, R.**, The expression of myosin heavy chain isoforms in normal and hypertrophied chicken slow muscle, *J. Cell. Biol.*, 103, 977, 1986.

67. **Cartwright, I.L., Abmayr, S.M., Fleischmann, G., Lowenhaupt, K., Elgin, S.C.R., Keene, M.A., and Howard, G.C.**, Chromatin structure and gene activity in the role of non-histone chromosomal proteins, *CRC Crit. Rev. Biochem.*, 13, 186, 1982.

68. **Darnell, J., Lodish, H., and Baltimore, D.**, *Molecular Cell Biology*, Sci. Amer. Books., New York, 1986.

69. **Anapassenko, G.L.**, The problem of interpretation of mechanisms of postexercise recovery, *Teor. Prakt. Fiz. Kult.*, 6, 49, 1985 (in Russian).

70. **Ingwall, J.S., Morales, F., and Stockdale, F.E.**, Creatine and the control of myosin synthesis in differentiating skeletal muscle, *Proc. Natl. Acad. Sci. USA*, 69, 2250, 1972.

71. **Ingwall, J.S., Weiner, C.D., Morales, F., Davis, E., and Stockdale, F.E.**, Specificity of creatine in the control of muscle protein synthesis, *J. Cell. Biol.*, 63, 145, 1974.

72. **Silber, M.L., Pliskin, A.V., Pshedin, A.I., and Rogozkin, V.A.**, A study of the creatine action on transcription in isolated skeletal muscle nuclei, *Cytologia*, 16, 779, 1974 (in Russian).

73. **Silber, M.L., Litvinova, V.N., Morozov, V.I., Pliskin, A.V., Pshedin, A.I., and Rogozkin, V.A.**, Effect of creatine on synthesis of proteins and ribonucleic acids in growing myoblast culture of chickens embryon, in *Biochemical Ways for Enhanced Effectiveness of Sports Training*, Yakovlev, N.N., Ed., Leningrad Res. Inst. of Phys. Cult., Leningrad, 1974, 110 (in Russian).

74. **Ingwall, J.S., and Wildenthal, K.**, Role of creatine in the regulation of cardiac protein synthesis, *J. Cell. Biol.*, 68, 159, 1976.

75. **Fulks, R.M., Li, J.B., and Goldberg, A.L.**, Effect of insulin, glucose, and amino acids on protein turnover in rat diaphragm, *J. Biol. Chem.*, 250, 290, 1975.

76. **Buse, M.G.**, *In vivo* effects of branched amino acids on muscle protein synthesis in fasted rats, *Horm. Metab. Res.*, 13, 502, 1981.

77. **Hedden, M., and Buse, M.G.**, Effects of glucose, pyruvate, lactate, and amino acids in muscle protein synthesis, *Am. J. Physiol.*, 242, E184, 1982.

78. **Fry, M.D., and Morales, M.F.**, A reexamination of the effects of creatine on muscle protein synthesis in tissue culture, *J. Cell. Biol.*, 84, 294, 1980.
79. **Ööpik, V., Viru, M., Timpmann, S., Medijainen, L., and Viru, A.**, Lack of stimulation of protein synthesis in skeletal muscles by creatine administration in rats, *Acta Comment. Univ. Tartuensis*, 958, 16, 1993.
80. **Volkov, N.I.**, *Legitimacies of Biochemical Adaptation in the Process of Sports Training*, State Centr. Inst. Phys. Cult., Moscow, 1986 (in Russian).
81. **Greenhaff, P.L., Casey, A., Short, A.H., Harris, R., Söderlung, K., and Hultman, E.**, Influence of oral creatine supplementation of muscle torque during repeated bouts of maximal voluntary exercise in man, *Clin. Sci.*, 84, 565, 1993.
82. **Viru, M., and Nurmekivi, A.**, Action of creatine intake on performance capacity of middle-distance runners, *Acta Comment. Univ. Taruensis*, 958, 31, 1993.
83. **Harris, R.C., Söderlund, K., and Hultman, E.**, Elevation of creatine in resting and exercised muscle of normal subjects by creatine supplementation, *Clin. Sci.*, 83, 367, 1992.
84. **Tischler, M.E., Desautels, M., and Goldberg, A.L.**, Does leucine leucyl-tRNA, or some metabolite of leucine regulate protein synthesis and degradation in skeletal and cardiac muscle? *J. Biol. Chem.*, 257, 1613, 1982.
85. **Garlick, P.J., McNurlan, M.A., and Fern, E.B.**, Does leucine regulate muscle protein synthesis *in vivo*? in *Nitrogen Metabolism in Man*, Waterlow, J.C. and Stephen, J.M.L., Eds., Applied Science Publishers, London, 1981, 125.
86. **Sugden, P.H., and Fuller, S.J.**, Regulation of protein turnover in skeletal and cardiac muscle, *Biochem. J.*, 273, 21, 1991.
87. **Li, J.B., and Jefferson, L.S.**, Influence of amino acid availability on protein turnover in perfused skeletal muscle, *Biochim. Biophys. Acta*, 544, 351, 1978.
88. **Viru, A., and Seli, N.**, 3-Methylhistidine excretion in training for improved power and strength, *Sports Med. Training Rehab.*, 3, 183, 1992.
89. **Yakovlev, N.N.**, Ornithine metabolism and adaptation to increased muscular activity, *Sechenov Physiol. J. USSR*, 65, 979, 1979 (in Russian).
90. **Tabor, C.W., and Tabor, H.**, 1,4-Diaminobutane (putrescine), spermidine, and spermine, *Annu. Rev. Biochem.*, 45, 285, 1976.
91. **Yakovlev, N.N.**, Formation of polyamines and development of work hypertrophy of skeletal muscles in their increased activity, *Sechenov Physiol. J. USSR*, 66, 525, 1980 (in Russian).
92. **Vaughan, M.H., and Hansen, B.S.**, Control of initiation of protein synthesis in human cells, Evidence for a role of uncharged transfer ribonucleic acid, *J. Biol. Chem.*, 248, 7087, 1973.
93. **Meerson, F.S.**, *General Mechanism of Adaptation and Prophylaxis*, Medicina, Moscow, 1973 (in Russian).
94. **Bylund-Fellenius, A.-C., Ojama, K.M., Flaim, K.E., Li, J.B., Wassner, S.J., and Jefferson, L.S.**, Protein synthesis versus energy state in contracting muscles of perfused rat hind limb, *Am. J. Physiol.*, 246, E297, 1984.
95. **Rapoport, E., and Zamecnik, P.C.**, Presence of diadenosine 5,5‴-P^1,P^4-tetraphosphate (A$_{P4}$A) in mammalian cells in levels varying widely with proliferative activity of the tissue: a possible positive 'pleiotypic activator', *Proc. Natl. Acad. Sci. USA*, 73, 3984, 1976.
96. **Tischler, M.E., and Fagen, J.M.**, Relationship of the reduction-oxidation state to protein degradation in skeletal and atrial muscle, *Arch. Biochem. Biophys.*, 217, 191, 1982.
97. **Booth, F.W., and Watson, P.A.**, Control of adaptation on protein levels in response to exercise, *Fed. Proc.*, 44, 2293, 1985.
98. **Buresova, M., Gutmann, E., and Klicpera, M.**, Effect of tension upon rate of incorporation of amino acids into protein of cross-striated muscles, *Experimentia*, 25, 144, 1969.
99. **Brevet, A., Pinto, E., Peacock, J., and Stockdale, F.E.**, Myosin synthesis increased by electrical stimulation of skeletal muscle cell culture, *Science*, 193, 1152, 1976.
100. **Baracos, V.E., and Goldberg, A.L.**, Maintenance of normal length improves protein balance and energy status in isolated rat skeletal muscle, *Am. J. Physiol.*, 251, C588, 1986.
101. **Vandenburgh, H.H., Hatealudy, S., Karlisch, P., and Shansky, J.**, Skeletal muscle growth is stimulated by intermedient stretch-relaxation in tissue culture, *Am. J. Physiol.*, 256, C674, 1989.
102. **Booth, F.W.**, Time course of muscular atrophy during immobilization of hind limbs of rats, *J. Appl. Physiol.*, 43, 656, 1977.
103. **Goldberg, A.L.**, Influence of insulin and contractile activity in muscle size and protein balance, *Diabetes*, 28 (Suppl. 1), 18, 1979.
104. **Millward, D.J., Bates, P.C., Laurent, G.J., and Lo, C.C.**, Factors affecting protein breakdown in skeletal muscle, in *Protein Turnover and Lysosome Function*, Segal, H.L., Ed., Academic Press, New York, 1978, 619.
105. **Vandenburgh, H.H., and Kaufman, S.**, Stretch-induced growth of skeletal myotubes correlated with activation of the sodium pump, *J. Cell. Physiol.*, 109, 205, 1981.
106. **Etlinger, J.D., and Matsumoto, K.**, Interaction of calcium, cyclic AMP and tension in the regulation of protein degradation in muscle, in *Metabolic and Functional Changes during Exercise*, Semigonovsky, B. and Tucek, S., Eds., Charles University, Prague, 1982, 57.

107. **Kameyama, T., and Etlinger, J.D.,** Calcium-dependent regulation of protein synthesis and degradation in muscle, *Nature*, 279, 344, 1979.

108. **Rodemann, H.P., and Goldberg, A.L.,** Arachidonic acid, prostaglandin E_2 and F_2 influence rates of protein turnover in skeletal and cardiac muscle, *J. Biol. Chem.,* 257, 1632, 1972.

109. **Smith, R.H., Palmer, R.M., and Reeds, P.J.,** Protein synthesis in isolated rabbit fore limb muscle, *Biochem. J.,* 214, 153, 1983.

110. **Vandenburgh, H.H., Shansky, J., Karlish, P., and Solerssi, R.L.,** Mechanogenic second messengers in stretch-induced skeletal muscle growth, *8th Int. Biochem. Exerc. Conf.,* Nagoya, 1991, 47.

111. **Palmer, R.M., Reeds, P.J., Atkinson, T., and Smith, R.H.,** The influence of changes in tension on protein synthesis and prostaglandin release in isolated rabbit muscle, *Biochem. J.,* 214, 1011, 1983.

112. **Hatfaludy, S., Shansky, J., and Vanderburgh, H.H.,** Metabolic alterations induced in cultured skeletal muscle by stretch-relaxation activity, *Am. J. Physiol.,* 256, C175, 1989.

113. **Rodermann, H.P., Waxman, L., and Goldberg, A.L.,** The stimulation of protein degradation in muscle by Ca^{2+} is mediated by prostaglandin E_2 and does not require the calcium-activated protease, *J. Biol. Chem.,* 257, 8716, 1982.

114. **McMillan, D.H., Reeds, P.J., Lobley, G.E., and Palmer, R.M.,** Changes in protein turnover in hypertrophying plantaris muscles of rats: effect of fenburen — an inhibitor of prostaglandin synthesis, *Prostaglandins,* 34, 841, 1987.

115. **Shephard, J.R.,** Difference in the cyclic adenosine 3'5'-monophosphate levels in normal and transformed cells, *Nature (New Biol.),* 236, 14, 1972.

116. **Xenophontos, X.P., Watson, P.A., and Chua, B.H.L.,** Increased cyclic AMP content accelerates protein synthesis in rat hearts, *Circ. Res.,* 67, 647, 1989.

117. **Minty, A., and Kedes, L.,** Upstream region of the human cardiac actin gene that modulates the transcription in mouse cells: presence of an evolutionary conserved repeated motif, *Mol. Cell. Biol.,* 6, 2125, 1986.

118. **Miwa, T., Boxer, L.M., and Kedes, L.,** CArG boxes in human cardiac α-actin gene are core binding sites for positive transacting regulatory factors, *Proc. Natl. Acad. Sci. USA,* 84, 6702, 1987.

119. **Breitbart, R.E., and Nadal-Ginard-B.,** Developmentally induced muscle-specific trans factors control the differential splicing of alternative and constructive troponin T exons, *Cell,* 49, 793, 1987.

120. **Murre, C., McCaw, P.S., Vaessin, M., Caudy, M., Jan, L.Y., Jan, Y.N., Cabrera, C.L., Buskin, J.N., Hauschka, S.D., Lassar, A.B., Weintraub, H., and Baltimore, D.,** Interactions between heterologous helix-loop-helix proteins generate complexes that bind specifically to a common DNA sequence, *Cell,* 58, 537, 1989.

121. **Robertson, M.,** More to muscle than MyoD, *Nature,* 344, 378, 1990.

122. **Eftimie, R., Brenner, H.R., and Buonanno, D.,** Myogenin and MyoD join a family of skeletal muscle genes regulated by electrical activity, *Proc. Natl. Acad. Sci. USA,* 88, 1349, 1991.

123. **Benezra, R., Davis, R.L., Lockshon, D., Turner, D.L., and Weintraub, H.,** The protein Id: a negative regulator of helix-loop-helix DNA binding proteins, *Cell,* 61, 49, 1990.

124. **Gundersen, K., and Merlie, J.E.,** Id and muscle fiber size in transgenic mice, in *Baltic/Scandinavian Physiology Meeting*, Tartu, 1993, C19.

125. **Florini, J.R.,** Hormonal control of muscle growth, *Muscle Nerve,* 7, 577, 1987.

126. **Florini, J.R., Ewton, D.Z., and Magri, K.A.,** Hormones, growth factors, and myogenic differentation, *Annu. Rev. Physiol.,* 53, 201, 1991.

127. **Kraemer, W.J., Gordon, S.E., Fleck, S.J., Marchitelli, L.J., Mello, R., Dziadas, J.E., Friedl, K., Haeman, E., Maresh, C., and Fry, A.C.,** Endogenous anabolic hormonal and growth factor responses to heavy resistance exercise in males and females, *Int. J. Sports Med.,* 12, 228, 1991.

128. **Mauro, A.,** Ed., *Muscle Regeneration*, Raven Press, New York, 1979.

129. **Mauro, A.,** Satellite cell of skeletal muscle fibers, *J. Biophys. Biochem. Cytol.,* 9, 493, 1961.

130. **Appell, H.-J.,** Mechanismen und Grenzen der Muskelwachstums, *Kölner Beitr. Sportwiss.,* 12, 7, 1983.

131. **Gonyla, W.,** Role of exercise in inducing increases in skeletal muscle fiber number, *J. Appl. Physiol.,* 48, 421, 1980.

132. **Darr, K.C., and Schultz, E.,** Exercise-induced satellite cell activation in growing and mature skeletal muscle, *J. Appl. Physiol.,* 63, 1816, 1987.

133. **Umnova, M.M., and Seene, T.P.,** The effect of increased functional level on the activation of satellite cells in the skeletal muscle of adult rats, *Int. J. Sports Med.,* 12, 501, 1991.

134. **Appell, H.-J., Forsberg, S., and Hollmann, W.,** Satellite cell activation in human skeletal muscle after training: evidence for muscle fiber neoformation, *Int. J. Sports Med.,* 9, 297, 1988.

135. **Kraus, W.E., Bernard, T.S., and Williams, R.S.,** Interactions between sustained contractile activity and β-adrenergic receptors in regulation of gene expression in skeletal muscle, *Am. J. Physiol.,* 256, C506, 1989.

136. **Goldfarb, A.H., Bruno, J.F., and Buckenmeyer, F.J.,** Intensity and duration of exercise effects on skeletal muscle cAMP, phosphorylase, and glycogen, *J. Appl. Physiol.,* 66, 190, 1989.

137. **Fitts, R.H., Booth, F.W., Winder, W.W., and Holloszy, J.O.,** Skeletal muscle respiratory capacity, endurance, and glycogen utilization, *Am. J. Physiol.,* 228, 1029, 1975.

138. **Palmer, W.K., Studney, T.A., and Doukas, S.**, Exercise-induced increases in myocardial adenosine-3'5' cyclic monophosphate and phosphodiesterase activity, *Biochim. Biophys. Acta,* 672, 114, 1981.

139. **Ji, L.L., Lennon, D.L.F., Kochan, R.G., Nagle, F.J., and Lardy, H.A.**, Enzymatic adaptation to physical training under β-blockade in the rat: evidence of a β_2-adrenergic mechanism in skeletal muscle, *J. Clin. Invest.,* 78, 771, 1986.

140. **Harri, M.N.E.**, Physical training under the influence of beta-blockade in rats. III. Effects on muscular metabolism, *Eur. J. Appl. Physiol.,* 45, 25, 1980.

141. **Svedenhag, J., Hendriksson, J., and Juhlin-Dannfeldt, A.**, β-adrenergic blockade and training in human subjects: effects on muscle metabolic capacity, *Am. J. Physiol.,* 247, E305, 1984.

142. **Williams, R.S., Caron, M.G., and Daniel, K.**, Skeletal muscle β-adrenergic receptors: variations due to fiber type and training, *Am. J. Physiol.,* 246, E160, 1984.

143. **Williams, R.S.**, Role of receptor mechanisms in the adaptive response to habitual exercise, *Am. J. Cardiol.,* 55, 680, 1985.

144. **Juhlin-Dannfeldt, A.**, β-Adrenoreceptor blockade and exercise: effects on endurance and physical training, *Acta Med. Scand. Suppl.,* 672, 49, 1983.

145. **Holloszy, J.O., and Coyle, E.F.**, Adaptation of skeletal muscle to endurance exercise and their metabolic consequences, *J. Appl. Physiol.,* 56, 831, 1984.

146. **Fell, R.D., Terblanche, S.E., Winder, W.W., and Holloszy, J.O.**, Adaptive responses of rats to prolonged treatment with epinephrine, *Am. J. Physiol.,* 241, C55, 1981.

147. **Chira, Y., Wakatsuki, T., Inoke, N., Kanazaki, M., and Holloszy, J.O.**, Non-exercise related stimulation of mitochondrial protein synthesis in creatine-depleted rats, *8th Int. Biochem. Exerc. Conf.,* Nagoya, 1991, 61.

148. **Holloszy, J.O., and Winder, W.W.**, Induction of δ-aminolevulinic acid synthase in muscle by exercise or thyroxine, *Am. J. Physiol.,* 236, R180, 1979.

149. **Poortmans, J.R.**, Protein metabolism, in *Principles of Exercise Biochemistry,* Poortmans, J.R., Ed., Karger, Basel, 1988, 164.

150. **Tipton, C.M., Struck, P.-J., Baldwin, K.M., Matthes, R.D., and Dowell, R.T.**, Response of adrenalectomized rats to chronic exercise, *Endocrinology,* 91, 573, 1972.

151. **Viru, A., Smirnova, T., Seene, T., Tomson, K., and Eller, A.**, Participation of glucocorticoids in development of physical working capacity, *Sechenov Physiol. J. USSR,* 65, 1790, 1979 (in Russian).

152. **Viru, A., and Seene, T.**, Peculiarities of adaptation to systematic muscular activity in adrenalectomized rats, *Endocrinologie,* 80, 235, 1982.

153. **Viru, A.**, The role of adrenocortical reactions to exercise in the increase of body working capacity, *Byull. Eksp. Biol. Med.,* 82, 774, 1976 (in Russian).

154. **Kraus, H., and Kinne, R.**, Regulation der bei langandeuerndem körperlichen Adaptation and Leistungssteigerrung durch Thyroid-hormone, *Pflügers Arch. ges. Physiol.,* 321, 332, 1970.

155. **Seene, T., Alev, K., Tomson, K., and Viru, A.**, The role of thyroid gland in adaptation of skeletal muscles to physical activity, *Sechenov Physiol. J. USSR,* 67, 299, 1981 (in Russian).

156. **Gollnick, P.D., and Ianuzzo, C.D.**, Hormonal deficiencies and the metabolic adaptations of rats to training, *Am. J. Physiol.,* 223, 278, 1972.

157. **Derevenco, P., Baciu, I., Stoica, N., Sovrea, I., Vitebski, V., Vaida, A., and Zdrenghea, V.**, Action of 6-hydroxydopamine on two parameters of motor learning, *Rev. Roum. Morphol. Embryol. Physiol.,* 17, 211, 1980.

158. **Goldberg, A.L.**, Work-induced growth of skeletal muscle in normal and hypophysectomized rats, *Am. J. Physiol.,* 213, 1193, 1967.

159. **Goldberg, A.L.**, Role of insulin in work-induced growth of skeletal muscle, *Endocrinology,* 83, 1071, 1968.

160. **Ianuzzo, C.D., and Armstrong, R.B.**, Short-term compensatory growth of normal and diabetic rat skeletal muscle, *Med. Sci. Sports,* 27, 65, 1975.

161. **Terjung, R.L., and Koerner, J.E.**, Biochemical adaptation in skeletal muscle of trained thyroidectomized rats, *Am. J. Physiol.,* 230, 1194, 1976.

162. **Noble, E.G., Ianuzzo, C.D., Hamilton, N., and Dabrowski, B.**, The influence of training on skeletal muscle enzymatic adaptation in normal and diabetic rats, *Med. Sci. Sports Exerc.,* 14, 173, 1982.

163. **Henriksson, J., Svedenhag, J., Richter, A., Christensen, N.J., and Galbo, H.**, Skeletal muscle and hormonal adaptation to physical training in the rat: role of the sympatho-adrenal system, *Acta Physiol. Scand.,* 123, 127, 1985.

164. **Baldwin, K.M., Ernst, S.B., Herrick, R.E., Hooker, A.M., and Mullin, W.J.**, Exercise capacity and cardiac function in trained and untrained thyroid-deficient rats, *J. Appl. Physiol.,* 49, 1022, 1980.

165. **Seene, T., Alev, K., Tomson, K., and Viru, A.**, Adaptation of hypo- and athyroid rat heart and skeletal muscles to physical exercise, *Vopr. Med. Khim.,* 20, 20, 1982 (in Russian).

166. **Vesselkin, N.Y., and Yakovlev, N.N.**, Role of sympathetic innervation for efficiency of muscle training, *Trans. Leningrad Res. Inst. Phys. Cult.,* 3, 252, 1940 (in Russian).

167. **Yakovlev, N.N.**, The role of sympathetic nervous system in the adaptation of skeletal muscles to increased activity, in *Metabolic Adaptation to Prolonged Physical Exercise,* Howald, H. and Poortmans, J., Eds., Birkhäuser, Basel, 1975, 293.

168. **Kuuskela, P., Kukkonen, K., Rauramaa, R., Hietanen, E., and Hänninen, O.**, Long-term physical training in old streptozotocine diabetic rats, *Acta Endocrinol.*, 94 (Suppl. 237), 49, 1980.

169. **Gillespie, C.A., and Edgerton, V.R.**, The role of testosterone in exercise-induced glycogen supercompensation, *Horm. Metab. Res.*, 2, 364, 1970.

170. **Morkin, E., Garrett., J.C., and Fishman, A.P.**, Effects of actinomycin D and hypophysectomy on development of myocardial hypertrophy in the rat, *Am. J. Physiol.*, 214, 6, 1968.

171. **Tipton, C.M., Terjung, R.L., and Barnard, R.J.**, Response of thyroidectomized rats to training, *Am. J. Physiol.*, 215, 1137, 1968.

172. **Booth, F.W., and Tipton, C.M.**, Effects of training and 17β-estradiol upon heart rates, oxygen weight, and ligamentous strength of female rats, *Int. Z. angew. Physiol.*, 27, 187, 1969.

173. **Viru, A.**, *Hormones in Muscular Activity,* Vol. 2. Adaptive Effects of Hormones in Exercise, CRC Press, Boca Raton, FL, 1985.

174. **Rogozkin, V.A.**, Metabolic effects of anabolic steroids on skeletal muscle, *Med. Sci Sports,* 11, 160, 1979.

175. **Lamb, D.R.**, Anabolic steroids and athletic performance, in *Hormones and Sport,* New York, 1989, 257.

176. **Hickson, R.C., Heusner, W.W., Van Huss, W.D., Jackson, D.E., Anderson, D.A., Jones, D.J., and Psaledas, A.T.**, Effect of dianabol and high-intensity sprint training on body composition of rats, *Med. Sci. Sports,* 8, 191, 1976.

177. **Stone, M.H., and Lipner, H.**, Responses to intensive training and methandrostenedione administration. Contractile and performance variables, *Pflügers Arch. ges. Physiol.*, 375, 141, 1978.

178. **Viru, A., and Kôrge, P.**, Role of anabolic steroids in the hormonal regulation of skeletal mucle adaptation, *J. Steroid Biochem.*, 11, 931, 1979.

179. **Brison, G.R.**, Ergogenic use of growth hormone, *Sci. Sports,* 4, 1, 1989.

180. **Goldberg, A.L., and Goodman, H.M.**, Relationship between growth hormone and muscular work in determining muscle size, *J. Physiol.*, 200, 655, 1969.

181. **Kurowski, T.T., Chatterton, R.T., and Hickson, R.C.**, Glucocorticoid-induced cardiac hypertrophy: additive effects of exercise, *J. Appl. Physiol.*, 57, 514, 1984.

182. **Hickson, R., and Davis, J.**, Partial prevention of glucocorticoid-induced muscle atrophy by endurance training, *Am. J. Physiol.*, 241, 226, 1981.

183. **Sccne, T., and Viru, A.**, The catabolic effect of glucocorticoids on different types of skeletal muscle fibres and its dependence upon muscle activity and interaction with anabolic steroids, *J. Steroid Biochem.*, 16, 349, 1982.

184. **Czerwinski, S.M., Kurowski, T.G., O'Neill, T.M., and Hickson, R.C.**, Initiating regular exercise protects against muscle atrophy from glucocorticoids, *J. Appl. Physiol.*, 63, 1504, 1987.

185. **Fimbel, S., Abdelmalki, A., Mayet, B., Sempore, R., and Favier, R.J.**, Exercise training fails to prevent glucocorticoid-induced muscle atrophy, *8th Int. Biochem. Exer. Conf.*, Nagoya, 1991, 146.

186. **Minelli, R., and Riccardi, L.**, Mechanism of development of myocardial hypertrophy from training, in *Sports Cardiology,* Vol. 2, Lubich, T., Venerando, A., and Zeppilli, P., Eds., Aulo Caggi, Bologna, 1983, 29.

187. **Yampolskaya, L.J.**, Supercompensation of glycogen content in muscles during restitution period after exercises of various rhythms and durations, *Sechenov Physiol. J. USSR,* 36, 749, 1950 (in Russian).

188. **Chagovets, N.R.**, Biochemical changes in the muscle in repeated exercises on dependence of rest duration between repetitions, *Ukr. Biokhim. Zh.*, 30, 661, 1958 (in Russian).

189. **Chagovets, N.R.**, Biochemical changes in the muscle caused by a single repeated exercise of long duration, *Ukr. Biokhim. Zh.*, 31, 204, 1959 (in Russian).

190. **Krestovnikov, A.N.**, *Survey on Physiology of Physical Exercises,* FiS, Moscow, 1951 (in Russian).

Chapter 9

GENDER DIFFERENCES IN TRAINING EFFECTS

Results from recent years indicate that on the top level the gender differences in sports performance are declining in various events. In Figure 9-1 the dynamics of the 100- and 1500-m world records are presented for example.[1] Thereby, it is justified to ask if there are any differences in training effects between male and female athletes at all. Taking into consideration the fact that the adaptive protein synthesis is induced by metabolites and hormones, the search for sex differences has to be concentrated on the gender-related peculiarities in the hormonal responses to exercise as well as in the tissues' responsiveness to hormones.

METABOLIC CAPACITIES IN MALE AND FEMALE ATHLETES

There is no reason to believe the existence of differences in the metabolic pathways used, and accordingly in the metabolite accumulation during exercises between men and women. If such differences exist, they have to be based on the different exercises and their intensities. When the exercises performed are the same, the metabolic responses may moderately vary only in the quantitative aspect due to the differences in fitness levels and the relation of the performed exercise to previous adaptation (training). Nevertheless, there is a possibility that in case of all-out exercise based on simultaneous high activity of both anaerobic and aerobic energy processes, the ratio between these processes may not be the same in male and female athletes. The examples are running races of 400 to 5000 m. The corresponding differences, if they appear, might be related to (1) various running velocities (probably due to differences in body build, e.g., ratio of leg length to body length), and thus to differences in the absolute intensity of exercises, and (2) the individual meaning of the absolute intensity of these exercises in terms of the percent of maximal capacities used. On the one hand, the lower absolute intensity of exercise (running velocity) makes the exercise 'more aerobic'. On the other hand, the lower levels of aerobic power (VO_2max) and particularly of anaerobic threshold cause an increased contribution of anaerobic processes at the same absolute intensity. If the anaerobic capacity is not highly developed, these peculiarities in energy metabolism become in turn a responsible factor, limiting the absolute intensity of exercise. However, in highly qualified female athletes these differences are not so much pronounced as in less trained women.

In highly qualified endurance athletes VO_2max values as high as 77 ml·min⁻¹·kg⁻¹ in an individual case[2] and 68.2 ml·min⁻¹·kg⁻¹ as a mean value of the team[3] were recorded. In both cases the female sportsmen were Nordic skiers. In 15 female elite runners of middle distances the mean value of 68 ml·min⁻¹·kg⁻¹ was found with an individual highest value of 73 ml·min⁻¹·kg⁻¹.[4] Instead of the difference of 30 to 35% between sedentary men and women,[2,5] in endurance-trained persons this difference is reduced to 10 to 20%[6-8] and relative to lean body mass to 5 to only 10%.[1,6,7] The lower hemoglobin level[2] and blood volume as well as smaller maximal stroke volume[9] may account for gender differences in the ability to transport O_2. However, training diminishes these differences.[7] In female athletes the exercise intensity corresponding to anaerobic threshold may lag behind in comparison with highly qualified male athletes.[1,10] However, an analysis showed that it is not clear whether males and females,

Time (s)

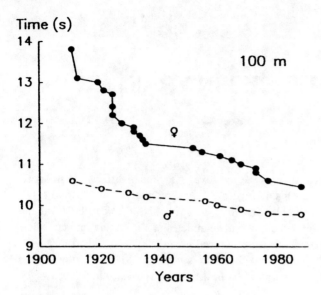

Time (s)

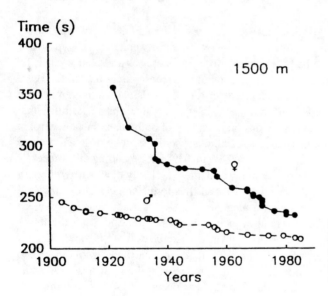

FIGURE 9-1. Progress in world records in 100-m and 1500-m run for female and male athletes.[1] (From Cerretelli, P., Marzorati, M., and Marconi, C., *Med. Sport,* 45, 39, 1992. With permission.)

matched by maximal aerobic power, differ consistently in anaerobic threshold or in variables that determine this quality.[5] In well-trained male and female runners approximately the same VO_2 was found during running with speeds of 202, 215, and 268 m·min^{-1} despite the VO_2max of 74 ± 5 in males and 60 ± 4 ml·min^{-1}·kg^{-1} in females. The activity of oxidation enzymes in muscles does not markedly differ between sexes, and the capillary supply (number of capillaries per square unit muscle tissue) is similar in both sexes.[11] The relative slow-twitch fiber volume (volume of ST fibers per unit muscle volume) as well as intercellular triglyceride store are even larger in females than in males.[12]

Differences were found in the skeletal muscle lactate dehydrogenase isozyme content. When male and female marathon runners with similar VO_2max (62 ± 5 and 61 ± 10 ml·min^{-1}·kg^{-1} respectively) and percent of slow-twitch muscle fibers ($71 \pm 10\%$ and $61 \pm 10\%$, respectively) were compared, the activity of isozymes 1 and 2 was higher in males, but the activity of isozymes 4 and 5 was higher in females.[13]

A comprehensive study by W. Kindermann and J. Keul[14] showed a pronounced increase in the blood lactate level and a drop of the blood pH value in female athletes at the finish of running races for 400 and 800 m. These changes were much more pronounced in male athletes. Later it was calculated that the maximal capacity of anaerobic glycogenolysis in qualified female rowers is approximately 170 cal·kg^{-1}, compared to 250 cal·kg^{-1} in male rowers.[15] The lower anaerobic capacity in female athletes was confirmed in other studies.[16,17] However, differences in the highest power output and glycolytic capacity disappeared when calculations were made in relation to lean body mass.[17] Activities of contractile and glycolytic enzymes are lower in female muscles than in male ones.[12] However, the maximal power output, evaluated by Margaria's staircase test is approximately the same in relation to the body mass.[1,15] The greater portion of body fat and the smaller relative lean body mass plays a decisive role in limiting the peak anaerobic alactic performance of sedentary women.[1]

ENDOCRINE SYSTEMS IN EXERCISE IN WOMEN

The differences in hormonal inductors may be related to (1) various hormonal responses to exercise in men and women, (2) the dependence of hormonal responses to exercise on the phases of the ovarian-menstrual cycle, (3) the decreased amount of testosterone in the female organism, which exerts a strong anabolic influence on muscle tissue, (4) gender differences in tissue sensitivity to hormones, and (5) relations between female sex hormones to the effect of other hormones.

HORMONAL RESPONSES TO EXERCISE IN WOMEN

The main determinants of hormonal responses to exercise are exercise intensity threshold and exercise duration threshold, which both depend on the degree of adaptation to the corresponding exercises. Additionally, a number of hormonal responses are related to the homeostatic needs during exercise (see Chapter 2). If we take into consideration the mentioned factors, no significant gender peculiarities can be revealed by cross-sectional comparison of data obtained in male and female persons.[18,19] Testosterone level is lower in women but relative changes are rather similar.[18] Also, during performance of strength exercises the relative increase of blood testosterone was rather similar: in males by 21.6% and in females by 16.7%. The androstenedione concentration increased significantly in both gender groups without difference in the magnitude of the response. In both groups during the first two post-exercise hours a high level of androstenedione persisted while the testosterone concentration returned to pre-exercise values within 30 min.[20]

Apart from these results, a testosterone response to programs of heavy resistance exercises was found in men but not in women in a study. Heavy resistance exercises caused in men a more pronounced rise in the blood testosterone level than in women, despite the 10- to 18-times higher initial level in males. The initial level as well as the exercise-induced rise in the somatotropin concentration were higher in females. The somatomedin-C (insulin-like growth factor 1) concentration in the blood increased in both gender groups when more repetitions were performed and when rest periods between repetitions were shorter. When heavy resistance protocol consisted of less repetitions, heavier weight and longer rest intervals, the somatomedin-C response was observed in males just after the exercise session, and in females 60 min after the end of the exercise.[21] These data indicate a possibility of sex differences in the somatotropin-somatomedin system response to strength exercises. It is not excluded that the somatotropin-somatomedin system may, to a certain extent, compensate for the lower anabolic effect in females due to the reduced levels and responses of testosterone.

Swimming until exhaustion (against incremental resistance provided by a weighted pulley device) caused a decrease in the blood testosterone concentration in 14- to 15-year-old swimmers. In girls the mean testosterone decline was 39% while in boys it was 19%.[22]

OVARIAN-MENSTRUAL CYCLE AND HORMONAL RESPONSES TO EXERCISE

The dynamics of female sex hormone production during the ovarian-menstrual cycle cause different ratios between sex and other hormones in various phases of the cycle. Therefore, a possibility exists that in various phases of the cycle the hormonal responses to exercise may differ. However, in most studies insignificant or only modest differences were found.[19,23-27] In some studies more pronounced hormone responses were observed in the post-ovulatory phase compared to pre-ovulatory phase.[18] The progesterone increase in response to exercise is mainly found in the luteal phase.[23,25,28] The exercise-induced increase in melatonin concentrations was almost the same in various phases of the ovarian-menstrual cycle.[30] Thus the possible suppressive action of melatonin remains the same throughout the cycle.

The question arises, are there any changes in the hormone-receptor interrelation during the ovarian-menstrual cycle? The background for this question is the competition between progesterone and glucocorticoids as well as between estrogens and other steroid hormones at the receptor level. When adrenalectomized rats were treated with a high dose of progesterone, glucocorticoid administration failed to increase their working capacity.[31]

A high level of progesterone, typical for the luteal phase of the ovarian-menstrual cycle, may change the sensitivity of carbohydrate metabolism to hormonal influence. In the luteal phase after an oral glucose load (1 g/kg b.w.) the insulin increase as well as the insulin/glucose ratio were bigger than in the follicular phase. No significant phase differences were found for the glucose response.[32] However, A. Bonen et al.[25] did not observe a menstrual phase difference in the insulin response to oral glucose load.

In the luteal phase at maximal exercise duration (at 60% VO_2max), glycogen depletion during exercise and glycogen repletion rate after exercise were greater than in the follicular phase.[29]

In regard to the influence of high levels of estrogens it may be indicated that ovulation may induce a decrease in physical working capacity.[18] At 30- to 60-min exercises the ratings of perceived exertion were higher in the ovulatory than in the mid-follicular or mid-luteal phases. The ovulatory phase was characterized by enhanced fat utilization and the mid-follicular phase by preferred carbohydrate utilization.[33]

Alterations in female athletes' adaptability were obtained due to the use of contraceptive preparations containing estrogens.[34,35] Users of oral contraceptive agents exhibited lower static muscle endurance[36] and more pronounced glucocorticoid level in the blood before and after exercise[37] than nonusers. No increments in progesterone, estradiol, or cortisol occurred in users during exercise.[38] The effect of contraceptive preparations might be compensated to a certain extent by a significant decrease of the levels of endogenous estradiol and prolactin in users.[38,39] By the results of a study, women soccer players using oral contraceptives had less traumatic sports injuries than nonusers.[40]

TRAINING INFLUENCE ON THE FEMALE REPRODUCTIVE SYSTEM

Training may change the production of sex hormones in various phases of the ovarian-menstrual cycle. This is revealed not only in the hormone levels, but also in menstrual disorders and delayed menarche. In resting conditions during the early follicular phase the pulsatile release of lutropin was suppressed in eumenorrhic women runners compared with sedentary women.[41] However, the results of another study indicated a suppression of lutropin level in the blood during the luteal phase. This study demonstrated a more pronounced increase of estradiol level in trained eumenorrhic subjects in the follicular phase.[19,24] In contrast to these results, high intensity training of runners was associated with a decreased concentration of follitropin in the middle of the follicular phase, of estradiol and testosterone during the ovulation and luteal phase, and of progesterone at the end of the luteal phase. Jogging did not alter the concentration of these hormones.[42] Accordingly, it is assumed that the subtle but reversible alterations in the regulation of the hypothalamic-pituitary-gonadal function occur in many women undergoing a strenuous endurance training program.[43] It is likely that these changes in hypothalamic-pituitary-gonadal regulation, and, thus, the ovarian-menstrual cycle variations, take place in every demanding training that causes an increased secretion of antireproductive hormones. Among them an essential role may belong to catecholamines.[44]

A most common effect of strenuous training on the ovarian-menstrual cycle is the diminished duration of the luteal phase.[26,43,44] In addition, approximately one third of the competitive female long-distance runners between ages 12 and 45 experience amenorrhea or oligomenorrhea for at least brief periods. This phenomenon appears more frequently in those women with a late onset of menarche who have not experienced pregnancy or who have taken contraceptive hormones.[45,46] However, the basal estrogen, progesterone, prolactin, and thyroid hormone levels were normal and so were lutropin and follitropin responses to gonadoliberin in female endurance athletes with menstrual disorders.[47] The changes in gonadal functions were believed to be due to disorders located in the hypothalamic regulating centers.[47] In amenorrheic athletes the capacity of the anterior pituitary to secrete corticotropin and endorphins in response to exercise to 80 or 100% VO_2max does not significantly differ from that in amenorrheic athletes.[48] In amenorrheic runners a 10-min cycling exercise induced a more pronounced response of testosterone but a less pronounced response of estrone than in normally cycling runners. Responses of lutropin, follitropin, and cortisol were similar.[49] Serum prolactin and somatotropin increased severalfold in response to progressive exercise test without significant differences in sedentary women and female runners with normal and abnormal menstrual cycles. No changes in follitropin, lutropin, and estradiol were observed in any group.[50]

Menstrual disorders were also found in female weight-lifters and competitive body-builders.[51] By the view of H.A. Keizer and A.D. Rogol[44] the amenorrhea is a result of short-term overtraining.

A well-known result of training at an early age is delayed menarche.[52-56] In young female rats the pulsatile secretion of lutropins and somatotropin were completely blocked by prolonged exercise to obtain food. Levels of gonadoliberin in the hypothalamus and lutropin in the pituitary were unchanged. Pulsatile infusions of gonadoliberin remained normal, but pubertal development and ovulation were restricted by prolonged exercise in growing rats.[57]

Does the action of physical training on the female reproductive system influence the adaptive protein synthesis as well? No results were available to confirm this possibility. Therefore, it seems suggestive that there are no substantial gender differences in metabolic and hormonal factors controlling the adaptive protein synthesis in training. The only exception is the lower level of testosterone in the female organism. Thereby, the adaptive synthesis of myofibrillar proteins in strength training may be less stimulated in females.

TRAINING EFFECTS ON MUSCLE STRENGTH AND HYPERTROPHY

A general sex difference is a less developed musculature in women as compared to men. The same difference is obvious in most species of mammals and birds. The overall strength of women averages about two-thirds of that of men.[58,59] In women strength tests for upper body muscle revealed an average of only 54% of that of men, as contrasted by 68% of male strength in the lower body muscles.[60] When body size is eliminated as a factor by relating strength to body weight or lean body mass, the sex difference in total strength decreases to about 20%.[7]

Biopsy studies proved larger muscle fibers in men,[61] the difference being most pronounced in fast-twitch fibers.[12] In sedentary populations, women's slow-twitch as well as fast-twitch fiber area amounts to only about two thirds that of the male, when the sampling site is the gastrocnemius muscle. In the vastus lateralis muscle the slow-twitch fibers area is almost equal, while the male fast-twitch fibers are about one third larger.[7]

Using minimal effective doses of isometric exercise, it was shown that the strength trainability increased after puberty in men. In young adult women the strength trainability amounted to only 60% of that in men. During subsequent decades of life the men's trainability decreases parallel to the reduction in 17-ketosteroid excretion. In ages over 60 the trainability of men and women is almost equal.[62] The strength training used was far different from that used in various sports in its amount of performed exercises. Therefore, these results may not agree with the results of actual strength training in female athletes. The subsequent studies with higher exercise loads and using mainly dynamic resistance exercise indicated the effectiveness of strength training in women. However, despite apparently similar increases in strength, muscle hypertrophy resulting from weight training occurred to a smaller extent in women than in men.[63-65] The cross section of fibers of the biceps brachii muscle in elite male body-builders was 9.6 μm^2 while in elite female body-builders it was 5.4 μm^2.[66] These differences have been assumed to be due to the lower blood testosterone concentration in women.[9] It has been assumed that women gain strength primarily from neural adaptation with minimal hypertrophy.[65] Some years later it was concluded that the relative contribution of neural and hypertrophic adaptations to strength changes in men and women were similar.[67] However, both conclusions may be valid, depending on the training methodology used.

Predominating neural adaptation in women is demonstrated in regard to power training. With this kind of training program, the time of force production shortened and the average forces increased in the beginning of the force-time curve of the leg extensor muscles. These changes were accompanied by an increase in the neural activation of the trained muscles. Hypertrophic changes, as judged from muscle fiber area of both fast- and slow-twitch fibers, were only slight. No significant changes occurred during training in the mean concentration of serum testosterone, free testosterone, follitropin, lutropin, cortisol, progesterone, estradiol, and sex hormone-binding globulin. However, the individual mean serum levels of both total and free testosterone correlated with the individual changes during the training in the force-time curve of the trained muscles.[68]

In rodents no sex difference has been found in compensatory muscle hypertrophy.[69-73] Taking into account various results, it was argued that there was virtually no direct information supporting the contention that lower blood androgen levels in women prevented muscle hypertrophy from occurring to the same extent as in men.[74,75]

More recently, it was demonstrated that women, like men, can increase muscle fiber size and strength when the training intensity and duration are sufficient.[59,76,77] As with men, women are capable of increasing the cross-sectional area of all three major fiber types.[77] However, the fast-twitch fibers appear to be affected to the greatest extent in both men and women.[76,77] When after 30 to 21 weeks of detraining a subsequent retraining followed for 6 weeks, a rapid muscular adaptation occurred in women. Detraining had relatively little effect on fiber cross-sectional area. Detraining for 6 weeks resulted in significant increase in the cross-sectional areas of both fast fiber types compared with detraining values.[78] A 16-week weight training with 70 to 90% of maximum voluntary contraction significantly increased the strength of various muscles in female as well as in male persons. Absolute changes were significantly greater in males than in females in two of the four tests whereas percentage-wise, changes were not significantly different. Muscle cross-sectional area in the upper arm, estimated by computed tomography scanning, increased in males by 15.9% and in females by 22.8%.[76]

Strength training effect on muscular hypertrophy in female persons was confirmed by measuring with an ultrasonic apparatus the cross-sectional area of the quadriceps femoris muscle before, during, and after a 10.5-week training period. The cross-sectional area increased in male persons by 13.6% and in female persons by 11.3%. Noteworthy is the correlation ($r = 0.76$, $P < 0.05$) between the individual mean serum level of testosterone and the individual change in maximal force.[79]

The overall increases in concentric and eccentric peak torque, in response to 12 weeks of accomodated resistance training, occurred at a rate that was independent of sex. The torque-velocity relationship however appears to change in males. Results were obtained suggesting a relatively greater enhancement of maximum voluntary force in the slow-speed, high-force region.[80]

Nevertheless, a comparison of muscle strength in untrained men and female athletes did not provide evidence that weight training can eliminate gender difference in absolute strength.[81]

The effectiveness of resistance training in female athletes in regard to muscle strength as well as in regard to muscle hypertrophy suggests that in the female organism the lower level of testosterone is effectively compensated. On one hand, it may be related to the increased sensitivity of skeletal muscles of women to the anabolic action of testosterone. In female rats the enhanced anabolic effect of testosterone was evidenced. Ovariectomy and adrenalectomy eliminated the enhanced anabolic effect of testosterone. In the castrated male rat the enhanced anabolic effect of testosterone was evoked by administration of estradiol.[82] Another possibility for compensation for the low level of testosterone exists in the form of the enhanced response of somatomedin-c and other growth factors to exercises for improved strength.[21]

TRAINING EFFECTS ON AEROBIC WORKING CAPACITY

Sports practices as well as numerous studies prove the effectiveness of endurance training in female persons. Females respond to systematically performed endurance exercises in much the same manner as males.[83-85] In cases of similar training programs the percent increase in VO_2max, V_{Emax}, and heart volume are almost equal, but the increase in blood volume in women is less pronounced than in men.[7] Increases in maximal values of stroke volume and cardiac output are also detected in women.[86] In female athletes, a strenuous training seems not to be necessary to increase the heart performance. Echocardiographic evaluation of left ventricular dimensions, wall thickness, and stroke volume failed to reveal any significant differences between a group of highly trained and a group of moderately trained female distance runners.[87]

The iron status may become a factor reducing the efficiency of endurance training in women. Women lose approximately 1.5 mg of iron per day, twice as much as men. Therefore, a high daily allowance of iron in the diet of women athletes is recommended.[88]

In women a progressive running program (weekly distance increased to 48 or 80 km over the usual running distance) caused a slight decrease of plasma levels of triiodothyronine and reverse-triiodothyronine, and an exaggerated thyrotropin response to thyroliberin when the weekly distance increased by 48 km.[89] With more prolonged training (weekly distance increased by 80 km), there were pronounced increases in thyroxine, reverse triiodothyronine, and unstimulated thyrotropin concentrations, while the ratios of thyroxine/reverse triiodothyronine and triiodothyronine/reverse triiodothyronine and the response of thyrotropin to thyroliberin decreased significantly.[90] Taking into consideration the activation of thyroid function by endurance training as well as the significance of thyroid hormones in adaptive synthesis of mitochondrial proteins, it is possible to suggest effective stimulation of improvements at the mitochondrial level by endurance training also in women. The reflection of this has to be the increased level of exercise intensity at the anaerobic threshold.

In male rats swimming training during 8 weeks resulted in an increase of glycogen store in the liver, red vastus lateralis and gastrocnemius muscles. In regard to the liver and gastrocnemius muscle the same results were obtained in normal female and ovariectomized rats. However, in the vastus lateralis muscle the glycogen content increased in ovariectomized but not in normal female rats.[91] In the available literature there are no results about a gender difference in endurance training action on skeletal muscle glycogen store in humans. By the above-mentioned result, obtained in ovariectomized rats, it is possible to speculate that at least during the time period when the estrogen level is high (pre-ovulatory and ovulatory days) the effectiveness of endurance training in augmentation of muscle glycogen is low.

Using dual photon absorbitiometry to measure the bone mineral content in female athletes, results were obtained suggesting that weight training may provide a better stimulus for increasing the bone mineral content than running and swimming training in normally menstruating females.[92]

SUMMARY

There are no essential reasons to believe the existence of pronounced gender differences in adaptive protein synthesis in training (Figure 9-2). A single real reason for this difference is the lower testosterone level in females. However, possibilities exist for compensation of this difference. Nevertheless a number of questions remain that need further systematic studies. An example of such questions is the gender peculiarities in the relation between androgen anabolic and glucocorticoid catabolic action in women. Attention has to be paid also to the interference of high estradiol level during ovulation as well as of high progesterone level in the luteal phase to the adaptive protein synthesis.

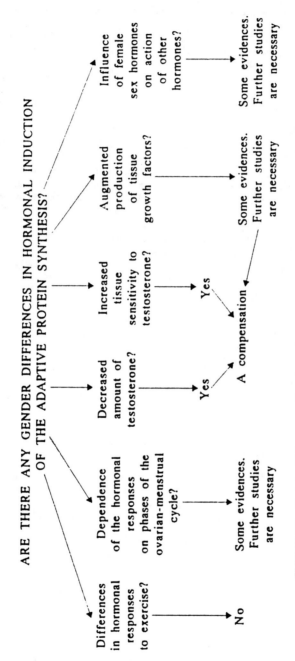

FIGURE 9-2. Factors which may contribute to gender differences in the adaptive protein synthesis in training.

REFERENCES

1. **Cerretelli, P., Marzorati, M., and Marconi, C.,** La donna e lo sport. Gli aspetti fisiologici generali, *Med. Sport,* 45, 39, 1992.
2. **Åstrand, P.-O., and Rodahl, K.,** *Textbook of Work Physiology,* 3rd ed., McGraw-Hill, New York, 1986.
3. **Rusko, H., Havu, M., and Karvinen, E.,** Aerobic performance capacity in athletes, *Eur. J. Appl. Physiol.,* 38, 151, 1978.
4. **Pate, R.R., Sparling, P.B., Wilson, G.E., Cureton, K.G., and Miller, B.J.,** Cardiorespiratory and metabolic responses to submaximal and maximal exercise in elite women distance runners, *Int. J. Sports Med.,* 8 (Suppl. 2), 91, 1987.
5. **Pate, R.P., and Kriska, A.,** Physiological basis of the sex differences in cardiorespiratory endurance, *Sports Med.,* 1, 87, 1984.
6. **Sparling, P.B.,** A meta-analysis of studies comparing maximal oxygen uptake in men and women, *Res. Q.,* 51, 542, 1980.
7. **Drinkwater, B.,** Training in female athletes, in *The Encyclopaedia of Sports Medicine. Vol. 1. The Olympic Book of Sports Medicine,* Dirix, A., Knuttgen, H.G., and Tittel, K., Eds., Blackwell Scientific Oxford, 1988, 309.
8. **Jordanskaya, F.A., Kuzmina, V.N., Murav'yeva, L.F., and Solovyov, V.A.,** Diagnostics and comparative evaluation of functional capacities of female and male athletes, *Teor. Prakt. Fiz. Kult.,* 5, 2, 1991 (in Russian).
9. **Wells, C.L.,** *Women, Sport, and Performance. A Physiological Perspective,* Human Kinetics, Champaign, 1985.
10. **Föhrenbach, R., Mader, A., and Hollmann, W.,** Determination of endurance capacity and prediction of exercise intensities for training and competition in marathon runners, *Int. J. Sports Med.,* 8, 11, 1987.
11. **Daniels, J., Krahenbuhl, G., Foster, C., Gilbert, J., and Daniels, S.,** Aerobic responses of female distance runners to submaximal and maximal exercise, *Ann. N.Y. Acad. Sci.,* 301, 726, 1977.
12. **Nygaard, E.,** Women and exercise — with special reference to muscle morphology and metabolism, in *Biochemistry of Exercise IVB,* Poortmans, J. and Niset, G., Eds., University Park Press, Baltimore, 1981, 161.
13. **Apple, F.S., and Rogers, M.A.,** Skeletal muscle lactate dehydrogenase isozyme alterations in men and women marathon runners, *J. Appl. Physiol.,* 61, 477, 1986.
14. **Kindermann, W., and Keul, J.,** *Anaerobic Energiebereitstellung im Hochleistungssport,* Hofmann Verlag, Schorndorf, 1977.
15. **Kots, Y.M.,** *Sports Physiology,* FiS, Moscow, 1986 (in Russian).
16. **Mayhew, J.L., and Salm, P.C.,** Gender differences in anaerobic power tests, *Eur. J. Appl. Physiol.,* 60, 133, 1990.
17. **Maud, P.J., and Shults, B.B.,** Gender comparisons in anaerobic power and anaerobic capacity tests, *Br. J. Sports Med.,* 20 (2), 51, 1986.
18. **Viru, A.,** *Hormones in Muscular Activity.* Vol. 1, Hormonal Ensemble in Exercise, CRC Press, Boca Raton, 1985.
19. **Keizer, H.R.,** Ed., Hormonal responses in women as a function of physical exercise and training, *Int. J. Sports Med.,* 8 (Suppl. 3), 137, 1987.
20. **Weiss, L.W., Cureton, K.J., and Thomson, F.N.,** Comparison of serum testosterone and androstenedione responses to weight lifting in men and women, *Eur. J. Appl. Physiol.,* 50, 413, 1983.
21. **Kraemer, W.J., Gordon, S.E., Fleck, S.J., Marchitelli, L.J., Mello, R., Dziados, J.E., Friedl, K., Harman, E., Maresh, C., and Fry, A.C.,** Endogeneous anabolic hormonal and growth factor responses to heavy resistance exercise in males and females, *Int. J. Sports Med.,* 12, 228, 1991.
22. **Cumming, D.C., Wall, S.R., Quinney, H.A., and Belcastro, A.N.,** Decrease in serum testosterone levels with maximal intensity swimming exercise in trained male and female swimmers, *Endocrin. Res.,* 13, 31, 1987.
23. **Jurkowski, J.E., Jones, N.L., Walker, W.C., Younglai, E.V., and Sutton, J.R.,** Ovarian hormonal responses to exercise, *J. Appl. Physiol.,* 44, 109, 1978.
24. **Keizer, H.A.,** *Hormonal Respones in Women as a Function of Physical Exercise and Training,* Uitgeverij de Vrieseborch, Haarlem, 1983.
25. **Bonen, A., Haynes, F., Watson-Wright, W., Sopper, M., Pierce, G., Low, M.P., and Grahan, T.W.,** Effects of menstrual cycle on metabolic responses to exercise, *J. Appl. Physiol.,* 55, 1506, 1983.
26. **Bonen, A.,** Endocrine alterations with exercise and training. in *The Menstrual Cycle and Physical Activity,* Piehl, J.J. and Brown, C.H., Eds., Human Kinetics, Champaign, 1986, 81.
27. **Lavoie, J.-M., Dionne, N., Helie, R., and Brisson, G.R.,** Menstrual cycle phase dissociation of blood glucose homeostasis during exercise, *J. Appl. Physiol.,* 62, 1084, 1987.
28. **Mastrogiacomo, I., Toderini, D., Bonanni, G., and Bordin, D.,** Gonadotropin decrease induced by prolonged exercise at about 55% of the VO$_2$max in different phases of the menstrual cycle, *Int. J. Sports Med.,* 11, 198, 1990.

29. **Nicolas, B.J., Hackney, A.C., and Sharp, R.L.**, The menstrual cycle and exercise: performance, muscle glycogen, and substrate responses, *Int. J. Sports Med.*, 10, 204, 1989.

30. **Ronkainen, H., Vakkuri, O., and Kauppila, A.**, Effects of physical exercise on the serum concentration of melatonin in female runners, *Acta Obstet. Gynecol. Scand.*, 65, 827, 1986.

31. **Viru, A., and Smirnova, T.**, Involvement of protein synthesis in action of glucocorticoids on the working capacity of adrenalectomized rats, *Int. J. Sports Med.*, 6, 225, 1985.

32. **Hackney, A.C., Cyren, C.H., Brammeier, M., and Sharp, R.L.**, Effect of menstrual cycle phase on the glucose-insulin relationship at rest and during exercise, *Biol. Sport*, 10, 73, 1993.

33. **Hackney, A.C., Curley, C.S., and Nicolas, B.J.**, Physiological responses to submaximal exercise of the mid-follicular ovulatory and mid-luteal phases of the menstrual cycle, *Scand. J. Med. Sci. Sports*, 1, 94, 1991.

34. **Schwartz, R., Göretzlehner, G., and Hamann, O.**, Der Einfluss des Menstruationzyklus and versciedener hormonaler Kontrazeptika auf Parameter des Kohlenhydratstoffwechsels bei Ausdauerbelastung, *Med. Sport*, 19, 369, 1979.

35. **Haynes, F., Sopper, M., Wright, W.W., Low, M., Pierce, G., Graham, T., and Bonen, A.**, Substrate and hormonal responses during exercise in users and nonusers of oral contraceptives, *Med. Sci. Sports Exerc.*, 13, 105, 1981.

36. **Wirth, J.C., and Lohman, T.G.**, The relationship of static muscle function to use of oral contraceptives, *Med. Sci. Sports Exerc.*, 14, 16, 1982.

37. **Neumann, G., and Saloman, B.**, Der Einfluss von Antikonzeptika auf die Konzentration der unkonjugierten 11-Hydrokortikosteroide im Plasmas, *Med. Sport*, 19, 366, 1979.

38. **Bonen, A., Haynes, F.W., and Graham, T.E.**, Substrate and hormonal responses to exercise in women using oral contraceptives, *J. Appl. Physiol.*, 70, 1917, 1991.

39. **Gürtler, H., Göretzlehner, G., Brünnler, H., and Pohlentz, H.**, Der Einfluß der hormonalen Kontrazeption auf ausgewöhlte sport-artspecifische and hormonale Untersuchungsergebnisse, *Med. Sport*, 30, 233, 1990.

40. **Möller-Nielsen, J., and Hammar, M.**, Women's soccer injuries in relation to the menstrual cycle and oral contraceptives, *Med. Sci. Sports Exer.*, 21, 126, 1989.

41. **Cumming, D.C., Vickovic, M.M., Wall, S.R., and Fluker, M.R.**, Defects in pulsatile LH release in normally menstruating runners, *J. Clin. Endocrin.*, 60, 810, 1985.

42. **Ronkainen, H., Pakarinen, A., Kirkinen, P., and Kauppila, A.**, Physical exercise-induced changes and season-associated differences in the pituitary-ovarian function of runners and joggers, *J. Clin. Endocrin.*, 60, 416, 1985.

43. **Prior, J.C., Camoron, K., HoYuen, B., and Thomas, J.**, Menstrual cycle changes with marathon training: anovulation and short luteal phase, *Can. J. Sports. Sci.*, 7, 173, 1982.

44. **Keizer, H.A., and Rogol, A.D.**, Physical exercise and menstrual cycle alterations. What are mechanisms? *Sports Med.*, 10, 218, 1990.

45. **Dale, E., Gerlach, D.H., Martin, D.E., and Alexander, C.D.**, Physical fitness and reproductive physiology of the female distance runners, *Phys. Sportmed.*, 7, 83, 1979.

46. **Dale, E., Gerlach, D.H., and Withite, A.L.**, Menstrual dysfunction in distance runners, *Obstet. Gynecol.*, 54, 47, 1979.

47. **Wakat, D.K., Sweeney, K.A., and Rogol, A.D.**, Reproductive system function in women cross-country runners, *Med. Sci. Sports Exerc.*, 14, 263, 1982.

48. **Hohtari, H., Elovainio, R., Salminen, K., and Laatikainen, T.**, Plasma corticotropin-releasing hormone, corticotropin, and endorphins at rest and during exercise in eumenorrheic and amenorrheic athletes, *Fertil. Steril.*, 50, 233, 1988.

49. **Cumming, D.C., and Rebar, R.W.**, Hormonal changes with acute exercise and with training in women, *Semin. Reprod. Endocrin.*, 3, 55, 1985.

50. **Chang, F.E., Dodds, W.G., Sullivan, M., Kim, M.H., and Malarkey, W.B.**, The acute effects of exercise on prolactin and growth hormone secretion: comparison between sedentary women and women runners with normal and abnormal menstrual cycles, *J. Clin. Endocrin.*, 62, 351, 1986.

51. **Walberg, J.L., and Johnston, C.S.**, Menstrual function and eating behavior in female recreational weight lifters and competitive body builders, *Med. Sci. Sports Exerc.*, 23, 30, 1991.

52. **Warren. W.P.**, The effect of exercise on pubertal progression and reproductive function in girls, *J. Clin. Endocrin. Metab.*, 51, 1150, 1980.

53. **Frisch, R.E., Gotz-Welbergen, A.V., McArthur, J.W., Albright, T., Witschi, J., Bullen, B., Birnholz, J., Reed, R.B., and Hermann, H.**, Delayed menarche and amenorrhea of college athletes in relation to age of onset of training, *JAMA*, 246, 1559, 1981.

54. **Malina, R.M.**, Menarche in athletes: a synthesis and hypothesis, *Ann. Hum. Biol.*, 1, 1, 1983.

55. **Stager, J.M., and Hatler, L.K.**, Menarche in athletes: the influence of genetics and prepubertal training, *Med. Sci. Sports Exerc.*, 20, 369, 1988.

56. **Stager, J.M., Wigglesworth, J.K., and Hatler, L.K.**, Interpreting the relationship between age of menarche and prepubertal training, *Med. Sci. Sports Exerc.*, 22, 54, 1990.

57. **Manning, J.M., and Bronson, F.H.**, Suppression of puberty in rats by exercise: effects on hormone levels and reversal with GnRH infusion, *Am. J. Physiol.*, 260, R717, 1991.

58. **Laubach,. L.L.**, Comparative muscular strength of men and women: a review of the literature, *Aviat. Space Environ. Med.*, 47, 534, 1976.

59. **Holloway, J.B., and Baechle, T.R.**, Strength training for female athletes. A review of selected aspects, *Sports Med.*, 9, 216, 1990.

60. **Heyward, V.H., Johannes-Ellis, S.M., and Romer, J.F.**, Gender differences in strength, *Res. Q.*, 57, 154, 1986.

61. **Edström, L., and Nyström, B.**, Histochemical types and sizes of fibres in normal human muscles. A biopsy study, *Acta Physiol. Scand.*, 45, 257, 1969.

62. **Hettinger, T.**, *Physiology of Strength*, Charles C. Thomas, Springfield, 1961.

63. **Brown, C., and Wilmore, J.H.**, The effects of maximal resistance training on the strength and body composition of women athletes, *Med. Sci. Sports*, 6, 174, 1974.

64. **Mayhew, J.H., and Gross, P.**, Body composition changes in young women with high resistance weight training, *Res. Q.*, 45, 433, 1974.

65. **Wilmore, J.H.**, Alterations in strength, body composition, and anthropometric measurements consequent to a 10-week weight training program, *Med. Sci. Sports*, 6, 133, 1974.

66. **Alway, S.E., Grumbt, W.H., Gonyea, W.J., and Stray-Gundersen, J.**, Contrasts in muscle and myofibers of elite male and female body-builders, *J. Appl. Physiol.*, 67, 24, 1989.

67. **Moritani, T., and DeVries**, Neural factors vs. hypertrophy in the time course of muscle strength gain, *Am. J. Phys. Med.*, 58, 115, 1979.

68. **Häkkinen, K., Pakarinen, A., Kyröläinen, S., Cheng, D., Kim, H., and Komi, P.V.**, Neuromuscular adaptations and serum hormones in females during prolonged power training, *Int. J. Sports Med.*, 11, 91, 1990.

69. **Mackova, E., and Hnik, P.**, Time course of compensatory hypertrophy of slow and fast rat muscles in relation to age, *Physiol. Bohemoslov.*, 21, 9, 1972.

70. **Ianuzzo, C.D., and Chen, V.**, Metabolic character of hypertrophied rat muscle, *J. Appl. Physiol.*, 46, 738, 1979.

71. **Marchetti, M., Figura, F., Candeloro, N., and Favilli, S.**, Effect of testosterone on compensatory hypertrophy of rat skeletal muscles, *J. Sports Med.*, 20, 13, 1980.

72. **Max. S.R., and Rance, N.E.**, No effect of sex steroids on compensatory muscle hypertrophy, *J. Appl. Physiol.*, 56, 1589, 1984.

73. **Timson, B.R., Bowlin, B., Dudenhoeffer, G.A., and George, J.B.**, Fiber number, area, and composition of mouse soleus following enlargement, *J. Appl. Physiol.*, 58, 619, 1985.

74. **Lamb, D.R.**, Anabolic steroids, in *Ergogenic Aids in Sport*, Williams, M.H., Ed., Human Kinetics, Champaign, 1983.

75. **Westerlind, K.C. Byrnes, W.C., Freedson, P.S., and Katch, F.I.**, Exercise and serum androgens in women, *Phys. Sportmed.*, 15, 87, 1987.

76. **Cureton, K.J., Collins, M.A., Hill, D.W., and Mclehannon, F.M.**, Muscle hypertrophy in men and women, *Med. Sci. Sports Exerc.*, 20, 338, 1988.

77. **Staron, R.S., Melicky, E.S., Leonardi, M.J., Falkel, J.E., Hagerman, F.C., and Dudley, G.A.**, Muscle hypertrophy and fast fiber type conversions in heavy resistance-trained woman, *Eur. J. Appl. Physiol.*, 60, 71, 1989.

78. **Staron, R.S., Leonardi, M.J., Karaponde, D.L., Malicky, E.S., Falkel, J.E., Hagerman, F.C., and Hikinda, R.S.**, Strength and skeletal muscle adaptations in heavy-resistance-trained women after detraining and retraining, *J. Appl. Physiol.*, 70, 631, 1991.

79. **Häkkinen, K., Pakarinen, A., Komi, P.V., Ryushi, T., and Kauhanen, H.**, Neuromuscular adaptations and hormone balance in strength athletes, physically active males and females during intensive strength training, in *12th Int. Congr. Biomech., Congr. Proc.*, Gregor, P.J., Zernicke, R.F., and Whiting, W.C., Eds., 1989, 8.

80. **Colliander, E.B., and Tesch, P.A.**, Responses to eccentric and concentric resistance training in females and males, *Acta Physiol. Scand.*, 141, 149, 1990.

81. **Morrow, J.R., and Hosler, W.W.**, Strength comparison in untrained men and trained women athletes, *Med. Sci. Sports Exerc.*, 13, 194, 1981.

82. **Danhaive, P.A., and Rousseau, G.G.**, Evidence for sex-dependent anabolic response to androgenic steroids mediated by glucocorticoid receptors in the rat, *J. Steroid. Biochem.*, 29, 575, 1988.

83. **Drinkwater, B.L.**, Physiological responses of women to exercise, *Exerc. Sport Sci. Rev.*, 1, 125, 1973.

84. **Pollock, M.L.**, The quantitation of endurance training programs, *Exerc. Sport Sci. Rev.*, 1, 155, 1973.

85. **Lamb. D.R.**, *Physiology of Exercise: Responses and Adaptations*, Macmillan, New York., 1978.

86. **Kilbom, A.**, Physical training in women, *Scand. J. Clin. Lab. Invest.*, 28 (Suppl. 119), 1971.

87. **Pollak, S.J., McMillan, S.T., Mumpower, E., Eharff, R., Knopf, W., Felner, J.M., and Yaganathan, A.P.**, Echocardiographic analysis of elite women distance runners, *Int. J. Sports Med.*, 8 (Suppl. 2), 81, 1987.

88. **Haymes, E.M.**, Nutrition for the female distance runners, in *Female Endurance Athletes*, Drinkwater, B.L., Ed., Human Kinetics, Champaign, 1986.

89. **Boyden, T.W., Pamenter, R.W., Stanforth, P., Rotkis, T.C., and Wilmore, J.H.**, Evidence for mild thyroid impairment in women undergoing endurance training, *J. Clin. Endocrin.*, 54, 53, 1982.

90. **Boyden. T.W., Pamenter, R.W., Rotkis, T.C., Stanforth, P., and Wilmore, J.H.**, Thyroid changes associated with endurance training in women, *Med. Sci. Sports Exerc.*, 16, 243, 1984.

91. **Riggs, C., and Kilgour, R.**, Role of ovarian hormones in the glycogenic response to endurance training, *J. Sports Med. Phys. Fitness*, 26, 241, 1986.

92. **Heinrich, C.H., Going, S.B., Pamenter, R.W., Perry C.D., Boyden, T.W., and Lohman, T.G.**, Bone mineral content of cyclically menstruating female resistance and endurance trained athletes, *Med. Sci. Sports Exerc.*, 22, 558, 1960.

Chapter 10

PHYSIOLOGICAL ASPECTS OF SELECTED PROBLEMS OF TRAINING METHODOLOGY (TRAINING TACTICS)

The final two chapters are dedicated to the problem of possible practical benefits of analysis of the adaptation processes in training. However, the practical aspects of training methodology are so capacious that it is impossible to treat this topic within one or two chapters. The methodology of every sports event is rather specific. In a general manner we can discuss those problems if we consider the background that makes possible more or less well-founded solutions. Nevertheless, even this approach needs a special volume or volumes to attempt a complete treatment of the topic. Therefore, in the last two chapters only selected methodological problems will be discussed, considering mainly those which are closely related to the problems of adaptation presented in the previous chapters. The problems of training tactics and training strategy will be distinguished according to the definition presented in Chapter 1. The approach presumes the consideration of changes in the organism's adaptivity when any of the training tasks is to be solved.

CHOICE OF TRAINING EXERCISES

EXERCISE AND TRAINING METHOD

The term 'tactics' means a concordant plan to achieve a certain goal. The training tactics determine the action for the body and conditions for their actualization. The matter of training tactics is the choice of exercises and training methods as well as organization of training sessions and microcycles (Figure 10-1).

Exercise is the main tool of training. Depending on the aim, exercises vary by the amount and localization of muscles used, degree of force and power output of muscle contractions, velocity and amplitude of movements, character of muscle contraction (isometric or auxotonic, eccentric or concentric), intensity and duration of activity, and peculiarities of coordination of the whole muscular activity as well as the activity of various motor units. These discriminants are the main factors determining the dominant metabolic pathways and activation of cellular structures in most active organs and muscle fibers. These same factors are the main determinants of the adaptive protein synthesis. In turn, the activation of adaptive protein synthesis depends on the accumulation of metabolic inductors and the stimulation of hormone responses necessary to amplify the transcription process as well as translational and post-translational control. For this reason a single exercise bout is usually insufficient. To obtain sufficient action, a certain number of repetitions have to be performed during a training session. In other cases the training effect is based on the insufficient duration of rest intervals between exercise bouts, which causes the actions of subsequent exercise bouts to add up. The third possibility is that a long duration of exercise will lead to the training effect. Accordingly, three principles may be discriminated by which exercises will achieve sufficient actions and will have training effect:

1. Principle of repetition
2. Principle of summation
3. Principle of duration

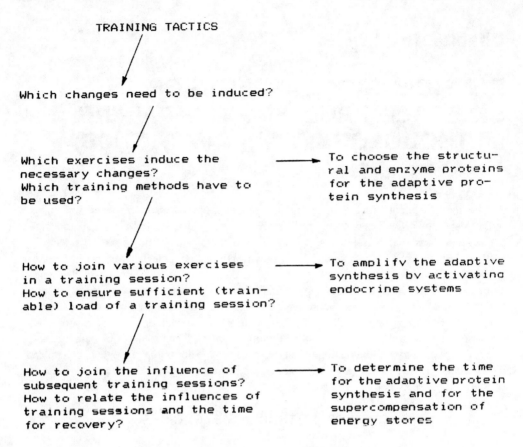

FIGURE 10-1. Training tactics.

In the literature on training methodology a great number of various training methods have been proposed. However, if we take into consideration the three above-mentioned principles as the reason for substantially different adaptation, the number of substantially different methods is rather limited. It seems reasonable to discriminate only the following training methods:

1. *Method of repeated exercises (repetition method).* This method consists of repeated performance of the same exercise. The characteristic sign of this method is sufficiently long rest intervals between repetitions to avoid accumulation of fatigue manifestations and to achieve complete restitution for the beginning of the next exercise bout (or readiness to perform the next exercise bout).

2. *Method of continuous (steady) training.* The main distinctive signs of this method are the long duration of the steady exercise and its continuous performance without interruption or change in the intensity and character.

3. *Method of intermittent training.* The whole duration of exercise may be rather long, but instead of steady activity various changes in the exercise intensity or its character are expected.

4. *Interval method.* The distinctive sign of this method is the insufficient duration of rest intervals between exercise repetitions. Therefore, (a) the action of subsequent exercise bouts adds up, and (b) the high metabolic and functional activity during the rest intervals gives them a significance in achievement of the peculiarities of the training effect.

5. *Method of circuit training.* This is a combination of the method of repeated exercises and the method of intermittent training. Similar to the repetition method a number of

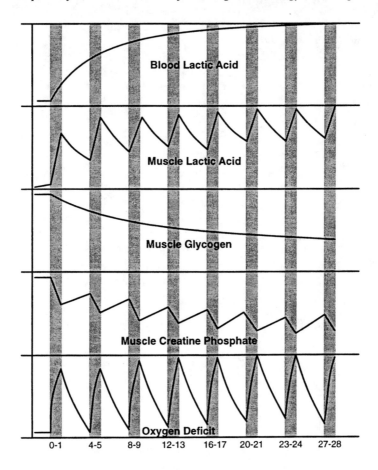

FIGURE 10-2. Changes in blood and muscle lactate, muscle glycogen, muscle creatine phosphate, and oxygen deficit during an intensive anaerobic interval training session. (From Lamb, D.R., *Physiology of Exercise*, Macmillan, New York, 1978. With permission.)

exercises will be performed subsequently. Differently from the repetition method and similar to the method of intermittent training, the subsequent exercises are different. When the time intervals between the subsequent exercises are small, this method acquires an effect similar to the interval method.

The principle of repetition is used in all methods except the method of continuous training. The principle of summation is used in the interval method and the method of intermittent training. It may also be used in certain cases of the circuit method. Figure 10-2 gives a generalized example of the acute effect of interval training on energy metabolism.[1] Figure 10-3 adds information on the dependence of these changes on the ratio between exercise and rest duration.[2] This ratio determines the main energy mechanism, influenced by the interval method[3] (Table 10-1).

The area of action of the principle of duration is not only the method of continuous training, but also the method of intermittent training, the interval method, and the method of circuit training. A way of using the principle of duration is performance of exercise up to exhaustion. These all-out exercises may consist of a steady performance (method of continuous training) or of maximal number of repetitions (methods of repeated exercises, interval training, or circuit training). In these cases the exercise intensity is usually prescribed. In cases of so-called tempo training not only the exercise intensity, but also the distance or performance time is prescribed.

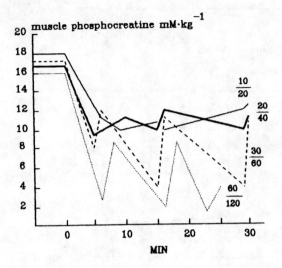

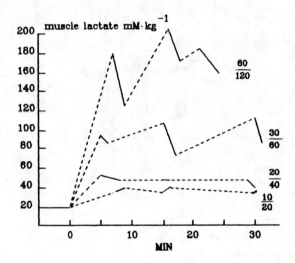

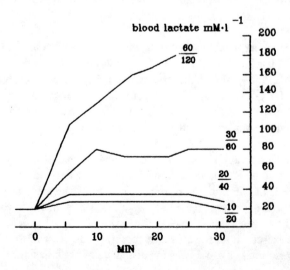

FIGURE 10-3. Dependence of changes of blood and muscle lactate and muscle phosphocreatine on the ratio between durations of exercise and relief period (indicated by the ratio exercise(s)/relief(s)). (From Rusko, H., in *Suomalainen Valmennusoppi, Harjoittelu,* Kantola, H., Ed., Gummerus Kirjapaino OY, Jyväskylä, 1989, 151. With permission.)

Table 10-1.   Variants of the Interval Method for Influence of Different Energy Mechanisms in Runners

Main mechanism for ATP resynthesis	Time of each running set	Repetitions per training session	Sets per training session	Repetitions per set	Running to rest (relief) ratio	Type of relief
Phosphocreatine mechanism	10 s	50	5	10		Rest relief (walking, flexing)
	15 s	45	5	9	1:3	
	20 s	40	4	10		
	25 s	32	4	8		
Phosphocreatine + anaerobic glycogenolysis	30 s	25	5	5	1:3	Work relief (light to mild jogging)
	40–50 s	20	5	5		
	60–70 s	15	3	5	1:2	
	80 s	10	2	5		
Anaerobic glycogenolysis + oxidative phosphorylation	1:30-2 min	8	2	4	1:2	Work relief
	2:10-2:40 min	6	1	6	1:1	Rest relief
	2:50-3 min	4	1	4		
Oxidative phosphorylation	3–4 min	4	1	4	1:1	Rest relief
	4–5 min	3	1	3	1:0.5	

From Fox, E.L., and Mathews, D.K., *Physiological Basics of Physical Education and Athletics,* 3rd ed. W.B. Saunders, Philadelphia, 1981. With permission.

An additional training method is the competition method. It consists of exercise performance in a competitive situation. The method implies the use of the related emotional state for a more complete mobilization of the organism's motor potential.

MANIFESTATIONS OF TRAINING SPECIFICITY IN EXERCISES FOR IMPROVEMENT OF THE MAIN QUALITIES OF THE HUMAN PHYSICAL WORKING CAPACITY

As with the model characteristics of the top athlete, the specific link between exercise and the induced change may be analyzed in fine detail or in a generalized manner. For practical considerations, the latter has to be discussed in the first place. Against the background of the results presented in the previous chapters, the following generalized schemes may be proposed (Table 10-2).

In addition, it is very useful to know that the recruitment of muscle fibers of various types depends on the exercise intensity[4] (Figure 10-4). The dependence of recruitment of muscle fibers on the muscle force application is probably analogous.

The principal difference between strength and power exercises and their effects is determined by the force-velocity relationship (Figure 10-5). The dependence of the training result on the force-velocity characteristics has been confirmed in various studies.[5-7]

Exercises for improved power have to be divided into two groups. One group consists of jumping exercises. Here the highest possible acceleration has been given to a heavy mass (the sportsman's body). In the other group the acceleration is transferred to a light mass (javelin, discus, shot, etc.). Accordingly, there must exist a substantial difference in the action of these two groups of exercises. It may be supposed that for acceleration of a heavy mass the force/velocity ratio must reflect the application of a higher force than in exercises for acceleration of a light mass. Therefore in the first case a greater stimulation of muscle hypertrophy may be expected. However, sports practice proves the opposite. A common feature is that power exercises do not stimulate hypertrophy. The pronounced muscular hypertrophy in all power athletes except jumpers is most likely the result of widely used strength exercises. In jumpers, muscular hypertrophy is not a favorable adaptation because it means an additional weight.

Table 10-2.   A Generalized Scheme of the Specificity of Action of Exercise for Improved Qualities of Human Physical Working Capacity

Site of action	Aerobic endurance	Anaerobic endurance	Speed	Power	Strength
Recruitment of motor units	Minimization of the number of recruited motor units	Choice of optimal number of simultaneously recruited motor units			Maximization of the number of simulataneously recruited motor units
Action on muscle fibers of various types	Slow-twitch oxidative, fast-twitch oxidative-glycolytic	Fast-twitch oxidative-glycolytic, fast-twitch glycolytic (at the very beginning of post-exercise recovery, also action on slow-twitch fibers)	Fast-twitch glycolytic	Fast-twitch glycolytic, fast-twitch oxidative glycolytic	Fast-twitch glycolytic (also fast-twitch oxidative-glycolytic and slow-twitch oxidative)
Within muscle fibers	Mitochondria, oxidative enzyme, glycogen store	Intensity of glyco-genolysis, glycogen store, glycose transport, buffer capacity	SR, phosphocreatine, ATP cycling, phosphocreatine store	Myofibrils, SR	Myofibrils
Cardio-vascular system	Heart hypertrophy, functional capacity, muscle blood flow, capillarization of skeletal and heart muscles, lung alveoles	Heart hypertrophy, cardiac functional capacity, muscle blood flow, capillarization of skeletal and heart muscles, lung alveoles			Heart hypertrophy
Blood	Blood volume, total hemoglobin	Buffer capacity			
Liver	Glycogen store, intensity of glycogenolysis	Intensity of glycogenolysis			
Adipose tissue	Mobilization and utilization of lipids				

Therefore, experienced coaches and athletes avoid exercises stimulating muscle hypertrophy. The effectiveness of the so-called 'plyometric' exercises is indicated for improvement of the vertical jump performance.[8-10] A different situation occurs in the case of discus throwers and shot-putters. In these events the high body mass helps to give greater acceleration to the discus or shot. Javelin throwers are in an in-between position.

Table 10-3 presents differences in the action of isometric, isotonic, and isokinetic exercies[1,11,12] and Table 10-4 presents the dependence of strength gain on the rate of exercise performance.[113] In regard to the action of exercises for improved strength on neural adaptations vs. muscle hypertrophy, the intensive and extensive training programs are differentiated (Figure 10-6) in Table 10-5.

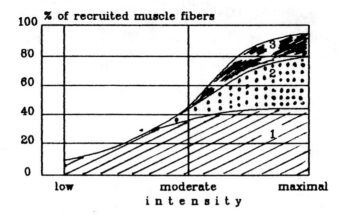

FIGURE 10-4. Recruiting of muscle fibers of various types in dependence of exercise intensity. 1 — SO, 2 — FOG, 3 — FG fibers. (From Costill, D., Sharp, R., and Troup, J., *Biokinetic Strength Training,* 1, 55, 1980. With permission.)

The final effect of exercise depends on the principle of action and the training method used. Therefore, for further evaluation of the choice of various exercises an additional approach is given in Table 10-6.

TRAINING SESSION

While the choice of exercises determines the accumulation of metabolites acting as inductors of the adaptive protein synthesis or as factors controlling post-transcriptional processes, the total load of a training session is the main determinant of the activation of the endocrine function. Thereby, the hormonal amplification of the adaptive protein synthesis is related to the load of a training session to a great extent. On the one hand, the total load of a training session is the sum of the influences of all exercises performed during the session. On the other hand, the total load also depends on the rest intervals betweeen the exercises. When a normally ineffective exercise follows a more strenuous one after a short rest interval, it may become effective in inducing training effects.

The total load of a training session can be divided into: (1) *excessive load*, which surpasses the functional capacity of the organism and causes overstrain phenomena, (2) *trainable load*, which causes specifically directed adaptive protein synthesis and thereby induces the training effects, (3) *maintaining load*, which is insufficient to stimulate adaptive protein synthesis but sufficient to avoid the detraining effect, (4) *restitution load*, which is insufficient to avoid the detraining effect but favors promotion of the recovery processes after a previous trainable load, and (5) *useless load* (Figure 10-7).

Taking into consideration these different levels of loads, at least three groups of criteria are necessary for detailed analysis of a training session's influence: (1) criteria for the highest possible trainable load, (2) criteria for the trainable (training) effect of the session, and (3) criteria for the minimum load possessing a maintaining effect. In the literature on sports medicine one can find numerous criteria for overstrain phenomena. The highest load that does not cause overstrain manifestations is the highest trainable load. However, practically, it means that only negative consequences will teach the sportsmen. Of course, it would be more desirable to have criteria that detect the highest load immediately preceding overstrain.

POWER TRAINING

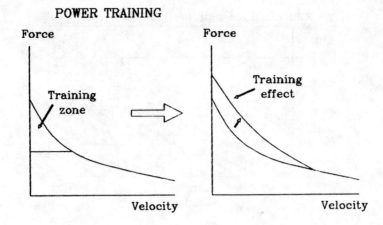

HEAVY RESISTANCE TRAINING

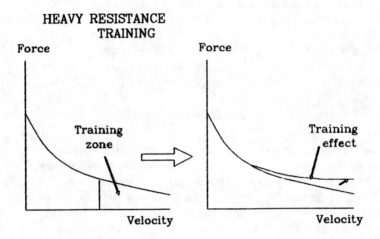

FIGURE 10-5. Specific changes in the force-time curve depending on the area of the curve used in training exercises. (From Komi, P.V., and Häkkinen, K., in *Olympic Book of Sports Medicine,* Dirix, A., Knuttgen, H.G., and Tittel, K., Eds., Blackwell Scientific, Oxford, 1988, 181. With permission.)

Table 10-3. Advantages of Isokinetic, Isotonic, and Isometric Training Exercises

Criterion	Isokinetic	Isotonic	Isometric
Rate of strength gain	Superior	Intermediate	Inferior
Strength gain	Excellent	Good	Poor
Time per training session	Intermediate	Inferior	Superior
Expense	Inferior	Intermediate	Superior
Ease of performance	Intermediate	Inferior	Superior
Ease of progress assessment	Expensive equipment required	Excellent	Dynamometer required
Adaptability to specific movement	Superior	Intermediate	Inferior
Probability of soreness	Small	Large	Small
Probability of injury	Slight	Moderate	Slight
Cardiac risk	Some	Slight	Moderate
Skill improvement	Some	Slight	None

From Lamb, D.R., *Physiology of Exercise,* Macmillan, New York, 1978. With permission.

Table 10-4. Strength Gain Dependence on the Rate of Exercise Performance

Rate of exercise	Mean ± S.E.M. strength gain in 10 weeks (kg)
High	9.0 ± 0.9
Intermediate	16.3 ± 0.5
Slow	9.5 ± 0.8
Varying	22.2 ± 0.6

From Vorobyer, A.N. *Weight-Lifting Sport. Survey on Physiology and Sports Training,* FiS, Moscow. 1977. With permission.

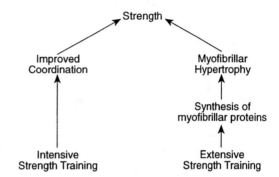

FIGURE 10-6.   Factors of improved strength in training.

Table 10-5.   Intensive and Extensive Strength Training Programs

Main action	Intensive training Neural adaptation	Extensive training Muscle hypertrophy
Percent of force application from 1RM	80–90 or 95–97	60–80
Number of repetitions in a series	2–4	5–15
Number of series per training session	6	3
Rest intervals between series	3–5 min	1–3 min
Number of exercises for improved strength of different muscle groups per training session	6	2–3
Number of training sessions in a micro-cycle	3–4	2–4

From Matveyev, L.P., *Foundations for Sports Training,* FiS, Moscow, 1977. With permission.

Unfortunately, such criteria have not yet been elaborated. We were not able to find in the available literature precisely measurable criteria for the minimal maintaining load either. In most cases both the highest trainable load and the minimal maintaining load are judged by experience and the sportsmen's feelings. Analysis of practical experience led to the following suggestions. For swimmers the change in swimming skill (technique) was recommended as a criterion for the highest possible load.[15] Proposed criteria for the whole scale of loads for swimmers and runners are presented in Tables 10-7 and 10-8. When cross-country skiers use the method of continuous training at the speed of 87% of competition velocity, the criterion for the highest trainable load was recommended to be a substantial drop of skiing velocity. The maintaining load constitutes 40 to 75% of that. It was thought that in cross-country skiers the trainable load begins at the moment when the skiing velocity can be maintained only with the aid of increasing stride frequency.[17]

CRITERIA OF THE TRAINABLE EFFECT OF TRAINING SESSIONS

Metabolites

Practically, the most important thing is to know whether the training session warrants a trainable effect or not. With the hypothesis of the adaptive protein synthesis as a foundation

Table 10-6.   An Advisable Scheme of Exercise Usage to Obtain Various Goals

Exercise	Goal	Principle of action	Methods	Site of adaptive protein synthesis
For improved skills	New coordinations or new coordination mechanisms, stabilization	Repetition (summation)	Repetition method A special variant of the interval method	Nervous tissue
For improved speed	Improved function of SR, lability of neuromuscular apparatus, power and capacity of phosphocreatine mechanism	Repetition	Repetition method	SR, mainly in fast-twitch glycolytic fibers
For improved strength	Creation of strength potential of muscles, reduction of the strength deficit	Repetition (summation)	Repetition method, circuit method, a special variant of the interval method	Myofibrillar proteins
For improved power	Application of the strength potential in a limited time	Repetition	Repetition method, Circuit method	Myofibrillar proteins, SR
For improved endurance	Improved O_2 transport, oxidation capacity of muscles, energy stores, functional stability	Duration (summation)	Method of continuous training, method of intermittent training, interval method	Mitochondria in skeletal muscle, myocardial proteins, new capillaries
For improved anaerobic endurance	Improved capacity and intensity of anaerobic glycogenolysis	Summation	Interval method, method of intermittent training	Buffer systems, pH resistive myocardial proteins
For improved flexibility	Increased elasticity of connective tissue structures, increased motility in joints	Repetition (summation)	Repetition, a special variant of the interval method	Connective tissue

for training effect, it means knowing whether or not the training session causes the critical metabolic and hormonal changes necessary to induce alterations in protein metabolism (Figure 10-8). Therefore, in the first place the criteria for the trainable effect should be found in the accumulation of certain metabolites and changes in the hormone level. In regard to corresponding indices, a number of problems arise. The most serious among these are

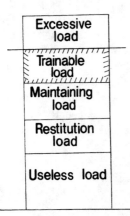

FIGURE 10-7. Load of training sessions.

Table 10-7.   Discrimination of Various Levels of Training Session Load in Swimmers

Load	Main characteristics	Action
Very heavy	Causes pronounced fatigue (a drop of working capacity)	Trainable load
Heavy	60–75% of the amount of exercises up to the drop in working capacity. The main influence is achieved by exercising at the level of compensated fatigue	Trainable load
Moderate	40–60% of the amount of exercises up to the drop in working capacity	Maintaining load
Light	15–20% of the amount of exercises up to the drop in working capacity	Restitution load

From Platonov, V.M., and Vaitsekhovsky, S.M., *Training of High Class Swimmers,* FiS, Moscow, 1985. With permission.

Table 10-8.   Various Zones of the Intensity of Training Session Load in Long-Distance Runners

Zones of load	Time for 1 km run (min:s) during prolonged running	Heart rate	Running velocity in relation to the individual best result
I — restitution load	4:30-5:00	130	
II — maintaining load	4:00-4:30	130–150	
III — trainable load	3:30-4:00	150–170	
IV — highly trainable load	3:00-3:00	170–190	80 %
V — sprints, accelerations, uphill running			81–95 %
VI — jumping, competition running			100 %

From Doroshenko, N.I., A study of Training and Competition Leads in Runners for Middle and Long Distances, Thesis acad. diss., Central Inst. Phys. Cult., Moscow, 1976. With permission.

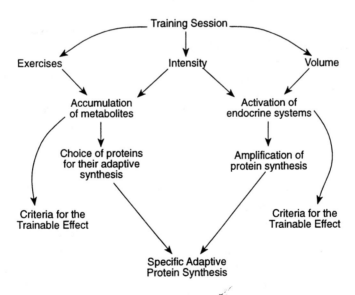

FIGURE 10-8.   Metabolic and hormonal criteria of the trainable effect.

methodological complications, the necessity of obtaining body fluids or tissue samples for analysis, as well as the necessity of using complicated biochemical methods. The metabolic changes controlling transcriptional and translational events are intracellular. Even with the use of the biopsy method, discriminating intracellular and total tissue changes in metabolic processes is not a simple task.

The main way is to check the metabolic changes by blood or urine analysis. In this case it is possible to evaluate the general alterations in the metabolic status and the accumulation of metabolites causing outflow from the intracellular compartment. Regrettably, we still do not know what the actual metabolic inductors causing the main training effects are. Nor do we know how great the accumulation of metabolites has to be. There is also the question of how the necessary intracellular accumulation of metabolites relates to their measurable outflow from the intracellular compartment. Consequently, the metabolic indices are still usable only for detecting general alterations in the metabolic status.

For assessment of the utilization of anaerobic capacity in energy metabolism the lactate level in the blood is widely used.[18-20] There are certain limitations in precise quantitative estimation of the amount of anaerobic glycogenolysis used by the accumulation of lactate in the blood. The most significant limitation arises due to the transfer of lactate from the blood to tissues where it is oxidized during exercise. A problem arises also due to the fact that a part of pyruvate, accumulated as a result of anaerobic glycogenolysis, is used for alanine formation. Further, when an exercise is performed by glycogen-depleted muscles due to previous prolonged exercises or due to a carbohydrate-poor diet, lactate concentrations are reduced at identical submaximal workload, while maximal performance and lactate production are diminished.[21,22] This leads to overestimation of the aerobic endurance capacity, if estimated by calculation of the anaerobic threshold based on fixed lactate values (4 mmol·l^{-1}), or to underestimation of exercise intensity in the monitoring of training.[20] The former will not occur if the calculations use the individual anaerobic threshold measured from the lactate kinetics during incremental exercise and recovery, which is not influenced by glycogen depletion.[22]

According to a number of papers, the blood lactate assay does not always give a dependable assessment of training intensity or current performance ability.[23-26] In negative results, a substantial contribution may belong to the above-mentioned limitations. Additionally, the assessment of the intensity of training sessions by lactate depends on (1) the duration of relief intervals between highly intensive exercise sets, (2) the time interval between the last intensive exercise and blood sampling for lactate determination, and (3) in short-term sprint exercise, despite the highest intensity, the lactate response is moderate due to the ATP resynthesis mainly on account of phosphocreatine breakdown.

Anyway, during strenuous anaerobic exercises the rise in the blood lactate is so tremendous that there is no reason to doubt the value of 'semiquantitative' evaluation of the used anaerobic capacity by blood lactate. In middle- and long-distance runners, significant correlations were found between the behavior of lactate during training sessions and the individual anaerobic threshold or percentage of speed at the individual anaerobic threshold in treadmill running.[27]

However, we do not know exactly how high the lactate level or for how long the increased lactate levels have to be maintained to achieve an effective stimulus for improved anaerobic capacity. In issues of training methodology, suggestions can be found that minimal doses of exercises for stimulation of the improved anaerobic capacity can be given by those causing the blood lactate level to be over 4 mmol·l^{-1}. However, these minimal doses are effective only in untrained persons. For qualified sportsmen the minimal effective exercise dose is thought to be characterized by rises in the blood lactate level over 11 mmol·l^{-1}. For elite sportsmen a blood lactate rise of up to 19 to 22 mmol·l^{-1} is supposed to be necessary. In all these cases the training effect increases with the duration of the period during which the lactate concentration persists at or surpasses the indicated levels.

One may argue whether these high lactate levels are indeed necessary for stimulating anaerobic capacity even in elite sportsmen. There are three principal ways to put a strong demand on the anaerobic glycogenolysis. When very intensive exercises are performed, high lactate levels may be caused, but only for a short time period. When the same amount of exercise is performed in parts, using the interval method, lactate concentration increases. The final lactate level may be the same or even higher, but the time period during which the increased lactate level persisted is more prolonged. There also exists a possibility that in case of using the interval method the blood lactate concentration levels off at a comparatively high value and persists for a time longer than in the previously mentioned cases. Are the training effects of these variants of training sessions the same or is it possible by using these variants to improve different forms of the use of anaerobic capacity (rapid use during a short time or gradual use during a prolonged time)? To get an answer, special investigation is needed.

Exercise intensity is indicated also by rise in the blood ammonia,[20] formed in the hydrolysis of AMP to IMP. Because increased ammonia production is considered to be specifically linked to fast-twitch glycolytic fibers, measurements of ammonia taken during training could provide clues as to the fiber types predominantly recruited.[28,29] The blood ammonia response may be different in sportsmen with identical aerobic capacity. However, a positive correlation was found between anaerobic power (measured in all-out 60-s tests) and the ammonia/lactate ratio during standardized exercise.[30]

About 20 years ago there appeared a widespread tendency to use blood urea in evaluation of the load of a training session and of the recovery processes.[31-35] It is thought that a pronounced increase in the the urea concentration indicates a strong influence of a training session and thereby suggests the existence of trainable effect. The normalization of the urea level in the blood is used as an index of time to perform subsequent strenuous training sessions. Nevertheless, links between exercise-induced blood urea changes and stimulation/actualization for the adaptive protein synthesis have not yet been established. In experiments with rats a disaccordance was found between blood urea changes and other indices of protein metabolism during a short-term training cycle[36] (Figure 10-9). Therefore the urea may not exactly express the actual alterations in the status of protein metabolism in training. The limitations for the use of urea levels are the suppression of urea production in exercises inducing high lactate levels[37] as well as the possibility of altered urea elimination during and after exercise (see Chapter 4).

In biochemical experiments the liberation of free tyrosine is used as an index of protein catabolism. However, the methodological complications obviously did not allow the use of the level of free tyrosine in the blood or urine in monitoring of a training session's effect.

A specific index of the catabolism of muscle contractile proteins is 3-methylhistidine excretion. When the actual excretion of 3-methylhistidine was corrected by subtraction of exogeneous 3-methylhistidine from the total value, the exercise-induced changes during and after a training session for improved power were identical with those obtained in case of the same training sessions performed after 3 days of meat-free diet.[38] Thus, the use of the corrected 3-methylhistidine excretion gives a possibility for avoiding the influence of intake of products whose digestion liberates 3-methylhistidine. Data obtained in humans as well as rats (see Chapter 4) indicated that after exercise, the 3-methylhistidine excretion increases gradually. Both in sportsmen and untrained persons the highest concentration was observed in urine collected 12 to 24 h after exercise.[38] Hence, if the training session takes place before noon, the urine collected during the following night expresses the most intensive 3-methylhistidine excretion caused by the training. The corrected 3-methylhistidine excretion during the night following a training session was significantly correlated both with the highest level of corrected excretion and with the total corrected excretion of 3-methylhistidine measured 48 h after a training session. Therefore, the use of the night 3-methylhistidine excretion value is suitable for studying the effect of serial training on excretion.

In order to find a relationship between 3-methylhistidine excretion and training effects, the excretion of 3-methylhistidine was measured in young men during an 8-week training period for improved power or strength. In both cases one group of persons used training exercises of 70% of one repetition maximum (1RM), and the other group 50% 1RM. Power training caused a significant improvement in the 30-m dash, vertical jump, standing long jump, standing triple jump, and squat lift if the exercise loads were 70% 1RM (in 50% 1RM exercise the effect was

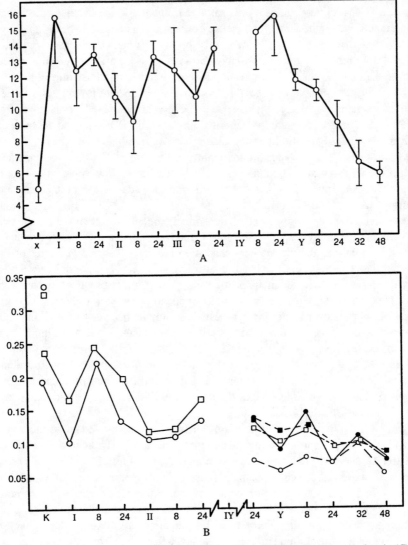

FIGURE 10-9. Dynamics of blood urea (A), synthesis rate of myofibrillar (B) and sarcoplasmic (C) proteins, muscle glycogen (D), and free tyrosine (E) during a training microcycle: ●—● FOG fibers of quadriceps muscle, ○—○ FG fibers of quadriceps muscle, □—□ gastrocnemius muscle, ■—■ SO fibers of soleus muscle. (From Ööpik, V., Alev, K., and Buchinskuyte, V., *Acta Comment. Univ. Tartuensis,* 814, 3, 1988. With permission.)

less pronounced). Heavy resistance training improved the results in vertical jump, standing triple jump, and most of all in squat lift. A very pronounced increase in a cross section of the thigh muscle (evaluated by X-ray photography) resulted from heavy resistance training with 70% 1RM exercise. In all groups a pronounced elevation of corrected 3-methylhistidine excretion was observed in the night urine during the first 3 weeks of training (Figure 10-10). The response was most pronounced and most durable in a group undergoing heavy resistance training with 70% 1RM exercise. In other groups, the degree of muscular hypertrophy and the duration of increased 3-methylhistidine excretion were smaller. In power training with 70% 1RM exercise, the mean 3-methylhistidine response approached the one observed in heavy resistance training when two persons who did not reveal an increase in a cross section of their thigh muscle with power training were excluded. Consequently, a relationship between training-induced muscular hypertrophy and 3-methylhistidine excretion was suggested.[38]

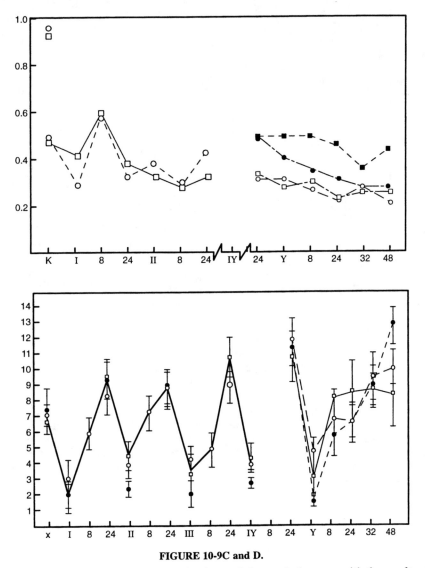

FIGURE 10-9C and D.

The increased 3-methylhistidine excretion in a training period agrees with the results of J.F. Hickson and collaborators,[39,40] who found significant increases in the metabolite excretion from the third day of progressive resistance training.

There are at least two ways to understand this relation. First, an increased 3-methylhistidine excretion during post-exercise recovery is assumed to express an enhanced turnover of contractile proteins (see Chapter 4). An enhanced protein turnover is an indispensable condition for muscular growth.[41] Thus, the increased 3-methylhistidine excretion is related to an overall condition of muscle protein anabolism, leading to muscular hypertrophy. On the other hand, an increased 3-methylhistidine production may describe a condition when inductor-metabolites for the synthesis of myofibrillar proteins accumulate. Either way, a high concentration of 3-methylhistidine excretion may be used as the index of training effectiveness in the stimulation of muscular hypertrophy.

During the late stage of training the increased 3-methylhistidine excretion disappeared (Figure 10-10). This was most likely related to adaptation to the given exercise stimulus. If this is the case, then at the end of the training period the training stimulus must have become insufficient to induce an anabolic response and should have been enhanced then.

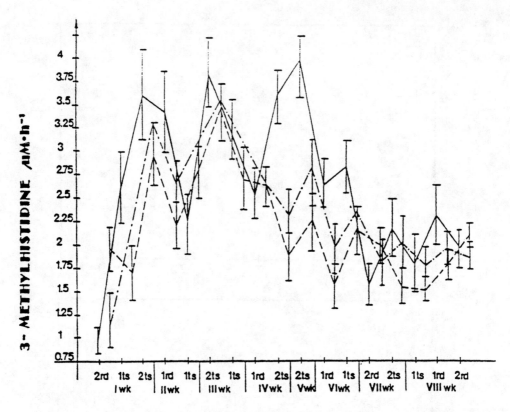

FIGURE 10-10. Excretion of 3-methylhistidine (μmol·h^{-1}) during a training period for improved strength (mean ± SE). Solid line — group exercised with 70% 1RM exercises, dashed line — group exercised with 50% 1RM exercises, dashed line with dots — group exercised with 50% 1RM exercises without two persons who did not have an increase in cross-section of the thigh muscle. On the abscissa, the time of sampling is indicated in the following manner: 1rd — night after one rest day, 2rd — night after two rest days, 1ts — night after one training day session, 2ts — night after 2 days of training session, wk — week of training. (From Viru, A., and Seli, N., *Sports Med. Training Rehabil.*, 3, 183, 1992. With permission.)

While 3-methylhistidine is derived from contractile proteins, its estimation may have significance in assessment of the trainable effect, first of all in heavy resistance or power exercises, acting on the myofibrillar size.

Hormones

The intensity of the training session is also expressed also by changes in blood catecholamine levels. When endurance running was performed at the level of the so-called aerobic threshold (a completely aerobic exercise), the change was modest and expressed mainly by an elevation of noradrenaline level. Running at the level of the individual anaerobic threshold caused a significant rise both in adrenaline and noradrenaline concentrations. The most pronounced rise in the blood level of catecholamine was observed after highly intensive anaerobic running.[20]

In regard to hormone inductors, most attention should be paid to the exercise-induced changes in testosterone and thyroxine + triiodothyronine levels in a training session for improved strength or endurance, respectively. However, neither the hormone basal levels nor the concentration just after exercise is informative, but the post-exercise dynamics are (see Chapter 4). The significance of a hormone's changes may be revealed in relation to the level of other hormones. Thus, statistically significant correlations were found between the testosterone concentration or testosterone/cortisol ratio and changes in strength and power during training periods up to a year.[42,43] However, exact estimation of these hormones in the blood needs vein punctuation and the use of radioimmunoassays. Therefore, this approach cannot be recommended for wide use.

Comparatively simple is the determination of 17-hydroxycorticoids (cortisol and its metabolites) in the urine. The cortisol response to exercise is necessary to obtain an improved working capacity (see p. 214). Moreover, the cortisol response indicates the activation of the mechanism of general adaptation, probably required to achieve the transition from acute adaptation to stable continuous adaptation. In female students an 8-week experimental training on a bicycle ergometer induced an increase in PWC_{170}. Simultaneously, an increased 17-hydroxycorticoid excretion was recorded as a response to training sets both in the first and last weeks of training.[44] In 15- to 17-year-old skiers the training sessions caused increased 17-hydroxycorticoid excretion when they skied at the velocity of 87 to 90% of competition velocity. When the skiing velocity used in training sessions corresponded to 81 to 83% of competition velocity, the increased 17-hydroxycorticoid excretion was found only at the end of a training microcycle. The improvement of performance was detected only in those skiers who used the higher velocity of skiing.[45]

In basketball players of a national or international level the 17-hydroxycorticoid excretion was determined on the first and fourth days of the training microcycle. Four variants of response were found: (1) activation of the adrenocortical function only at the end of a 4-day microcycle, (2) activation both on the first and last day of the microcycle, (3) activation on the first but suppression on the last day, and (4) suppression of adrenocortical function throughout the microcycle. In sportsmen revealing activation of adrenocortical activity throughout the microcycle, the VO_2max, PWC_{170}, as well as the playing effectiveness increased during the corresponding training stage. In those who did not exhibit adrenocortical activation, detraining manifestations were found: VO_2max, PWC_{170}, and playing effectiveness decreased. In cases of persisting suppression of adrenocortical activity, VO_2max did not change, PWC_{170} decreased, and in ECG, ST depression and isoelectric T were observed.[46,47]

Simplified Criteria

There are three groups of simpler criteria for the trainable effect of a session. The first one consists of the accomplishment of a certain task (to acquire skill, to perform perfect side splits, to increase the maximal number of repetitions, to run a certain distance at the prescribed speed etc.). Of course, the opportunities to use these criteria are rather limited because it must be proved if the accomplishment of the task means an actual stimulus for increased possibilities.

The second possibility is based on the assumption that the performance of competition exercises will warrant a stimulus for the improvement of the athlete's capacities. This assumption is undoubtedly correct in endurance events, but not in power events and sprint. It is doubtful that six long jumps, six maximal discus throws, or one to two times running for 100 m will warrant a training effect. In endurance events it may be suggested that the trainable effect appeared a little bit before the finish when the competition velocity was used. The effect increases when this velocity is maintained and the race is continued after the normal finish line (Figure 10-11). However, the possibilities for continuing the race at competition velocity are rather limited. Therefore, for skiers a velocity equal to 87 to 90% of the competition velocity is recommended to be maintained for the maximal possible time.[17]

Physiologically, this approach means maintaining a certain rate of energy expenditure for the time necessary to achieve the highest possible total expenditure at this rate. Both the rate and total energy expenditure are determined by actual demands of the competition exercise.

Heart Rate Studies

More profound criteria may be provided by assessment of functional strain in the organism. In endurance exercises (but not in power or strength exercises) the simplest and most sufficiently objective criterion is heart rate. The foundation for the use of heart rate is that there exists a linear relationship between the rate of energy expenditure and heart rate. However,

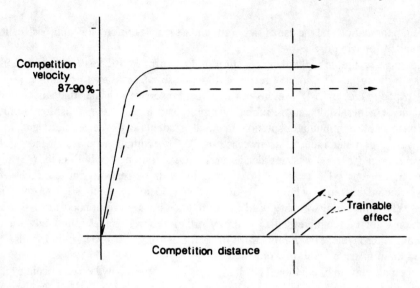

FIGURE 10-11.   An approach to evaluation of the trainable load in cross-country skiers on the basis of competition velocity (see the text).

this relationship exists only up to the anaerobic threshold. Hence, the main area for using heart rate in the control of training load is in exercises for improved aerobic endurance.

In these exercises the training stimulus is related both to the exercise intensity and duration: the higher the intensity, the shorter the time to achieve a stimulus for improvement of the aerobic capacity (Figure 10-12). At the same time this relationship differs between persons. Together with increased fitness, a more prolonged exercise is necessary at the same level of heart rate to achieve the stimulus for an improvement.

It is assumed that the minimal exercise intensity for stimulation of improved aerobic endurance corresponds to the heart rate of 130 beats/min (Figure 10-13). This suggestion is based on the fact that at a heart rate of 120 to 140 beats/min the stroke volume will rise to its maximum. Further increases in exercise intensity do not change the value of stroke volume up to the so-called 'critical heart rate' that may cause a reduction in the stroke volume. It was suggested that in order to stimulate the development of the functional capacity of the heart, it has to contract with the maximal stroke volume for a long time.[48] While this is fairly believable in regard to the improved functional capacity of the heart, further evidence is required in regard to the stimulation of the increase in energy stores, activity of oxidative enzymes, functional ability, etc. The results obtained in untrained students indicated that 8 weeks of exercising by the method of continuous steady training caused an increase in VO_2max when they ran at the heart rate level of 165 to 175 beats/min. However, this exercise regime was ineffective for elevation of the level of high density lipoproteins. When approximately the same total amount of energy was expended by running at the heart rate level of 140 to 150 beats/min, the increase of VO_2max was insignificant but the concentration of high density lipoproteins increased significantly (by 19%).[49]

A certain limitation for the use of heart rate will be caused by the dependence of exercise heart rates on emotional excitement and environmental factors (barometric pressure, temperature).

The best situation for the use of heart rate is when the method of continuous steady training is used. Complications arise with the method of intermittent training or when the training consists of various exercises (e.g., usual physical education lesson, circuit training session, training session in wrestlers or football players, etc.). In these cases an approach consists of taking into account the total time when the heart rate exceeded 130 or 170 beats/min (Figure 10-14). The number of minutes during which the heart rate was above 130 beats/min indicate

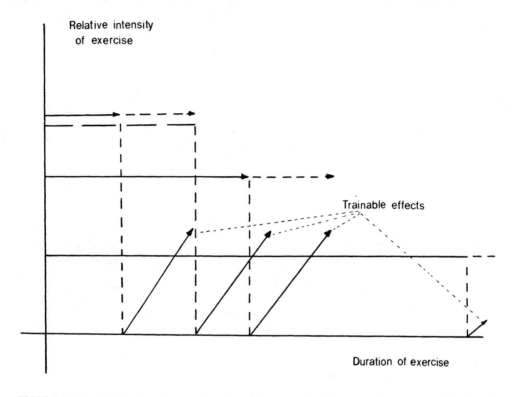

FIGURE 10-12.   Relationships between intensity and duration of continuous aerobic exercise and the trainable effect. The less intensive the exercise, the longer is the duration necessary to achieve the trainable effect.

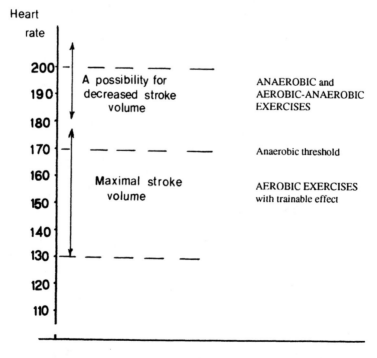

FIGURE 10-13.   Evaluation of exercise load by heart rate.

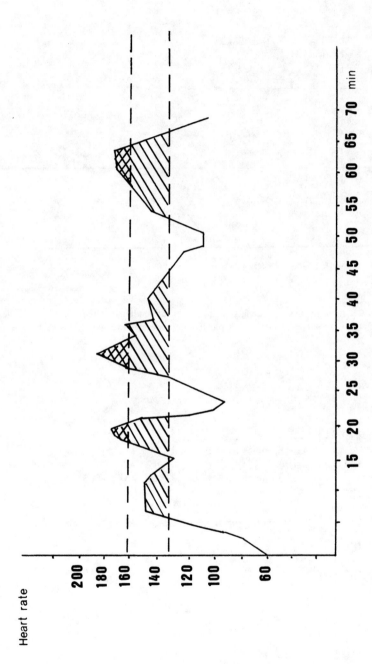

FIGURE 10-14. Evaluation of the trainable load by the time period during which the heart rate is over 130 beats/min (striated area). The time period during which the heart rate is over 180 beats/min (cross-striated area) indicates the time for exercises over anaerobic threshold.

Table 10-9.   Account of Exercise Intensity by Heart Rate in Wrestlers

Energy regimen of exercises	Heartbeats/min	Score
Aerobic	114	1
	120	2
	126	3
	132	4
	138	5
	144	6
	150	7
Aerobic-anaerobic	156	8
	162	10
	168	12
	174	14
	180	17
Anaerobic	186	21
	192	25
	198	33

Comment: For calculation of the criterion for total load of training session (1) each score is multiplied by the time (min) of the exercises at the corresponding intensity and (2) the sum of products of score-time gives the criterion.

From Sorvanov, V.A., *Teor. Prakt. Fiz. Kult.*, 2, 19, 1978. With permission.

the time of stimulation of the development of aerobic capacity. The time of heart rate above 170 beats/min expresses the duration of the influence on the anaerobic capacity. Another approach consists of the use of special scores (Table 10-9).

Middle- and long-distance runners have been recommended 30 to 60 min of running at the heart rate of 130 to 160 beats/min for stabilization of aerobic endurance, and 30 to 60 min of running at the heart rate of 170 beats/min for improved aerobic capacity.[51]

The evaluation of the exercise intensity by absolute values of heart rate may be incorrect if various sportsmen are compared due to differences in the resting heart rate.[26] To avoid this possible source of error, the intensity of exercise may be expressed as percent of heart rate reserve:[52]

$$\% \text{ of heart rate reserve } = \frac{(\text{training heart rate } - \text{ resting heart rate})}{(\text{maximum heart rate } - \text{ resting heart rate})} \times 100$$

It is recommended that the training target heart rate necessary to bring about a change in the anaerobic threshold is 85 to 90% of maximal heart rate.[53] Training heart rate may be expressed as percentage of race-pace heart rate as well.[54]

INTENSITY AND VOLUME OF TRAINING LOADS

The volume of training load is a quantitative characteristic. It may be measured in kilometers of the total distance covered during the session, total weight of resistance exercises, number of exercise repetitions, total time of exercising, etc. The intensity of load expresses the volume in a unit of time. The intensity of exercise load may be measured by the relative intensity of performed exercises, the mean level of power output during exercise, the percentage of exercise characteristics in regard to individual maximum or to characteristics of the competition exercise, or relation of volume indices to the expended time.

Table 10-10. Dependence of Exercise Influence on Its Intensity

$VO_2/l \cdot min^{-1}$	$VO_2/ml \cdot kg^{-1}$	Energy expenditure $(kcal \cdot min^{-1})$	MET	Heartbeats/min	Increase in blood lactate concentration	Maximal duration
		Aerobic exercise (oxidative phosphorylation)				
2.0–2.5	28–35	10.0–12.5	8–10×	140–160	1.5–2×	More than 40 min
		Aerobic-anaerobic (oxidative phosphorylation + anaerobic glycogenolysis)				
2.5–3.0	35–42	12.5–15.0	10–12×	160–180	2–6×	5–40 min
		Anaerobic-glycolytic (anaerobic glycogenolysis)				
3.0	42	15.0–62.0	12–48×	180–200	6×	0.5–5 min
		Anaerobic-alactatic (phosphocreatine mechanism)				
—	—	300	240×	150–170	2–3×	up to 10 s

It must be emphasized that the increase or decrease in exercise intensity does not always mean the enhanced or reduced influence in a certain direction. When the change in exercise intensity induces transition from one mechanism of ATP resynthesis to another, the physiological influence of the same exercise gains new features. The main characteristics of exercises influencing various mechanisms of ATP resynthesis are presented in Table 10-10.

In sports practice attempts have been made to increase the exercise load by running in deep water or snow, cycling against the wind or rowing upstream, addition of weight, etc. A special study of such approaches was made in regard to added weights. Endurance athletes wore a vest weighing 9 to 10% b.w. every day from morning to evening for 4 weeks including every (six athletes) or every other (also six athletes) training session. After 4 weeks the experimental group had significantly higher blood lactate and oxygen uptake during running at moderate speed and an increased blood lactate concentration after a short running test to exhaustion in comparison with the values obtained before the experimental period. Running velocity at anaerobic threshold did not change. Those athletes who used added loads during every training session had improved running time to exhaustion, improved vertical velocity when running up stairs, and an increased VO_2 during submaximal running after the added load period. It was concluded that the additional load increased anaerobic metabolism in the leg muscles during submaximal and maximal exercise, obviously due to increased recruitment and adaptation of the fast-twitch muscle fibers. The negative effects observed immediately after added load training disappeared, and maximal performance capacity improved during the subsequent 2 weeks of training in normal conditions.[55] These suggestions were justified in a rat experiment. The effect of running training with added load (20% b.w.) on citrate synthase, malate dehydrogenase and phosphofructokinase activities was pronounced in the white quadriceps but not in the red quadriceps and soleus muscles.[56] Thus, the added load changed the motoneuron coordination of the slow-twitch fibers to the fast-twitch glycolytic fibers.

SIGNIFICANCE OF EXERCISE SCHEDULE

Results were obtained by N.N. Yakovlev and collaborators[57] indicating the various influence of exercise in dependence of their place in the training session. First of all, the energy attained in various exercises depends on the activation of oxidative phosphorylation by previous exercises. This may be achieved with the aid of warm-up exercises. Studies in training sessions have showed that after a complex of warm-up exercises, rowing for 2500 m as well as running for 5000 m caused a less pronounced increase in lactate and pyruvate concentrations than without the warm-up exercises. In skiers two schedules of the same exercises (5 × 100 m, 4 × 200 m, 3 × 400 m, 1000 m, and 1500 m vs. 1500 m, 1000 m, 3 × 400 m, 4 × 2000 m, and 5 × 100 m) were compared. In both cases before the main 'anaerobic influence' (3 × 400 m) the lactate and glucose levels were the same. No significant difference was found in lactate and glucose response to 3 × 400 m either. However, in the first schedule the lactate and glucose level did not decrease toward the end of the session as was observed in the second exercise schedule. Obviously, the relation between lactate production and elimination favors the latter during the final part of the session in the second schedule.

For the stimulation of oxidative phosphorylation and, thereby, lactate elimination, an essential role may belong to a modest activation of anaerobic metabolism. In cyclists a short-term acceleration of the cycling tempo at the 2nd or 28th to 30th min caused a lower lactate level at the end of a 60 min of session than was detected after 60 min of steady cycling.[57]

Some significance should also be attributed to the fact that despite the similarity in the energy attained from various exercises, their influence may be different when one of them, but not others, correspond to the competition exercise. In rowers, running or rowing during the first half of the training session increased the blood lactate level. When during the second half of the session running was replaced by rowing, the lactate level decreased. However, when rowing was replaced by running, an elevated lactate level persisted. No differences in the dynamics of glucose or pyruvate levels were found. When after running or rowing weight lifting exercises were performed and after that rowing or running took place, respectively, the blood lactate dynamics were similar to those obtained in the first experiment: rowing during the final part of training induced a lower lactate level than did running. This was observed despite the fact that weight lifting after running increased the lactate level more than it did after rowing.[57]

Besides the differences in energy processes the exercise schedule, as well as the rest intervals between them, determine the changes in the excitability and lability of the central nervous system. One must take into consideration that in all cases when exercise is directed toward improvement of the coordination mechanism, its effectiveness depends on the optimal functional state of the nervous structures.

Endurance and Strength Exercises

One problem is the interaction of strength and endurance training. A general consensus is the incompatibility of these training modes:[58-62] strength training may inhibit endurance improvement[58] and endurance training may inhibit strength development.[60-62] However, a program of combined running and weight training during 12 weeks (3 days/week) caused in both male and female persons significant increases in VO_2max and strength as well as a decrease in body-fat percentage. The same, but less pronounced, changes were found after a program of circuit weight training.[63]

The results obtained indicated a possibility for increasing leg strength by 30% when heavy resistance training 3 days/week was added to endurance training (6 days/week) during a 10-week period. During this period fast- and slow-twitch fiber areas, citrate synthase activity, as well as VO_2max remained unchanged. However, short-term endurance (4 to 8 min) was increased by 11 and 13% during cycling and running, respectively. Long-term cycling to exhaustion at 80% VO_2max increased from 71 to 85 min. Thus, these data did not demonstrate any negative performance effects of adding heavy-resistance training to ongoing endurance-training regimes. It was suggested that certain types of endurance performance, particularly those requiring fast-twitch fiber recruitment, can be improved by strength training supplementation.[64]

It was demonstrated that high intensity endurance training (at 90% VO_2max) per se increased the isokinetic muscle power. A significant increase of isokinetic peak power of knee extension was found at lower test speeds (30, 60 and 120°·s^{-1}) but not at faster velocities of 120, 240 and 300°·s^{-1}.[65] According to the above-mentioned data it was found that peak torque increases were similar with concurrent endurance and velocity-controlled resistance training and resistance training only.[66] Using a single-leg training model, it was established that combined endurance and high resistance training did not impair the cellular adaptation or strength performance associated with training for strength or endurance separately.[67]

NECESSITY OF INCREASED LOAD (SATURATION PHENOMENON)

Repetition of one and the same exercise stimulates adaptation processes. The results are specifically related structural, metabolic, and functional changes. The expression of those results is an increase in related cellular structures as well as a decrease in functional and metabolic adjustments during this exercise. Collectively, it means that the organism has achieved a good adaptation to this exercise level, and the performance is increased in regard to this exercise. However, all those results cause a loss of stimulus for further development that was still exerted by this exercise. Consequently, the adaptation to one level of exercise makes it necessary to increase the exercise intensity or duration or to use more strenuous or complicated exercises.

The principle of increased training loads fits in well with the overload principle. The amount of exercise in a time unit was considered critical to reach a sufficient overload.[68] Accordingly, the stimulus for training effect is equal to the sum of training volume and intensity. Assuming that the training effect means an adaptation, the stimulus has to increase.[69]

The principle of increased training load is well recognized by anyone who has experience in physical training. Analyses of practical experiences of sportsmen as well as results of related investigations allowed J. Verhoshanski[70] to formulate the following four rules:

1. The trainable effect of exercise decreases with the increase of specific fitness of the sportsmen.
2. Training loads have to warrant the trainable effect in dependence on the status of the athlete's organism.
3. Remaining imprints from the action of the previous training session change the trainable effect of the session.
4. The trainable effect of an exercise complex is determined not by the sum of all stimuli, but by their interrelation, schedule, and time intervals between various stimuli.

An analysis of sports practice also led to a suggestion that the higher the functional reserve of the athlete, the larger the amount used to warrant the trainable effect.[71]

The main problem is how to increase the training load. Among other aspects of the problem there is the question of whether the loads have to be increased linearly from one training session to another. The alternative possibility is repetition of the same exercise load during a certain time to ensure complete adaptation to this level of exercise load, and only then do a transition to a higher load follow. In a model experiment on rats it was found that the increase of swimming duration only at the beginning of every week caused a more pronounced reduction in the utilization of glycogen and phosphocreatine stores, as well as in the lactate response during 15 min of swimming, than training with daily increased swimming duration. When the swimming duration was increased over 2 or 3 weeks, the training resulted in more pronounced increases in phosphocreatine, glycogen, total protein, activities of ATPase, cytochrome oxidase, and succinate dehydrogenase in muscles as well as P/O and maximal swimming duration than other training variants.[72-74] An analysis of the training-induced changes in cytochrome c confirmed the benefit of stepwise increased load.[75] The stepwise increase of training load is approved also in issues on training methodology.[14,15,76,77]

Evidence was provided that adaptation to endurance training is rapid. An exercise program consisting of 3 days of interval training and 3 days of continuous running or cycling weekly induced a VO_2max increase to a constant level with the half-time of the increase being 10.3 days. After elevation of training load a new increase in VO_2max was observed with the half-time of 10.8 days. The decrease in heart rate and blood lactate response to a standard submaximal exercise test also occurred within the first 2 to 3 weeks of each training period.[78] In rats after 9 weeks of gradually increased training load, the running time sharply rose from $60\,min\cdot d^{-1}$ to $120\,min\cdot d^{-1}$ in the first 2 days, to $240\,min\cdot d^{-1}$ in the next 2 days and to $360\,min\cdot d^{-1}$ in the final 2 days during the 10th week. An additional increase in oxidative capacity and citrate synthase activity was observed both in the soleus and the plantaris muscles with no change in the white vastus lateralis muscle. The liver but not muscle glycogen content increased as well. Peak tetanic tension in the gastrocnemius was not changed by the first part of training nor by the days of increased training load.[79]

In Figure 6-4 results were presented demonstrating the dependence of VO_2max improvement on the volume of endurance exercises in a year.[80] However, one must take into consideration that only previous adaptation makes it possible to increase the training volume. With the aid of mathematical modeling the optimal zones of volumes of endurance exercises for VO_2max improvement were established in a certain contingent. It follows that for long-distance runners separate training influences on the anaerobic glycogenolysis have to be no more than 30 h/year, i.e., 6% of the total volume.[80]

In a number of cases in the course of training the effectiveness of training decreases despite an increase in training loads. The rapid increase in glycogen and phosphocreatine in the early stage of training slows down afterwards. Later, despite the continued training, the energy stores level off.[72,73,81] Similar dynamics were found in VO_2max.[82] In these cases it is possible to suggest that the increase of exercise load (stimulus for improvement) was insufficient. However, a study of the dependence of increase in muscle succinate dehydrogenase activity on the training volume indicated that up to a certain volume of training (called saturation threshold) there exists a direct dependence of increase on the volume. Further increase in the volume induces a trend to reduction in enzyme activity. More strenuous training using the interval method resulted in the saturation phenomenon at lower training volume than continuous steady training method. However, the obtained highest levels of the enzyme activity were almost the same (Figure 5-7).[83]

In sportsmen the saturation phenomenon was revealed by plotting the increase in the oxygen supply of the organism to the total time expended for training by the interval method in runners for middle distances. It was found that the appearance of the saturation phenomenon depends on the previous fitness level: the higher the performance level, the larger the training volume to induce saturation (Figure 10-15).[83]

It may be speculated that the appearance of the saturation phenomenon is related to exhaustion of the organism's adaptivity (or adaptation energy, according to H. Selye[84]). If this is the case, the results in Figure 10-15 provide evidence that training increases adaptivity. Accordingly, it was suggested that in the training process the plastic reserve of the organism (adaptivity) is not only exhausted but also supercompensated.[85] Obviously, the art of training consists of ensuring purposeful utilization of the adaptive possibilities as well as of finding the time for restoration and supercompensation of these activities.

MICROCYCLE OF TRAINING

VARIANTS OF TRAINING MICROCYCLES

A limited number of training and rest days together constitute a training microcycle (Figure 10-16). This main element in training organization has to: (1) concert the action of subsequent training sessions, (2) determine the ratio between training time to rest hours, and (3) ensure the complete restitution for the onset of the next microcycle. For the latter, one or two rest or relief days usually terminate the training microcycle. Most often the microcycle structure is six and one, five and two, four and one, or three and one training and relief days, respectively. The time for actualization of the adaptive protein synthesis and supercompensation of energy stores is determined by the organization of training microcycles. While training exercises

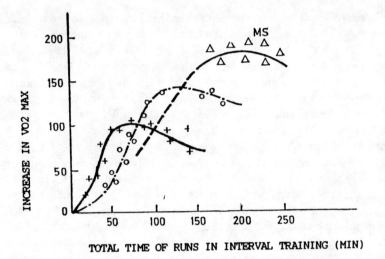

FIGURE 10-15. Increase of VO$_2$max in dependence of the volume of interval training. 1 — athletes of national level, 2 — athletes of medium level 3 — athletes of university level. Constructed by N. Volkov.[83]

decide the specificity of the adaptive protein synthesis and the load of training sessions ensures hormonal alterations for its amplification, the training microcycle determines the summing up or other interrelations between various influences on protein turnover.

In methodological issues a classification is proposed by which the microcycles are discriminated into:[14,15]

1. Development microcycles — to ensure the desired result(s) of training; (a) ordinary microcycle (the difference between total load of this and the previous microcycle is moderate), (b) 'blow' microcycle (the total load of microcycle is to a great extent larger in comparison with the previous ordinary microcycles)
2. Applied microcycle — to adjust the athlete's organism to training at the beginning of a training period, or to new training conditions (transition from outdoor to indoor conditions or vice versa, or from running to skiing, etc.) or to ensure immediate readiness for competition

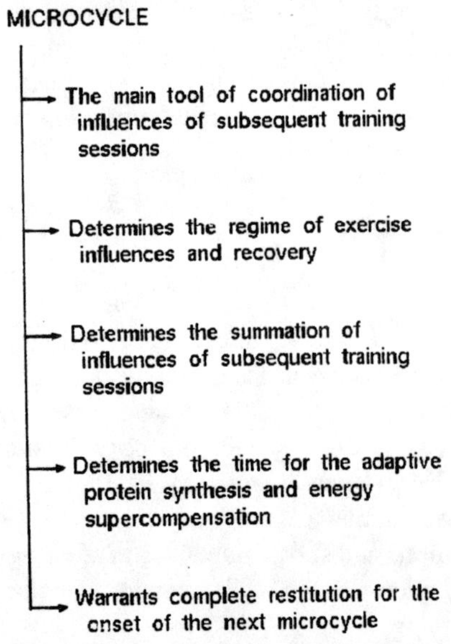

MICROCYCLE

→ The main tool of coordination of influences of subsequent training sessions

→ Determines the regime of exercise influences and recovery

→ Determines the summation of influences of subsequent training sessions

→ Determines the time for the adaptive protein synthesis and energy supercompensation

→ Warrants complete restitution for the onset of the next microcycle

FIGURE 10-16. Significance of the training microcycle.

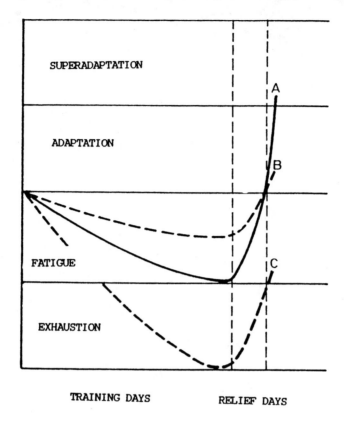

SUPERADAPTATION

ADAPTATION

FATIGUE

EXHAUSTION

TRAINING DAYS   RELIEF DAYS

FIGURE 10-17.   Three variants of summation of loads in training microcycle (see the text). Constructed by J.E. Counsilman.[87]

3.   Competition microcycle — from last day(s) before competition and days of competition
4.   Restitution microcycle — relief days or weeks just after the competition microcycle or after the 'blow' microcycle

In regard to ordinary microcycles, most decisive is the ratio of training loads to restitution between sessions.[86]

From the physiological point of view the ordinary microcycles have to be discriminated into microcycles with complete restitution to the next training set and into microcycles with summation of loads. The first type exists in physical education of adolescents as well as in training of beginners. In advanced sportsmen, especially in qualified athletes, this variant of ordinary microcycle means a waste of time. The summation of loads within a microcycle is caused by daily repetition of vigorous training sessions.

In these cases the following variants are possible:

•   Summation of the action of daily training sessions influencing the same functions (capacities)
•   Summation of the action of daily sessions influencing different functions (capacities)
•   Insertion of sessions with maintaining loads between trainable sessions
•   Insertion of sessions with restitution loads between trainable sessions

SUMMATION OF INFLUENCES OF SUBSEQUENT SESSIONS

Principally, the microcycles with summation of loads may cause three different results[87] (Figure 10-17): (1) summation of loads causes a general fatigue for the last training day(s);

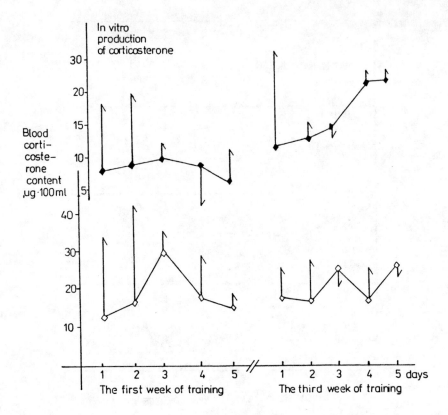

FIGURE 10-18. Changes in *in vitro* production of corticosterone (closed symbols) and blood corticosterone concentration (open symbols) in rats during two training microcycles. The symbols indicate the levels before exercise and the arrows the response to training exercises. (From Viru, A., Kostina, L., and Zhurkina, L., *Fiziol. Zh.*, 34(4), 61, 1988. With permission.)

during subsequent rest day(s) the recovery processes ensure the normalization of stores and functions as well as a moderate stimulus for further adaptation; (2) summation of loads causes a drop of body state until the borderline of dangerous exhaustion; this situation is a strong stimulus for adaptation processes and a state of 'superadaptation' will be achieved for the onset of the next microcycle; and (3) summation of loads gives such a demanding situation that a dangerous exhaustion (with overstrain phenomena) develops: now restitution days are necessary for treatment of overstrain phenomena, and the next microcycle begins from the level of decreased working capacity and persisting fatigue. In the latter case a restitution microcycle has to follow in order to avoid overstrain.

When 30 min of swimming was daily repeated in rats during 5 days, on the first day the adrenocortical activity increased in response to exercise (Figure 10-18). During further repetition of exercise a generally high level of adrenocortical activity persisted in the resting state as well as after exercise. It was followed by signs of subtotal depletion of the adrenocortical reserve (a decreased content of corticosterone in the adrenals and a low level of corticosterone production *in vitro*). On the fifth day of the training week a restoration of the normal level of activity was observed without any response to the same exercise load. Activation of the adrenocortical function was observed again when the load of training exercise was augmented and the same dynamics were repeated during the next training weeks.[88] These data suggest that adaptation to a concrete level of exercise load is achieved through a phase of subtotal depletion of the resources of the adrenal cortex. Obviously, an improvement in the apparatus of corticosteroid biosynthesis was necessary for the achievement of adaptation. In the third week of training a high level of corticosterone production *in vitro* was observed. This suggests that the glucocorticoid biosynthesis mechanism had reached a new augmented level.

This experiment was repeated using 90-min instead of 30-min swims. The corticosterone concentration in the adrenals increased significantly during the first 2 days in response to a swimming set with the highest level on the second day after exercise. On the third and fourth days the increase was insignificant. In the post-exercise recovery period the corticosterone concentration decreased, except for the second day. On the fifth day only a decrease in the corticosterone concentration was found. The blood corticosterone level increased in response to swimming on days one, two, three, and five. On the fourth day the corticosterone concentration decreased instead of increasing. On the fourth and fifth days the recovery period was characterized by drops of the hormone levels below the initial. During the 5 days of training the basal level of *in vitro* corticosterone production as well as the response to added corticotropin decreased.[89] These results also indicate that daily repetition of exercises during 5 days causes a subtotal exhaustion of the adrenal reserve. However, the adrenal responsiveness to corticotropin persisted.

Agreeing results were obtained in a group of middle- and long-distance runners. A strenuous daily training caused first a pronounced elevation of the cortisol resting level in conjunction with unusually high responses of cortisol and somatotropin to training exercises. Afterwards a high resting level of blood cortisol was accompanied by a reversed cortisol response and a low somatotropin level after exercise.[88]

In rats, daily swimming of 90 min during 5 days resulted in a pronounced and long-lasting suppression of the rate of synthesis of sarcoplasmic and myofibrillar proteins in the soleus, gastrocnemius, and both red and white portions of the quadriceps muscle. The decreased rate of protein synthesis persisted also during the two subsequent rest days. The blood urea level was elevated during exercise days. However, 32 h after the last swimming set it normalized despite the persisting diminished rate of protein synthesis in the muscles. The level of free tyrosine increased in the muscles during swimming sets. In muscles of predominantly red fibers the free tyrosine level usually normalized after 8 h of every exercise bout, and in muscles of predominantly white fibers the elevated content of free tyrosine persisted 24 h or more after exercise.[90] These results suggest that this regimen of the training microcycle was too exhaustive. However, glycogen reserves in the muscles and liver were replenished or even supercompensated during the 24-h recovery periods after every exercise bout.[36]

In another series of experiments the swimming duration was reduced by 60 min after the first 2 days of every week. In this case the protein synthesis was suppressed only on exercise days and it intensified to a level above control values during the days of recovery.[90] During 4 weeks of training the physical working capacity (maximal duration of swimming), glycogen reserves, activity of succinate dehydrogenase in red muscles and dry weight of the adrenals increased in both training regimes (Figure 10-19).[91] Hence, the overall suppression of protein synthesis in skeletal muscles did not exclude the increase in working capacity and in other training effects. The increased activity of the mitochondrial enzyme indicated that at least in regard to these enzymes the adaptive protein synthesis took place. This agrees with the previously noted fact that after an endurance exercise the main locus of elevated protein synthesis is mitochondrial proteins in the red fibers. The training effects were even more pronounced in cases of persisting suppression of protein synthesis than in a less strenuous training regime, leading to an elevated rate of protein synthesis during recovery after 5 days of training. This fact led us to the assumption that the overall suppression of protein synthesis excluded the competition between the synthesis of various proteins for 'building materials' and helped to concentrate the adaptive protein synthesis for the most responsible proteins.

Apart from the results obtained in rats, in regard to sportsmen it was demonstrated that daily repetition of vigorous training sessions may cause a gradual decrease of the muscle glycogen content (Figure 10-20).[92-95] In well-trained swimmers a sudden increase in the training load for

WORKING CAPACITY

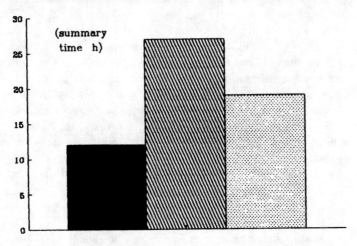

LIVER GLYCOGEN

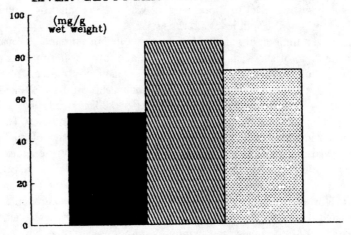

FIGURE 10-19.   Changes induced by 4 weeks of training in maximal duration of swimming, glycogen reserves, and activity of succinate dehydrogenase in various muscles. Dotted columns — sedentary control rats, striated columns — training without change of the load during a microcycle, black columns — training with a decrease of load after the first two sessions in each microcycle. (From Ööpek, V. and Viru, A., *Sports Med. Training Rehabil.*, 3, 55, 1991. With permission.)

10 consecutive days elicited symptoms of overstrain with marked reduction in the resting glycogen concentration.[96] This finding was confirmed in well-trained runners: increased training loads for 5 successive days caused an extensive glycogen depletion in both type I and type II fibers.[97] On the one hand, the low glycogen level will limit the working capacity. On the other hand, the glycogen level is one of the factors controlling energy metabolism in skeletal muscles. Hence, exercising at the decreased glycogen level induced certain peculiarities in metabolic regulation and, thereby, in training influence. When 10 min of cycling at 85% VO_2max was repeated four to seven times daily, after 3 days the decrease in the glycogen concentration was associated with reduced glycogen and enhanced lipid utilization during exercise.[98] When 60 min of running or cycling at 75% VO_2max was performed during three successive days, the degree of repletion of muscle glycogen during 24 h decreased from day to day in both types of exercise.[99]

CLYCOGEN CONTENT (mg/g wet tissue)

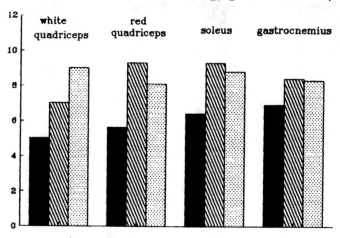

SDH ACTIVITY

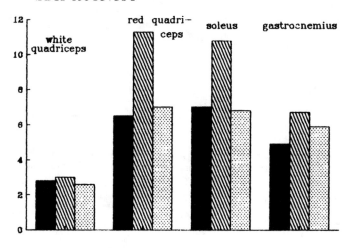

FIGURE 10-19 (continued)

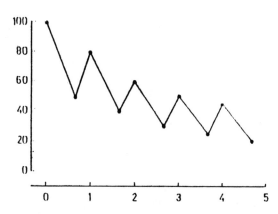

FIGURE 10-20. Gradual decrease in muscle glycogen during a strenuous microcycle. Constructed by H. Kantola and H. Rusko.[95]

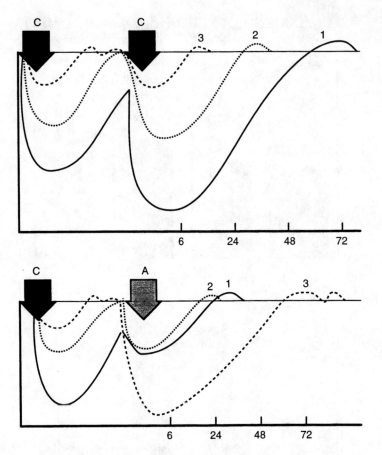

FIGURE 10-21. Dynamics of speed (1), anaerobic capacity (2), and aerobic capacity (3) in swimmers after two subsequent training sessions for improved speed (C) or improved aerobic capacity (A). Speed, anaerobic, and aerobic capacities were evaluated by swimming tests. Constructed by V. Platonov.[100]

Using various performance tests in swimmers, it was demonstrated that when training sessions of the same direction are repeated, the summation is revealed first of all in the performance capacity toward which the training influence was directed (Figure 10-21).[100] Even when the load of the subsequent training session of the same direction was moderate, a pronounced summing up of the influence was revealed in regard to trained performance capacity.

MICROCYCLES WITH VARIABLE TRAINING LOADS

The idea to use training sessions of alternating influences on different performance capacities is founded on the assumption that when a function has not yet recovered, it is possible to give a training influence on other functions that have already normalized. Indeed, the results obtained in swimmers indicated that in the case of alternating influences the summation of training sessions' actions gained a new character (Figure 10-21). When three different training sessions were subsequently performed, each of them induced a most pronounced drop in corresponding performance capacity (Figure 10-22). However, within 36 to 72 h after the last one, all capacities were at the initial level.[100]

The question arises whether alternating influences depend on the action that follows the previous one. The significance of this question is supported by results showing that resistance and endurance training performed on the same day impeded strength development in comparison to training for either on separate days.[101] When one group of persons performed concurrent

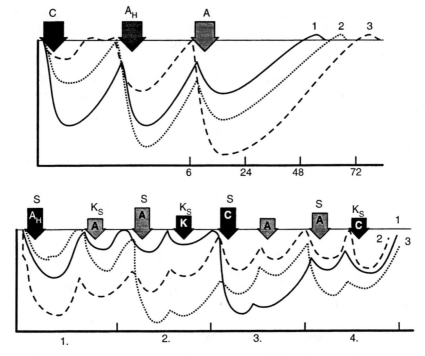

FIGURE 10-22. Dynamics of speed (1), anaerobic capacity (2), and aerobic capacity (3) in swimmers after three subsequent training sessions (upper panel) or in two training sessions daily (lower panel). C — training for improved speed, A_H — training for improved anaerobic capacity, A — training for improved aerobic capacity, S — session with a great load, K_S — sessions with a moderate load, V — session with a modest load. Constructed by V. Platonov.[100]

endurance training 3 days a week and low velocity resistance training on 3 alternate days, after 3 and 9 weeks they exhibited significant increase in the knee extensor peak torque, the total work during four maximal knee extensions, and in the cross-sectional area of the quadriceps. These increases were similar to the group performing only resistance training without any endurance exercise. During the 10th to 12th weeks the progress continued in the latter but not in the former group. Oxygen uptake, heart frequency, and blood lactate during 6 min of rowing at the power output of 125 W decreased in the first group progressively during the 12-week period.[102] The results indicate a possibility for inserting endurance exercises into the microcycles for improved strength. However, this is not yet a solution to the whole complicated problem.

TWO OR MORE DAILY TRAINING SESSIONS

In highly qualified sportsmen the training microcycles are characterized by two or even three training sessions daily. In track and field athletes of international level a microcycle consists of six to seven main and seven to twelve additional training sessions,[103] in swimmers of high qualification, a microcycle consists of two to four training sessions of great load and six to eight sessions of moderate loads.[15] Quite common is a combination of training sessions of high and moderate loads, i.e., one main and one or two additional sessions during a day. The summing up of the influences of subsequent training sessions becomes decisive.

Model experiments on rats showed that 1 h after a 30-min swim the muscle glycogen, as well as blood lactate and free fatty acid level were normalized, the phosphocreatine content was supercompensated, and cytochrome oxidase activity had increased in the muscles. At 2 h after swimming muscle glycogen was supercompensated as well as phosphocreatine stores, and liver glycogen normalized. An increased cytochrome oxidase activity persisted. Accordingly, when the same exercise was repeated four times over 2-h intervals, it was thought to be reasonable that at least the second exercise began from the level of supercompensation. In this case the decrease of muscle and liver glycogen as well as the rise in the blood lactate level were less pronounced, and the increase in the blood free fatty acid level was more pronounced in comparison with the action of 2 h of swimming without any interruption. Also, the activity of cytochrome oxidase was higher. One hour of restitution was enough for normalization of the muscle glycogen store and the blood lactate level in the first case but not in a 2-h swim without interruption.[104] These data indicate that the acute adaptation to 4 × 30 min swimming over 2-h rest periods proceeded more effectively than to a 2-h swim.

Training for 1 month with an increase of session load over a 10-day period induced more pronounced increases in skeletal muscle, myocardium and liver glycogen, skeletal muscle phosphocreatine, and cytochrome oxidase activity. An increase was also induced in the maximal duration of swimming when the daily load was divided into four parts and performed with 2-h periods of rest between them. These training effects became even more pronounced when in addition to the division the daily loads were varied (from 50 to 200% of the daily load for a corresponding period). When trained rats performed a swimming test for maximal duration the decrease of glycogen stores per exercise time and the rise in the blood lactate were less pronounced and the rise in the free fatty acid level was more pronounced in rats trained with four exercise sets daily, compared to rats trained once daily.[104]

In another experiment, increasing of the number of daily training sessions from one to three (saving the total daily load constant) resulted in increased training effects on the content of skeletal muscle proteins, synthesis rate of both microsomal and ribosomal RNA, and the stability of poly-A-containing mRNA. The synthesis of myofibrillar, sarcoplasmic, and myostromal proteins increased as well.[105]

Thus, adaptation is promoted by dividing the daily training load into parts. Accordingly, in male strength athletes (power-lifters and body-builders) dividing the amount of the daily training session into two created more effective training stimuli leading to further strength development. However, two training sessions daily caused a decrease in free testosterone concentration and an increase in cortisol concentration during the following relief days.[106]

In practice of top level sports, the idea of the increased number of daily sessions is not only to favor the adaptation, but also to increase the daily load. Practical experience justifies the possibility. The same may be demonstrated by the results of an investigation of training microcycle in swimmers. The data presented in Figure 10-22 indicate that when the training session varied by the load and the direction of influence, at the end of the microcycle a parallel recovery occurred in speed, anaerobic, and aerobic performance capacities.[100] After microcycles consisting of 6 or 11 training sessions, all tests provided evidence of the overall decrease of special working capacity in swimmers. Restitution was observed 48 h after the last training session. At 72 h after the last session a slight increase in special working capacity of swimmers was found.[107]

In cases of two training sessions daily the hormonal responses may change. In highly qualified weight-lifters both sessions caused decreases in voluntary strength and integral EMG. After the first session the blood levels of testosterone and cortisol were decreased, but after the second session they increased.[108] During subsequent days the response of testosterone and cortisol to morning and afternoon training sessions remained without substantial alterations in elite weight-lifters. The somatotropin response to the morning session was reduced after the first 3 days and then remained unchanged. The somatotropin response to the afternoon session did not change.[109] When speed skaters performed three training units with higher intensity on the first day, a decrease of the free testosterone/cortisol ratio followed the next day, showing the prevalence of catabolic over anabolic actions. This change was not observed in sportsmen performing less intensive training exercises as it was indicated by a less pronounced increase in the blood lactate concentration after training exercises.[30]

The use of microcycles with an increased training load and especially with an increased number of daily sessions makes it feasible to find help in tools for speeding up the recovery processes. The idea is that when the recovery processes are speeded up, higher loads may be used. However, one must not forget that any tool that influences the recovery rate may also influence the training effect. When the recovery processes are favored with the aid of exogeneous substrates or regulatory substances, the alleviation may decrease the stimulation of adaptive changes and, thereby, the training effect. All in all, any interference with the internal affairs of the organism causes an actual risk of confusing the normal regulative process.

In the case of the last microcycle before responsible competitions the repletion and supercompensation of energy stores becomes decisive. One way is to use the 'tapering' scheme, consisting of a voluminous training load together with a low-carbohydrate diet, followed by moderate loads and a high-carbohydrate diet. Aiming to achieve a high level of supercompensation on the competition day, it is thought to be useful for long-distance runners to perform 3 days before an anaerobic training, 2 days before an aerobic training, and 1 day before a speed training.[110]

THE MAIN PRINCIPLES OF TRAINING TACTICS

All questions related to training tactics may find worthwhile answers if at least five main principles of training organization are followed. These principles are:

1. The principle of systematic exercising
2. The principle of increased load
3. The principle of individualization of training actions
4. The principle of the use of maximal loads
5. The principle of cycling organization of training

The background for the first principle of the training effects results only from often-repeated exercises. Moreover, training effects are achieved if subsequent training sessions follow each other after optimal time intervals. This necessitates the use of imprints of the previous influence to have the most favorable condition to actualize the next influence. The phenomenon of detraining appearing after cessation of systematically repeated exercises (see p. 286–288) makes year-round systematic training necessary.

The significance of increased loads was discussed above (p. 262–263). The necessity of individualization of training actions, taking into consideration the age, sex, peculiarities of the genotype and phenotype, fitness level, previous experience etc. need no special argumen. The use of maximal loads is thought to be necessary to teach the body to mobilize the acquired motor potential. The principle of cyclic organization was already established in the 1960s against the background of analyses of training of sportsmen belonging to the international class.[111] Their training revealed that training influences and organizational forms repeat themselves at three levels. Accordingly, there are three groups of waves of training volume and intensity (Figure 10-23). The duration of waves of the first group is approximately a week. The waves of the second group sum up three to six waves of the first group. Last, all these waves constitute the greatest wave with the duration of a year or half of a year. Correspondingly, the training mezo- and macrocycles are distinguished.

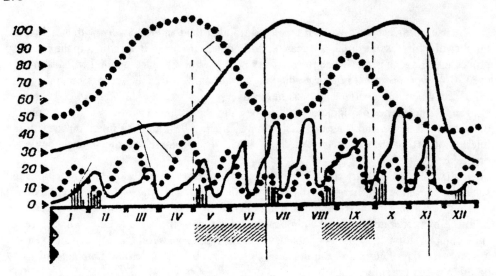

FIGURE 10-23. Three groups of waves of training loads of qualified athletes. The first two lines indicate the training macrocycle and the other two indicate the training mezocycle. Dotted lines — volume of training, solid lines — intensity of training. The volume of training per microcycle is indicated by short vertical lines. The competition periods are indicated by striated areas. Numbers under the abscissa show the months. (From Matveyev, P., *The Problem of Sports Training Periodicity*, FiS, Moscow, 1964. With permission.)

REFERENCES

1. **Lamb, D.R.**, *Physiology of Exercise*, Macmillan, New York, 1978.
2. **Rusko, H.**, Kestävys and sen harjoittaminen, in *Suomalainen Valmennusoppi. Harjoittelu*, Kantola, H., Ed., Gummerus Kirjapaino OY, Jyväskylä, 1989, 151.
3. **Fox, E.L., and Mathews, D.K.**, *Physiological Basis of Physical Education and Athletics.* 3rd ed., W.B. Saunders, Philadelphia, 1981.
4. **Costill, D., Sharp, R., and Troup, J.**, Muscle strength: contributions to sprint swimming, *Biokinetic Strength Training*, 1, 55, 1980.
5. **Komi, P.V., and Häkkinen, K.**, Strength and power, in *Olympic Book of Sports Medicine*, Dirix, A., Knuttgen, H.G., and Tittel, K., Eds., Blackwell Scientific, Oxford, 1988, 181.
6. **Caiosso, V.J., Perrine, J.J., and Edgerton, V.R.**, Training-induced alteration of the *in vivo* force-velocity relationship of human muscle, *J. Appl. Physiol.*, 51, 750, 1981.
7. **Coyle, E.F., Feiring, D.C., Rotkins, T.C., Cote, R.W., Roby, F.B., Lee, W., and Wilmore, J.H.**, Specificity of power improvements through slow and fast isokinetic training, *J. Appl. Physiol.*, 51, 1437, 1981.
8. **Brown, M.E., Mayhew, J.L., and Boleach, L.W.**, Effect of plyometric training on vertical jump performance in high school basketball players, *J. Sports Med. Phys. Fitness*, 26, 1, 1986.
9. **Masalgin, N.A., Verhoshansky, Y.V., Golovina, L.L., and Naraliyev, A.M.**, Action of plyometric training method on electromyographic parameters of explosive event, *Teor. Prakt. Fiz. Kult.*, 1, 45, 1987 (in Russian).
10. **Verhoshanski, Y.V.**, *Foundations for Specific Physical Conditioning of Sportsmen*, FiS, Moscow, 1988 (in Russian).
11. **Atha, J.**, Strengthening muscle, *Exerc. Sports Sci. Rev.*, 9, 1, 1981.
12. **Pipes, T.V., and Wilmore, J.H.**, Isokinetic vs. isotonic strength training in adult men, *Med. Sci. Sports*, 7, 262, 1975.
13. **Vorobyev, A.N.**, *Weight-Lifting Sport. Survey on Physiology and Sports Training*, FiS, Moscow, 1977 (in Russian).
14. **Matveyev, L.P.**, *Foundations for Sports Training*, FiS, Moscow, 1977 (in Russian).
15. **Platonov, V.M., and Vaitsekhovsky, S.M.**, *Training of High Class Swimmers*, FiS, Moscow, 1985 (in Russian).
16. **Doroshenko, N.I.**, A Study of Training and Competition Loads in Runners for Middle and Long Distances, Thesis acad. diss., Central Inst. Phys. Cult., Moscow, 1976 (in Russian).
17. **Baikov, V.M.**, Experimental Foundation of Regimes of Training Loads for Improved Endurance in Cross-Country Skiers, Thesis acad. diss., Tartu University, Tartu, 1975 (in Russian).
18. **Kindermann, W., Simon, G., and Keul, J.**, The significance of the aerobic-anaerobic transition for the determination of work load intensities during endurance training, *Eur. J. Appl. Physiol.*, 42, 25, 1979.

19. **Jacobs, I.**, Blood lactate: implications for training and sports performance, *Sports Med.*, 3, 10, 1986.
20. **Urhausen, A., and Kindermann, W.**, Biochemical monitoring of training, *Clin. J. Sports Med.*, 2, 52, 1992.
21. **Yoshida, T.**, Effect of dietary modifications on lactate threshold and onset of blood lactate accumulation during incremental exercise, *Eur. J. Appl. Physiol.*, 53, 200, 1989.
22. **Fröhlich, J., Urhausen, A., Seul, U., and Kindermann, W.**, Beeinflussing der individuellen anaeroben Schwelle durch kohlenhydraterne and -reiche Ernährung, *Leistungssport*, 19, 18, 1989.
23. **Stegemann, H., Kindermann, W., and Schnabel, L.**, Lactate kinetics and individual anaerobic threshold, *Int. J. Sports Med.*, 2, 160, 1981.
24. **Busse, M., Maassen, N., and Braumann, K.M.**, Interpretation of lactate values, *Mod. Athlete Coach*, 27, 26, 1989.
25. **Bueno, M.**, The anaerobic threshold: from euphoria to confidence crisis, *Mod. Athlete Coach*, 28(1), 8, 1990.
26. **Hopkins, W.G.**, Quantification of training in competitive sports, *Sports Med.*, 12, 161, 1991.
27. **Coen, B., Schwarz, L., Urhausen, A., and Kindermann, W.**, Control of training in middle- and long-distance running by means of the individual anaerobic threshold, *Int. J. Sports Med.*, 12, 519, 1991.
28. **Meyer, R.A., and Terjung, R.L.**, AMP deamination and reamination in working skeletal muscle, *Am. J. Physiol.*, 239, C32, 1980.
29. **Dudley, G.A., Staron, R.S., Murray, T.F., Hagerman, F.C., and Luginbuhl, A.**, Muscle fibre composition and blood ammonia levels after intense exercise in humans, *J. Appl. Physiol.*, 54, 582, 1983.
30. **Urhausen, A., Heckmann, M., and Kindermann, W.**, Ammoniakverhalten bei erschöpfender Ausdauerbelastung, *Dtsch. Z. Sportmed.*, 39, 354, 1988.
31. **Gorokhov, A., Krasnova, A., and Yakovlev, N.**, Dynamics of blood urea content and urinary excretion of catecholamines in sportsmen during physical exercises of various character, *Teor. Prakt. Fiz. Kult.*, 9, 34, 1973 (in Russian).
32. **Berg, A.**, Die aktuelle Belastbarkeit — Versuch ihrer Beuerteilung anhand von Stoffwechselgrößen, *Leistungssport*, 7, 420, 1977.
33. **Lorenz, R., and Gerber, G.**, Harnstoff bei körperlichen Belastunggen: Veränderung der Synthese, der Blutkonzentration and der Ausscheidung, *Med. Sport*, 19, 240, 1979.
34. **Voznesenskij, L., Zaleskij, M., Arzhamova, G., and Tôshkevich, V.**, Control by blood urea in cyclic sports events, *Teor. Prakt. Fiz. Kult.*, 10, 21, 1979 (in Russian).
35. **Zerbes, H., Kühne, K., and Götte, H.-C.**, Der Einfluss von körperlicher Belastung and Eiweissgehalt der Nahrung auf die Harnstoffproduction, -excretion and -retention, *Med. Sport*, 23, 299, 1983.
36. **Ööpik, V., Alev, K., and Buchinskayte, V.**, Dynamics of protein metabolism in skeletal muscle during daily repeated muscular work, *Acta Comment. Univ. Tartuensis*, 814, 3, 1988.
37. **Litvinova, L., and Viru, A.**, Urea metabolism in muscular activity, in *Biochemistry of Nutrition of Sportsmen*, Feldkoren, B. and Shishkina, N., Eds., Leningrad Res. Inst. Phys. Cult., Leningrad, 1989, 160 (in Russian).
38. **Viru, A., and Seli, N.**, 3-Methylhistidine excretion in training for improved power and strength, *Sports Med. Training Rehabil.*, 3, 183, 1992.
39. **Hickson, J.F., and Hinkelmann, K.**, Exercise and protein intake effects on urinary 3-methylhistidine excretion, *Am. J. Clin. Nutr.*, 41, 246, 1985.
40. **Pivornik, J.M., Hickson, J.F., and Wolinsky, I.**, Urinary 3-methylhistidine excretion increases with repeated weight training exercise, *Med. Sci Sports Exerc.*, 21, 283, 1989.
41. **Waterlow, J.C.**, Protein turnover with special reference to man, *Q. J. Exp. Physiol.*, 69, 409, 1984.
42. **Häkkinen, K., Pakarinen, A., Alen, M., Kauhanen, H., and Komi, P.V.**, Relationships between training volume, physical performance capacity, and serum hormone concentrations during prolonged training in elite weightlifters, *Int. J. Sports Med.*, 8 (Suppl. 1), 61, 1987.
43. **Busso, T., Häkkinen, K., Pakarinen, A., Carasso, C., Lacour, J.R., Komi, P.V., and Kauhanen, H.**, A system model of training responses and its relationsip to hormonal responses in elite weight lifters, *Eur. J. Appl. Physiol.*, 61, 48, 1990.
44. **Viru, E., Pärnat, J., Täll, S., and Viru, A.**, Influence of frequent short-term training session on physical working capacity of female students, *Acta Comment. Univ. Tartuensis*, 497, 12, 1979 (in Russian).
45. **Alev, M., and Viru, A.**, A study of the state of mechanisms of general adaptation by excretion of 17-hydroxycorticoids in young skiers, *Teor. Prakt. Fiz. Kult.*, 12, 16, 1982 (in Russian).
46. **Vigla, A., Viru, A., Karumaa, T., and Miil, T.**, Variants of dynamics of adrenocortical activity in sportsmen during training microcycle, in *Physiological Action of Extreme Factors on Animal and Plant Organisms*, Ksents, S.M., Ed., Tomsk University, Tomsk. 1984, 26 (in Russian).
47. **Jalak, R., and Viru, A.**, Adrenocortical activity in many times repeated physical exercises in a day, *Fiziol. Chel.*, 9, 418, 1983 (in Russian).
48. **Reindell, H., Roskham, H., and Gerschler, W.**, *Das Intervalltraining*, München, 1962.
49. **Jürimäe, T., Viru, A., and Pedaste, J.**, Running training, physical working capacity and lipid and lipoprotein relationships in man, *Finn. Sports Exerc. Med.*, 3, 104, 1984.
50. **Sorvanov, V.A.**, Indications of training tools of various intensity in sports wrestling, *Teor. Prakt. Fiz. Kult.*, 2, 19, 1978.

51. **Buono, M.**, Middle and long distance training concepts, *Track Tech. Annu.*, 83, 32, 1983.
52. **Karvonen, J., and Vuorimaa, T.**, Heart rate and exercise intensity during sports activities, *Sports Med.*, 5, 303, 1988.
53. **Powers, S., and Steben, R.E.**, Shifting the anaerobic threshold in distance runners, *Track Tech. Annu.* 83, 107, 1983.
54. **Spangler, D., and Hooker, G.**, Scientific training and fitness testing, *Cycling Sci.*, 2(1), 23, 1990.
55. **Rusko, H., and Bosco, C.**, Metabolic response of endurance athletes to training with added load, *Eur. J. Appl. Physiol.*, 56, 412, 1987.
56. **Rusko, H., Bosco, C., Komulainen, J., Leinonen, A., and Vihko, V.**, Muscle enzyme adaptations to added load during training and nontraining hours in rats, *J. Appl. Physiol.*, 70, 764, 1991.
57. **Yakovlev, N.N., Korobkov, A.V., and Jananis, S.V.**, *Physiological and Biochemical Foundations for Theory and Methodology of Sports Training*, FiS, Moscow, 1960 (in Russian).
58. **Maisuradze, M.I.**, Action of strength exercises on the development of endurance, *Teor. Prakt. Fiz. Kult.*, 11, 840, 1960 (in Russian).
59. **Zimkin, N.V.**, Qualitative features of muscular activity, in *Physiology of Muscular Activity Work and Sports*, Smirnov, K.M., Ed., Nauka, Leningrad, 1969, 377 (in Russian).
60. **Hickson, R.C.**, Interference of strength development by simultaneous training for strength and endurance, *Eur. J. Appl. Physiol.*, 45, 255, 1980.
61. **Dudley, G., and Djamil, R.**, Incompatibility of endurance and strength training modes of exercise, *J. Appl. Physiol.*, 59, 1446, 1985.
62. **Hunter, G., Demment, R., and Miller, D.**, Development of strength and maximum oxygen uptake during simultaneous training for strength and endurance, *J. Sports Med. Phys. Fitness*, 27, 269, 1987.
63. **Gettman, L.R., Ward, P., and Hagan, R.D.**, A comparison of combined running and weight training with circuit weight training, *Med. Sci. Sports Exerc.*, 14, 229, 1982.
64. **Hickson, R.C., Dvorak, B.A., Gorostiaga, E.M., Kurowski, T.T., and Foster, C.**, Potential for strength and endurance training to amplify endurance performance, *J. Appl. Physiol.*, 65, 2285, 1988.
65. **Tabata, I., Atomi, Y., Kanehisa, H., and Miyashita, M.**, Effect of high-intensity endurance training on isokinetic muscle power, *Eur. J. Appl. Physiol.*, 60, 254, 1990.
66. **Nelson, A., Conlee, R., Arnall, D., Loy, S., and Silvester, L.**, Adaptation to simultaneous training for strength and endurance, *Phys. Ther. Rev.*, 70, 281, 1990.
67. **Sale, D., MacDoughall, J., Jacobs, I., and Garner, S.**, Interaction between concurrent strength and endurance training, *J. Appl. Physiol.*, 68, 260, 1990.
68. **Hellebrandt, F.A., and Heutz, S.J.**, Mechanisms of muscle training in man: experimental demonstration of the overload principle, *Phys. Ther. Rev.*, 36, 371, 1956.
69. **Thayer, R.**, Planning a training program, *Track Tech. Annu.* 83, 4, 1983.
70. **Verhoshanski, J.V.**, *Foundations for Special Strength Training in Sports*, FiS, Moscow, 1977 (in Russian).
71. **Platonov, V.N.**, *Training in Qualified Sportsmen*, FiS, Moscow, 1986 (in Russian).
72. **Pyzova, V.A.**, Effect of the character of increase in physical exercise on adaptation to intense muscular activity, *Sechenov Physiol. J. USSR*, 58, 534, 1972 (in Russian).
73. **Pyzova, V.A.**, Analysis of the effect of physical loads increasing during the adaptation to muscular activity, *Sechenov Physiol. J. USSR*, 59, 428, 1973 (in Russian).
74. **Pyzova, V.A.**, The biochemical changes in albino rats due to maximum muscular work and their dependence on the way of adaptation, *Sechenov Physiol. J. USSR*, 59, 1087, 1973 (in Russian).
75. **Booth, F.**, Effects of endurance exercise on cytochrome c turnover in skeletal muscle, *Ann. N.Y. Acad. Sci.*, 301, 431, 1977.
76. **Ozolin, N.G.**, *Contemporary System of Sports Training*, FiS, Moscow, 1970 (in Russian).
77. **Kantola, H.**, Harjoittelun periaatteet, in *Suomalainen Valmendusoppi. Harjoittelu*, Kantola, H., Ed., Gummerus Kirjapaino OY, Jyväskylä, 1989, 123.
78. **Hickson, R.C., Hagberg, J.M., Ehsani, A.A., and Holloszy, J.O.**, Time course of the adaptive responses of aerobic power and heart rate to training, *Med. Sci. Sports Exerc.*, 13, 17, 1981.
79. **Kirwan, J., Costill, D.L., Flynn, M.G., Neufer, P.D., Fink, W.J., and Morse, W.M.**, Effects of increased training volume on the oxidative capacity, glycogen content and tension development of rat skeletal muscle, *Int. J. Sports Med.*, 11, 479, 1990.
80. **Volkov, N.I.**, *Human Bioenergetics in Strenuous Muscular Activity and Pathways for Improved Performance in Sportsmen*, Anokhin Res. Inst. Normal Physiol., Moscow, 1990 (in Russian).
81. **Kozenkova, Z.E.**, Biochemical changes in rats during muscular activity in different temperature conditions, *Sechenov Physiol. J. USSR*, 59, 1091, 1973 (in Russian).
82. **Henriksson, J., and Reitman, J.S.**, Time course of changes in human skeletal muscle succinate dehydrogenase and cytochrome oxidase activities and maximal oxygen uptake with physical activity and inactivity, *Acta Physiol. Scand.*, 99, 91, 1977.
83. **Volkov, N.I.**, The problems of biochemical assays in sports activities of man, in *Metabolism and Biochemical Evaluation of Fitness of Sportsmen*, Yakovlev, N.N., Ed., Leningrad Res. Inst. Phys. Cult., Leningrad, 1974, 213.

84. **Selye, H.**, *Physiology and Pathology of Exposure to Stress*, Medical Publishers, Montreal, 1950.
85. **Viru, A.**, Das Problem der Vergrösserung der plastishen Reserve der Organismus in Traninsprocess, *Leistungssport*, 4, 280, 1980.
86. **Harre, D.**, Zu den Beziehungen zwischen Belastung and Erholung im mikrozyklischen Aufbau das Trainings der Ausdauersportarten, *Teor. Praxis Körperkult.*, 33, 767, 1984.
87. **Counsilman, J.E.**, *The Science of Swimming*, Prentice-Hall, Engelwood Cliffs, NJ, 1968.
88. **Viru, A., Kostina, L., and Zhurkina, L.**, Dynamics of cortisol and somatotropin contents in blood of male and female sportsmen during their intensive training, *Fiziol. Zh.*, 34(4), 61, 1988 (in Russian).
89. **Ööpik, V., Port, K., and Viru, A.**, Adrenocortical activity during daily repeated exercise, *Biol. Sports*, 8, 187, 1991.
90. **Ööpik, V., and Viru, A.**, Specific nature of adaptive protein synthesis in systematic muscular activity, *Proc. Acad. Sci. Estonia. Biol.*, 37, 158, 1988.
91. **Ööpik, V., and Viru, A.**, Changes of protein metabolism in skeletal muscle in response to endurance training, *Sports Med. Training Rehabil.*, 3, 55, 1991.
92. **Hultman, E., and Bergström, J.**, Muscle glycogen synthesis in relation to diet studied in normal subjects, *Acta Med. Scand.*, 182, 109, 1967.
93. **Bergström, J., Hermansen, L., Hultman, E., and Saltin, B.**, Diet, muscle glycogen and physical performance, *Acta Physiol. Scand.*, 71, 140, 1967.
94. **Costill, D.L., Bowers, R., Graham, G., and Sparks, K.**, Muscle glycogen utilization during prolonged exercise on successive days, *J. Appl. Physiol.*, 31, 834, 1971.
95. **Kantola, H., and Rusko, H.**, *Sykettä ladulle*, Valmennuskirjat OY, Jyväskylä, 1985.
96. **Costill, D.L., Flynn, M.G., Kirwan, J.P., Houmard, J.A., Thomas, R., Mitchell, J., and Park, S.H.**, Effects of repeated days of intensified training on muscle glycogen and swimming performance, *Med. Sci. Sports Exerc.*, 20, 249, 1988.
97. **Kirwan, J.P., Costill, D.L., Mitchell, J.B., Houmard, J.A., Flunn, M.G., Fink, W.J., and Bettz, J.D.**, Carbohydrate balance in competitive runners during successive days of intense training, *J. Appl. Physiol.*, 65, 2601, 1988.
98. **Kots, Y.M., Vinogradova, O.L., Mamadu, K., and Danicheva, F.D.**, Redistribution in utilization of energy substrates in daily intensive exercises, *Teor. Prakt. Fiz. Kult.*, 4, 22, 1986 (in Russian).
99. **Pascoe, D.D, Costill, D.L., Robergs, R.A., Davis, J.A., Fink, W.J., and Pearson, D.R.**, Effects of exercise mode on muscle glycogen restorage during repeated days of exercise, *Med. Sci. Sports Exerc.*, 22, 593, 1990.
100. **Platonov, V.N.**, *Adaptation in Sports*, Zdorovya, Kiev, 1988 (in Russian).
101. **Sale, D., Jacobs, I., MacDoughall, J., and Garner, S.**, Comparison of two regimens of concurrent strength and endurance training, *Med. Sci. Sports Exerc.*, 22, 348, 1990.
102. **Bell, G., Petersen, S.R., Wessel, J., Bagnall, K., and Quinney, H.A.**, Physiological adaptations to concurrent endurance training and low velocity resistance training, *Int. J. Sports Med.*, 12, 348, 1991.
103. **Ozolin, N.G., and Khomenkov, L.C.**, Organizational and scientific foundations of training in athletes of international class, in *Textbook in Track and Field*, FiS, Moscow, 1982, 4 (in Russian).
104. **Yakovlev, N.N., Krasnova, A.F., and Gorokhov, A.L.**, The influence of physical load on the adaptation to muscular activity, *Sechenov Physiol. J. USSR*, 58, 401, 1977 (in Russian).
105. **Rogozkin, V.A.**, The effect of the number of daily training sessions on skeletal muscle protein synthesis, *Med. Sci. Sports*, 8, 223, 1976.
106. **Häkkinem, K., and Pakarinen, A.**, Serum hormones in male strength athletes during intensive short term strength training, *Eur. J. Appl. Physiol.*, 63, 194, 1991.
107. **Platonov, V.N.**, Training load as a tool for guidance with recovery processes and working capacity of sportsmen in training sessions and microcycles, in *Guidance of Recovery Processes in Sports Training*, Petrovsky, V.V., Ed., Kiev Inst. Phys. Ed., Kiev, 1973, 71 (in Russian).
108. **Häkkinen, K., Pakarinen, A., Alen, M., Kauhanen, H., and Komi, P.V.**, Neuromuscular and hormonal responses in elite athletes to two successive strength training sessions in one day, *Eur. J. Appl. Physiol.*, 57, 133, 1988.
109. **Häkkinen, K., Pakarinen, A., Alén, M., Kauhanen, H., and Komi, P.V.**, Daily hormonal and neuromuscular responses to intensive strength training in 1 week, *Int. J. Sports Med.*, 9, 422, 1988.
110. **Eynde, E.V.**, Training of long distance runners, *Mod. Athlete Coach*, 21(2), 35, 1983.
111. **Matveyev, L.P.**, *The Problem of Sports Training Periodicity*, FiS, Moscow, 1964 (in Russian).

Chapter 11

PHYSIOLOGICAL ASPECTS OF SELECTED PROBLEMS OF TRAINING METHODOLOGY (TRAINING STRATEGY)

The strategy determines a general design for purposeful activity. Training strategy depends on the final goal of achievement to which the training will be devoted during many years. During these years a general strategical design should guide the training from the beginner-teenager to the adult elite athletes. For that purpose four problems have to be solved: (1) which changes have to be induced in the trainee's organism, (2) of what length is the total time necessary to induce the changes, (3) when is the best time to stimulate each change, and (4) how to relate the maintenance and further development of the achieved changes with the other actions in the trainee's organism. (Figure 11-1)

TRAINING DESIGN FOR A PERIOD OF MANY YEARS

When the training goal is the top level of sports results, purposeful training may already begin at ages 8 to 12. A long time will elapse before the first outstanding results are achieved. Of course, more years are necessary to reach the peak of individual achievement (Tables 11-1 and 11-2). After the achievement of best results during a number of years a high level of mastery persists. This long time period is proposed to be divided into three stages:[1]

1. *The stage of fundamental preparation.* The main goals are to stimulate the concordant ontogenetic development, to elevate the fitness level, to create conditions for effectiveness in training influences on structure, metabolic processes, and functions, and to acquire a rich stock of various motor skills. It was thought that this stage would take 4 to 6 years.[1] The stage begins with a preliminary preparation for sports. The main attention is paid to the development of various motor coordinations and to the improvement of speed in association with a moderate endurance training to ensure health promotion and the development of the organism's adaptivity.[2] After 2 years a tentative specialization in a certain sports event follows. The technical skills for the corresponding event will be acquired. However, at least during the first 2 years the majority of exercises will serve the general fitness improvement.[2-4]

2. *The stage of maximal realization of the performance capacity of the sportsman's organism.* First, during 2 to 3 years a strong influence will be exerted for the development of metabolic capacities and functional systems limiting the performance in the corresponding event.[1,2] The opportunities for the adaptive protein synthesis will be utilized for increase of the most reponsible cellular structures and for augmentation of enzyme molecules of the most active metabolic pathways. However, a certain relationship between specific training and general fitness exercises has to be maintained. Otherwise, the risk of overstrain phenomena or overtraining will be rather high. One may speculate that the general fitness exercises serve to promote the organism's adaptivity. For the optimal age of highest sports performance, the sportsman has to be sufficiently prepared to tolerate the high loads necessary for realization

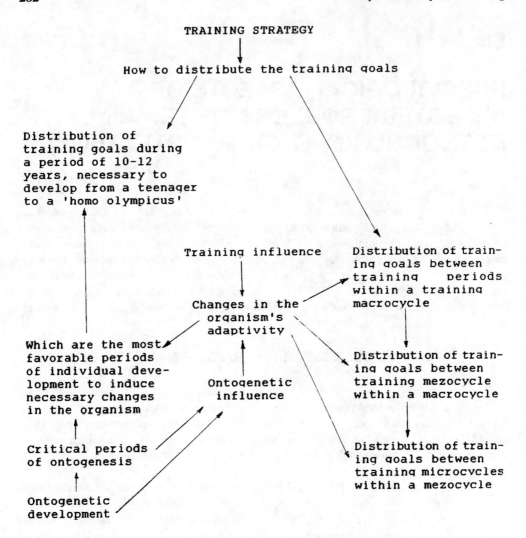

FIGURE 11-1. Training strategy.

of the maximum of the organism's capacities and, thereby, for achievement of the highest possible performance level.

3. *The stage of long-time sports mastery.*[1] The stage begins with the stabilization of results on a relatively high level without further progress in performance. Obviously, the potential for development of the body's faculties is exhausted. Does it reflect a certain 'fatigue' of the cellular genetic apparatus? Anyway, stabilization of performance shows that the adaptive protein synthesis proceeds at least sufficiently enough to ensure the effective renewal of responsible cellular structures. Accordingly, instead of the trainable loads, the main role will belong to maintaining loads. When the possibilities for maintaining high performance are also exhausted, the sportsman will drop from this level. However, continued training at lower levels of loads will help him to ensure good general fitness as well as health conditions for 2 to 3 decades. One must take into consideration that with a sudden cessation of training, the contrasting change from a high level of motor activity to sedentary life may become a pathogenic factor.

It is rather difficult to decide how to relate the maintenance and further development of achieved changes to other actions in the sportsman's organism. This question has been very

Table 11-1.   Ages of Success in Sports in Various Events in Male Athletes[3,45]

Event	First outstanding results	Top achievements	Maintaining of high level of mastery
		Age in years	
Running			
100 and 200 m	19–21	22–24	25–26
400 m	22–23	24–26	27–28
800 and 1500 m	21–23	25–27	28–30
5000 and 10000m	24–25	26–28	29–30
marathon	25–26	27–30	31–35
High jump	20–21	22–24	25–26
Long jump	21–22	23–25	26–27
Triple jump	22–23	24–27	28–29
Vault jump	23–24	25–28	29–30
Hurdle race			
110 m	23–24	24–26	27–28
400 m	22–23	24–26	27–28
3000 m	24–25	26–28	29–30
Walking			
20 km	25–26	27–29	30–32
50 km	26–27	28–30	31–35
Shot-put	22–23	24–25	26–27
Discus	23–24	25–26	27–28
Javelin	24–25	26–27	28–29
Hammer	24–25	26–30	31–32
Decathlon	23–24	25–26	27–28
Swimming			
100 to 400 m	17–18	19–22	22–25
800 and 1500 m	15–17	16–18	19–20
Gymnastics	18–20	21–24	25–26
Wrestling	19–21	22–26	27–30
Weight-lifting	19–21	21–24	25–27
Paddling, canoeing	18–21	21–26	26–28
Academic rowing	17–20	21–25	26–28
Basketball	19–21	22–25	26–28
Football	20–21	22–26	27–28
Figure skating	13–26	17–25	26–28
Skiing	20–22	23–28	29–30
Speed skating	18–19	20–24	25–28
Ice hockey	20–23	24–28	29–30
Cycling, trek	17–20	21–24	25–29
Cycling, road	17–19	20–24	25–28

poorly studied. It even seems that the sports practice ignores this question altogether. However, it is reasonable to believe that the lack of corresponding knowledge reduces the efficiency of sports training.

ONTOGENETIC ASPECTS

A quite believable suggestion exists, at least for a theoretical answer, as to when is the best time to stimulate each change that collectively constitute the foundation for performance. The ontogenetic development goes through the so-called critical (sensitive) periods. These are periods when a specific action on the developmental faculties of the organism induces the highest response.[5] It is assumed that in these periods new events are introduced by the genetic program.[6] In a number of studies periods of the highest rate of improvement of fitness indices have to be established.[7-11] These periods exist at different ages for various physical abilities.

Table 11-2. Ages of Success in Sports in Various Events in Female Athletes[3,45]

	Age in years		
Event	First outstanding results	Top achievements	Maintaining of high level of mastery
Running			
100 and 200 m	17–19	20–22	23–25
400 m	20–21	22–24	25–26
800 and 1500 m	20–23	22–26	27–28
High jump	17–18	19–22	23–24
Long jump	17–19	20–22	23–25
Hurdle-race for 80 and 100m	18–20	21–24	25–27
Shot-put	18–20	21–23	24–25
Discus	18–21	22–24	25–26
Javelin	20–22	23–24	25–26
Swimming			
100 to 400 m	14–16	17–20	21–23
800 and 1500 m	13–15	16–18	19–20
Cycling, trek	16–19	20–23	24–27
Gymnastics	13–15	16–18	19–20
Paddling	16–18	19–23	24–26
Basketball	16–18	19–24	25–26
Figure skating	13–15	16–24	25–26
Skiing	18–20	21–25	26–27
Speed skating	17–18	19–23	24–25

Note: Data of this and previous tables were obtained on the basis of analysis of sports biography of best sportsmen of the 1970s. Therefore, these data now indicate only general trends.

A comparison of related results of various authors suggests that the ages of the critical periods may depend on ethnic peculiarities. In our context, the most important fact is that the training effects on any physical ability of teenagers is the highest during the corresponding critical period.[8-10] In swimmers it was found that the training effect on VO_2max is the highest at the age of 13 to 15, but on indices of anaerobic working capacities it is highest at the age of 18 to 20[12] (Figure 11-2).

There are differences in factors limiting the performance in children. Therefore, the approaches to stimulating the performance improvement have to be different depending on the age. The best age for acquiring the sports skills is considered to be 8 to 12 for girls and 8 to 13 for boys.[13] However, until the age of 10 the acquired skills are rather unstable and children are less able to use the acquired elements of motor coordination for formation of a new skill. High possibilities for acquiring various motor skills are revealed at the ages of 10 to 12.[7,14] As a result of the corresponding training, 11- to 14-year-old children achieve a particularly high level of motor coordination. They can demonstrate very precise performance of motor tasks.[14] Afterwards the acquiring of motor skills is complicated by disorders in motor coordination during the high pubertal growth rate, and later by the formation of individual forms of motor coordination after puberty.[15]

Until puberty the possibilities for muscle hypertrophy are low and the improvement of strength is based mainly on neural adaptation.[7,11] The ineffectiveness of training to increase the muscle cross-sectional area of the extremities was attributed to a lack of circulating androgens in the prepubertal boys.[16] However, in a number of studies a significant increase in voluntary strength was obtained in prepubertal children following various resistance training programs.[17-19] In pre-pubertal boys a 20-week period of progressive resistance training

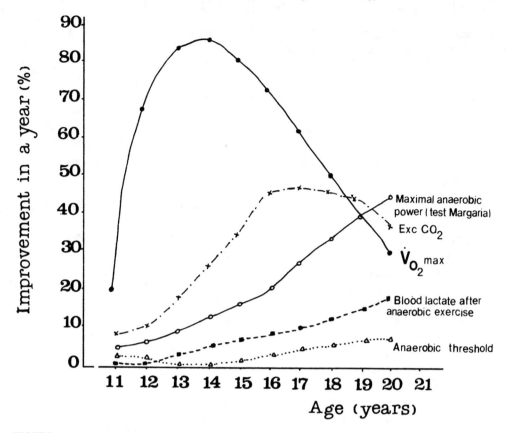

FIGURE 11-2. Annual gain in various characteristics of performance capacity in young swimmers. (From Voitenko, Y.L., *Dynamics of Training Loads and Working Capacities in Young Swimmers,* Thesis acad. diss., Cent. Inst. Phys. Cult., Moscow, 1985. With permission.)

increased muscle strength but not the muscle cross-sectional area and the percentage of motor unit activation.[20] Accordingly, it was suggested that the increased twitch torque was founded on the possible adaptation in the muscle excitation-contraction coupling.[20] After puberty, boys have an increased capacity of secreting testosterone. Thereby, a pronounced development of the muscle tissue occurs. The training becomes effective in stimulating muscle hypertrophy. In this connection the increase of the volume of resistance exercise and used weights must in postpubertal girls be lower than in boys.[13]

The speed of separate movements increases to its maximum by the age of 12 to 14, and the velocity of muscle contraction at the age of 15.[7] The most favorable age for increasing the speed of movements or their frequency with the aid of corresponding training is the age of 7 to 11. From the age of 12 to 15 and older, the speed of running increases no more due to stride frequency, but instead due to the increased length of stride. Thus, from this age on, the main tool for the improved speed of running and other cyclic activity is an increase in muscle power.[3]

The main factors limiting the endurance in preschool children and children of primary school years are peculiarities in circulation and energy metabolism. A child's heart is small, but the arterial vessels are large relative to heart volume.[7] This anatomical condition makes it difficult to increase pressure in the aorta and thereby to intensify the blood circulation during exercise. In this connection the blood pressure responses to exercise are only modest in children.[21] This difference disappears with puberty.[22,23] However, the training effect on myocardial hypertrophy has been recorded as early as the age of 8 to 10.[24,25]

The efficiency of oxygen transport function is also limited by the poor effectiveness of the respiration act and a relatively low hemoglobin content.[26] At the same time, the lower mechanical efficiency in children as compared with teenagers or adults results in an increased oxygen demand.[27] In children 5 to 7 years old the most economical exercise intensity (evaluated by oxygen demand per unit of mechanical work) is substantially lower than in older children.[28] A significant elevation of activity of muscle mitochondrial enzymes with age was not found until the age of 11 to 16 years.[29] Accordingly, the anaerobic threshold in expression of percent of VO_2max significantly increases from prepubertal to pubertal age.[30] Nevertheless, the maximal oxygen uptake per kilogram of body mass remains stable from the age of 9 to 11 up to the adult age.[29,31-33] Among preschool children a group was found having VO_2max per kilogram similar to children of 10 to 12 years.[34]

Studies in experimental training indicate the increase in VO_2max as a result of systematically performed endurance exercises already at 10 to 12 years[35-37] and even at 7 to 9 years of age.[38] In comparison with older children, a low trainability was found in children up to 10 years.[11] In children of 3 to 6 years systematical exercising failed to increase the aerobic working capacity.[39] The training effect on the anaerobic threshold was found in 11-year-old boys.[40] However, according to O. Bar-Or[41] the aerobic trainability of different maturation groups is still pending.

Anyway, from the second decade of life and beyond the oxygen transport function does not seem to impede the performance improvement in endurance events anymore. The most economical zone of exercise intensity is in 15- to 17-year-old adolescents approximately the same as in adult untrained persons.[28]

However, there remain other factors impeding a high endurance level. First of all, one must emphasize the low-rate development of anaerobic capacity. The content of phosphocreatine remains low as well as the capacity for anaerobic glycogenolysis in children of 7 to 12 years. At the age of 15 to 17 years the capacity for the phosphocreatine mechanism and anaerobic glycogenolysis increases, but the increases continue also during transition from adolescnece to adulthood.[29] The concentration of phosphofructokinase, the rate-limiting enzyme of glycogenolysis, is in teenagers lower than in adults.[29] The maximal level of blood lactate is inversely proportional to the age of up to 17- to 18-year-old teenagers.[27,42] When young sportsmen of 13 to 15 years performed exercises at the highest possible intensity, the lactate concentration in the working muscles rose up to 11 mmol·kg^{-1} vs. 17 mmol·kg^{-1} in adults. A child's organism is highly sensitive to changes in pH.[43] All these peculiarities eliminate possibilities for special training of anaerobic working capacity up to the age of 17 to 18.

A study of exercise-induced changes in the blood glucose level suggested a reduced effectiveness in mobilization of hepatic carbohydrate stores in teenagers in comparison with adults.[7] In prolonged exercises the reduction in steady levels of stroke volume, arterial pressure, and oxygen uptake occurs in teenagers earlier than in adults.[44] Hence, the functional stability improves up to adulthood.

YEAR-ROUND TRAINING

In methodological issues the year-round training, the training macrocycle, is considered to consist of three periods: preparatory period, competition period, and transition (relief) period.[1,45-47] Each of them in turn consists of mezocycles, which in turn consist of three to six microcycles. According to the common approach it is advised to increase the training volume during the preparatory period while a substantial increase in the training intensity begins to occur during the second half of the preparatory period and reaches the highest values in the competitive period. The ratio of specific exercise for improved faculties, necessary for performance at a competition, to exercises for general fitness is low at the beginning of the preparatory period and highest in the competition period. Practical actualization of these suggestions depends above all on the sports event.

Only two more general problems will be discussed: the interrelations between stimulation of various changes, and alterations in general adaptivity of the organism during the training year.

INTERRELATIONS BETWEEN VARIOUS TRAINING-INDUCED CHANGES

The effect of each exercise used in the induction of a certain change depends on the concentration of opportunities for the adaptive protein synthesis to related cellular structures and enzymes. When exercises for other changes are used simultaneously in the same training sessions or microcycles, then in some cases all tasks are performed relatively successfully. In other cases some exercises impede the positive effect of others. Accordingly, in sports practice two approaches are used: (1) attempts for simultaneous stimulation of induction of various necessary changes, and (2) a concentration of training influence on a certain direction to a limited time period. The first approach is widely used in the training of beginners and sportsmen of lower qualification. However, this approach becomes problematic in regard to the training of highly qualified sportsmen. Obviously, in the latter case the distribution of possibilities for the adaptive protein synthesis is rather limited. Earlier we referred to results of a model experiment on rats, indicating that the positive adaptive effect is achieved in a vigorous training regimen against the background of an overall suppression of protein synthesis in skeletal muscles (p. 267). As was suggested, the overall suppression of protein synthesis was necessary in order to concentrate the adaptive protein synthesis on a limited number of the most responsible proteins related to the positive effect.

However, the concentration of unidirectional training influences for a limited time period raises a question of how the results will be maintained later and how they are used for the competition performance.

In training, two different but interrelated tasks have to be completed: (1) to create an increased motor potential, and (2) to ensure opportunities for utilization of the increased motor potential in competition performance. The first is achieved through a certain quantitative volume of training loads. The latter needs an accomplishment of sports technique in order to adjust the skill to a new level of motor potential. The necessary volume of training load will cause a pronounced amount of fatigue, associated with reduced excitability and lability of the central nervous structures. The latter impede effective accomplishment of motor coordination to ensure the effective use of the increased motor potential. This contrariness is considered a reason for distributing the accomplishment of these two tasks among different time periods.[48]

THE STEADY TRAINING EFFECT

Figure 11-3 gives a typical picture of the dynamics of indices of faculties closely related to sports performance.[48,49] The main feature of the dynamics is an undulated pattern with a general trend to an increase. As a similar pattern was found in sportsmen performing in various events, it was concluded that in sports training the adaptation process is characterized by two types of indices. One group of them includes labile indices, revealing an undulated pattern. These are indices of various factors of functional capacities of the sportsman's organism (Figure 11-3, lines B and C). Pronounced waves were also found in the degree of actualization of the motor potential during competition (Figure 11-3, line D). Nevertheless, the dynamics of best performance represent a steadily increasing line (Figure 11-3, line A). Obviously, the adaptive alterations induced by training include temporary, rapidly reversible changes as well as stable, steady changes. Both of them have to be founded on the adaptive protein synthesis. The main difference is probably related to the stabilization of the increased cellular structures and concentration of enzymes in the latter case. It means that the cellular control mechanism,

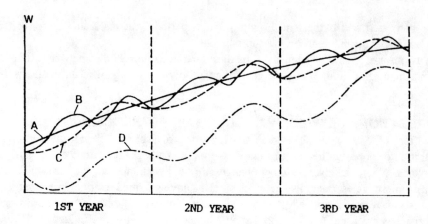

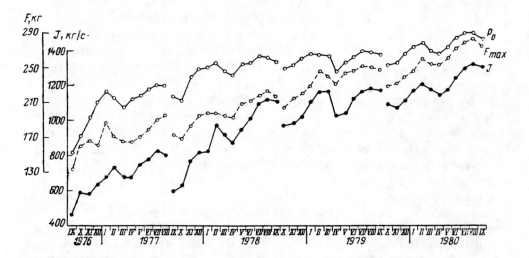

FIGURE 11-3. Upper panel: a generalized scheme of dynamics of characteristics of performance capacity in athletes during many years of training. A — dynamics of annual best performance, B,C — dynamics of various factors of functional capacities of sportsman's organism, D — degree of actualization of the motor potential in competition. I, II, III — years of training. Lower panel: dynamics of maximal voluntary strength (P_0), of maximum explosive strength (F_{max}), and of velocity of force development (kg/s. J) in a highly qualified triple-jumper. (From Verhoshansky, Y.I., and Viru, A., *Leistungssport*, 3, 10, 1990. With permission.)

avoiding the increase of protein structures, was reset on a new level. The sports practice suggests that for such resetting of the cellular control mechanism, repeated actions are necessary. It is quite plausible that these actions must be caused not only by trainable, but also by maintaining loads.

DETRAINING EFFECT

After cessation of exercising, results of the previous training disappear within a certain time period. The rate of detraining manifestations on the one hand, and retained adaptations when training is maintained at a reduced level, on the other hand, discriminate rapidly reversible temporary changes and the steady training effect.

After the cessation of training, reduction in exercise performance occurs within weeks. The losses in endurance performance coincide with declines in the cardiovascular function and the muscle oxidative potential.[50] Significant reductions in VO_2max have been reported to occur within 2 to 4 weeks of detraining.[51-56] Nine weeks of training caused a significant increase in VO_2max and the anaerobic threshold. After the following 9 weeks of detraining both indices decreased to the level found after 3 weeks of training.[57] In junior runners VO_2max increased from 65.4 to 75.5 ml·min^{-1}·kg^{-1} between ages 14.8 and 18.8 years. In those who discontinued training at the age of 18, VO_2max decreased to the level of ordinary schoolboys within a year.[58] Conversely, in runners who had training practice of 10 ± 3 years, during the following 84-day period of detraining, VO_2max did not change.[59]

Seven weeks of no training was sufficient to neutralize the effect of a conditioning program of similar duration to VO_2max. During the retraining period the training response was the same as in the first training period.[60]

The initial rapid decline in VO_2max seems to be related to a corresponding fall in maximal cardiac output, which, in turn, appears to be mediated by reduced stroke volume.[50]

Decreases in the left ventricular end-diastolic diameter, posterior wall thickness, and calculated left ventricular mass were reported in collegiate distance runners after only 4 days of detraining. However, the reduction of VO_2max was only 4%.[56] Other studies confirmed that detraining reduced the cardiac mass increased by training.[61,62] A significant role belongs to a decrease of both the total blood and plasma volume. When the blood volume was normalized by dexture infusion, stroke volume and cardiac output returned to values of before detraining.[54]

In male competitive distance runners 10 days of exercise cessation decreased the plasma volume and increased the maximum exercise heart rate but did not alter their cardiac dimensions or VO_2max.[63] Eight weeks of detraining after 8 weeks of endurance training eliminated the training-induced increased capillarization as well as the elevated activities of succinate dehydrogenase and cytochrome oxidase. Phosphofructokinase activity did not change during training but decreased during the following detraining.[52] The elimination of training effects on mitochondrial enzymes by detraining has been confirmed in humans.[55,64-66] In swimmers a reduction in respiratory capacity as well as in the glycogen content of the deltoid muscle occurred in as little as 1 to 4 weeks of inactivity after a vigorous training regimen.[65] In the vastus lateralis muscle the decrease in both succinate dehydrogenase and cytochrome oxidase activity is more rapid than in VO_2max, when a detraining period follows training.[55] Calculations made by F. Booth[67] showed that 3 weeks of retraining was necessary to overcome the decrease in cytochrome c concentration caused by 7 days of bed rest due to ankle injury (Figure 11-4).

Adaptation to aerobic training may be retained for at least several months when training is maintained at a reduced level[50]. VO_2max can be maintained by reduced training for 5 weeks (3 or 4 instead of 5 days/week). When the frequency of training sessions was reduced to 2 days/week, VO_2max was not maintained.[68] Increased VO_2max and some cardiac dimensions accompanying the exercise training of sedentary subjects were maintained despite a 33 or 67% reduction in training time.[69] Similarly, there is little change in VO_2max or the echocardiographic dimensions of competitive runners or cyclists during periods of reduced training.[70] After 10 weeks of an endurance exercise program of six training days weekly the frequency of training sessions was reduced either to four sessions or two sessions weekly for an additional 15 weeks. The intensity and duration of exercise sessions remained the same as in the tenth week of training. During the first 10 weeks VO_2max increased by 25% when measured during bicycle testing and by 20% when measured during treadmill testing. During the reduced training period the VO_2max remained essentially the same.[71,72] In highly trained runners a reduction of training load for 10 days (from 110 to 80 km·m^{-1}) neither sufficiently diminished nor improved the aerobic capacity or oxygen uptake during submaximal exercise or time of running to exhaustion.[73]

In male distance runners during 3 weeks of reduced training (running distance decreased from 81 ± 5 to 24 ± 2 km/week) the low resting level of blood testosterone persisted, but high serum creatine kinase activity decreased.[74]

The detraining effect is similar on muscle strength. The cessation of training induced a rapid decrease in the maximal isometric strength of various muscles, as well as in the speed

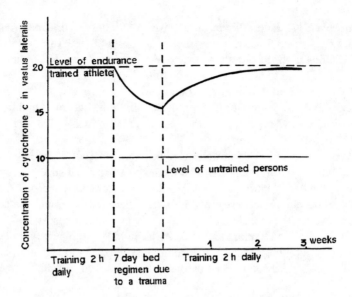

FIGURE 11-4. Decrease of concentration of cytochrome c in vastus lateralis muscle of an endurance trained athlete during 7 days of bed rest due to a trauma and recovery of the concentration during the following retraining. (From Booth, F., *Ann. N.Y. Acad. Sci.*, 301, 431, 1977. With permission.)

of movements and endurance. However, 9 months after detraining, levels over the results obtained before a 5-month training, were found. The beneficial training effect on the speed of movements persisted for a shorter time and on endurance for a longer time than training effects on muscle strength.[75] A one-leg model of resistance training indicated that only part of a 10-week training effect on the peak torque at two velocities was lost within 12 weeks of detraining. While training increased the cross-sectional area of fast-twitch glycolytic fibers by 18%, the following detraining eliminated only two thirds of this change.[76] After 18 weeks of variable resistance training the muscular strength was maintained during the following 12 weeks when instead of the previous three training days weekly, only one or two sessions were performed weekly. The subjects who stopped training lost 68% of the isometric strength gained during training.[77]

During the following 5 months of competitive training (9000 yards·d⁻¹, 6 days·week⁻¹), swimmers went through 4 weeks of either reduced training (3000 yards·session⁻¹, three sessions per week in one group or one session per week in the other) or inactivity. Measurement of muscular strength with the aid of a biokinetic swim bench showed no decrement in any group over the 4 weeks. In contrast, swim power (tethered swim) was significantly decreased in all groups. After a standard 200 yard front crawl swim the blood lactate level increased in all groups (most of all in the inactivity group and least of all in the group having three swimming sessions per week). Maximal oxygen uptake decreased significantly over the 4 weeks in the group of one training session weekly, but not in the group of three training sessions weekly. These results suggest that aerobic capacity is maintained over 4 weeks of moderately reduced training (three sessions weekly) in well-trained swimmers.[78]

Three general suggestions can be derived from the results of detraining effects. First, detraining manifestations develop with various speeds. An essential factor determining the involution velocity is probably the half-life of proteins of related structures and enzymes. Most rapid is the loss of increased activity in glycolytic enzymes having the shortest half-life. The reduction of activity in the mitochondrial enzymes occurs less rapidly. However, despite the drop in oxidation enzymes activity, the VO_2max may be maintained.[55,79] This indicates that protein structures of the cardiorespiratory system may be maintained longer than muscle

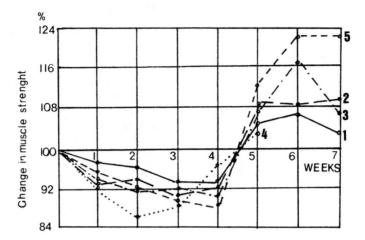

FIGURE 11-5. Changes in muscle strength of five high jumpers during 4 weeks of concentrated strength training and during the following 3 weeks of training for improved power and accomplished skills. (From Verhoshansky, Y.V., *Programming and Organization of Training Process,* FiS, Moscow, 1985. With permission.)

enzyme activities on the level obtained by adaptation to training exercises. A comparatively long half-life is common to myofibrillar proteins. This explains the possibility of maintaining the strength level for a certain time.

The second suggestion is the possibility that as a result of many years of training the training effects become more stable. This suggestion seems to be logical but there is no striking evidence of this possibility. Therefore, it is necessary to check the correctness of this suggestion.

The last suggestion is derived from experiments with the reduction of training volume or intensity. The related results are rather conclusive, suggesting that while a comparatively high level of training influences are needed to bring about adaptive alterations, a substantially lower level of muscular activity ensures the maintaining of these alterations. This conclusion gives a background for concentration of unidirectional training influences on a limited time period.

THE CONCENTRATED UNIDIRECTIONAL TRAINING

In jumpers a concentrated strength training during 4 weeks caused a rather pronounced decrease in the results of power tests (Figure 11-5). Then two restitution microcycles followed and afterward the training was changed to exercises for improved skills (sports technique). During these microcycles the power increased to a higher level than it was before the strength training block.[48] Y.V. Verhoshansky[48] considers such strength training blocks necessary for creating the motor potential in highly qualified sportsmen. According to his recommendation a strength training block has to include five to six ordinary or three to four 'blow' microcycles, followed by two restitution microcycles. He advised planning a strength training block for the first half of the preparatory period and another one close to the beginning of the competition period. When the rest time was used for power exercises and for improved technical skills, the highest levels of both power and strength were recorded during the competition period (Figure 11-6).

In a training experiment with untrained male persons a period of 7.5 weeks of high-resistance exercise with a low repetition number was followed by detraining for 5.5 weeks and then by low-resistance exercises with a high repetition number for 7.5 weeks. After the high resistance training a significant increase was observed in the cross-sectional area of IIA fibers of the vastus lateralis muscle. After low-resistance, high-repetition exercises the fiber size of all types was reduced. The maximal isometric strength increased after high-resistance training. The obtained level persisted up to the end of low-resistance training. When the training began

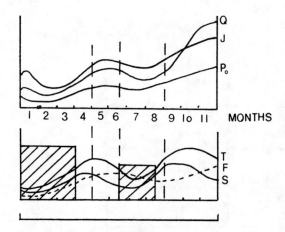

FIGURE 11-6. A model of training for athletes in power events. Upper panel: Q — explosive strength, J — force/time ratio, P_o — isometric strength. Lower panel: T — volume of training for accomplishment of performance technique (skills), F — volume of general fitness training, K — volume of speed exercises. Striated areas indicate the 'strength block', the height of columns indicate the volume of strength exercises. (From Verhoshansky, Y.V. *Programming and Organization of Training Process,* FiS, Moscow, 1985. With permission.)

with low-resistance high-repetition exercises, the first stage resulted in an increased cross-sectional area of all muscle fiber types (most of all in IIA fibers). The following second stage (high-resistance exercises) promoted further increase in fibers I and IIB. Training by this protocol indicated after the first stage an insignificant increase in maximal isometric strength, but a very pronounced strength increase after the second stage.[80]

Pedagogical experiments showed that including resistance and power exercises in the training program for certain periods favors training effects in year-round dynamics.[81]

Carrying out the strategy of the 'strength training blocks' presupposes the persistence of corresponding steady effects in training. On the other hand, the transition from heavy resistance to power training also presupposes a suitable schedule of influences exerted by heavy resistive and power exercises. The empirical experience of sports practice was generalized to a suitable schedule of corresponding exercises in the manner of a 'pyramid of power' training, consisting of seven 'floors': (1) strength endurance exercises (e.g., 3×10 repetitions of 50% 1RM), (2) base strength exercises (e.g., 4×4 repetitions of 80% 1RM) (3) power exercises (e.g., multiple hops, bounds, skips, and pumps), (4) absolute strength exercises (e.g., 4×1 repetitions of 1RM), (5) heavy power exercises (e.g., olympic lifts and explosive lifting), (6) dynamic power exercises (quick explosive hops, bounds, and vertical jumps), and (7) speed and quickness exercises (e.g., movement drills and block starts).[82]

It was found that in a suitable schedule of exercises the next one will potentiate the action of the previous one.[81]

The idea of concentration of unidirectional training influences has been supported and developed in various publications on training methodology.[4,83-85] Obviously, the experience in practical actualization of this idea has provided evidence of the correctness of this strategy. Figure 11-7 presents a possibility for the actualization of this strategy in endurance training.

ADAPTIVITY OF THE ORGANISM DURING THE TRAINING YEAR

The art of training consists of ensuring both purposeful utilization and restoration of the adaptive possibility. More than 30 years ago L. Prokop[86] pointed to the dependence of the performance dynamics on the exhaustion of adaptivity in sportsmen. According to him, a sportsman has to exhaust a great part of his adaptivity to reach the top performance. Thereafter a decrease in the performance level will follow. In this situation continuing training with high loads unduly magnifies the drop in performance while reduced training helps overcome the decrease in performance and ensures a new improvement. This consideration fits in with the experiments with sportsmen. Against this background reduced training is recommended when the top performance has been achieved.[1,4,45,46] Reduced training was recommended during the competition period between two or three most responsible competitions. In these cases three to six restitution microcycles (reduced training) was recommended after the first competition. During the following three to six microcycles the training loads have to be increased gradually

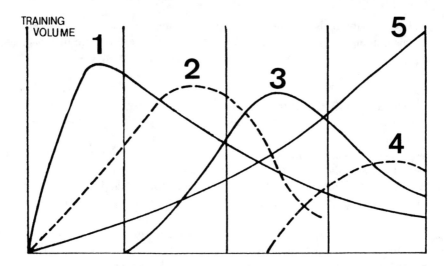

FIGURE 11-7. An example of concentration of exercises for improvement of various qualities needed for high performance in endurance athletes. 1 — continuous aerobic exercise, 2 — strength and strength endurance exercises, 3 — interval training, 4 — competition exercises, 5 — performance level.

in order to achieve the same level of training intensity that existed before the first competition.[87] Accordingly, in female rowers of the Dutch national team after a training camp and the Olympic qualifying race a decrease was found in training intensity, after which the sportsmen increased the training volume.[88]

A longitudinal observation on athletes combined with a computer-modeling of training confirmed that when after 30 days of hard training the 'training impulse' was reduced for 20 days, a pronounced increase appears in performance level.[89] When after 8 weeks of hard aerobic training the volume of each exercise session (duration of continuous cycling) was reduced for 4 or 8 days, power output at anaerobic threshold and muscle glycogen content increased. Continuation of training at the same level of loads caused decreases of anaerobic threshold and glycogen store. Eight days after complete disruption of training anaerobic threshold was retained and glycogen content increased similarly to reduced training. Activities of β-hydroxyacyl CoA dehydrogenase, and carnitine palmityltransferase, and cytochrome oxidase were maintained after reduced training on the level elevated by previous training. After training disruption the activities decreased.[90] Consequently, a reduced training ensures better actualization of previous training effects than a complete rest.

Another manifestation of reduced training, approved by sportsmen's experience, is the transition or relief period after the competition period. The data presented above suggest that the duration of the reduced training at that time must be adjusted to avoid too great a decrease in the function and metabolic faculties responsible for a high performance in sportsmen.

The reason for the exhaustion of the organism's adaptivity in training with high loads is not clear. One possibility is that a change occurs at the level of gene induction and/or expression that allows us to suppose the appearance of fatigue in the cellular genetic apparatus. It is not excluded that there exists a regulatory mechanism that eliminates the unidirectional adaptive protein synthesis after stimulating it for a while. There also exists an alternative possibility that the disappearance of training efficiency is related to the exhaustion of either the central nervous system or endocrine systems.

Anyway, physiological studies provide evidence of changes in endocrine functions in sportsmen as a result of prolonged periods of high-volume or -intensity training. Ten successive days of increased swimming training (daily swimming distance increased from 4.266 to 8.790 m, swimming intensity at 94% of VO_2max) did not cause a progressive change of swimming power, sprinting and endurance performance, aerobic capacity, and m. deltoid citrate synthase activity in eight highly trained male swimmers. Four swimmers were unable to tolerate this training. Together with a decreased swimming performance they had significantly reduced muscle glycogen values.[91] Serum cortisol and creatine kinase levels were elevated in all the subjects. Blood catecholamine levels were elevated insignificantly.[92] The swimmers' performance improved with a week of detraining, whereas muscle oxidative capacity fell by up to 50% during the same period.[93]

In eight experienced middle- and long-distance runners a sharp increase in the training volume during 4 weeks (from 85.9 to 174.6 km/week) did not improve the performance. None of them were able to reach their personal records during the subsequent competition sessions. Pronounced changes in the endocrine function were recorded. Plasma noradrenaline levels increased at the same submaximal work load during treadmill ergometry. Nocturnal excretion of dopamine, noradrenaline, and adrenaline fell to 28 to 30%, and the 24-h excretion of cortisol to 70% of baseline values.[94]

During a training year a significant strain of adaptation processes may be suggested in elite endurance athletes by increased level of blood cortisol.[95-99] The increased cortisol resting level was associated with extremely high cortisol and somatotropin concentrations after a 7-min simulated rowing test.[99] In the course of an intensive training, the first two microcycles were followed by some suppression of adrenocortical activity and the pituitary somatotropic function, reflected in lowered cortisol levels before training sessions and after rowing exercises, as well as in reduced somatotropin responses. On the fourth, fifth, and sixth microcycles cortisol and somatotropin responses to rowing were increased.[100]

The morning cortisol level in the blood increased during the first 4 weeks of high-intensity endurance training and then decreased during the following 3 weeks.[101]

In elite speed skaters low cortisol levels were found after 2 weeks of altitude training as well as after a high intensity training on ice before the competition period.[102] Could the low cortisol level be related to overstrain of adaptive mechanisms?

This possibility cannot be ignored. However, controversially, it is assumed that overstrain is related to a decreased free testosterone/cortisol ratio, suggesting the prevalence of catabolism over anabolism in the athlete's organism.

During 7 weeks of the competition period the serum testosterone level as well as the testosterone/cortisol ratio decreased in rowers. A week of regeneration phase in the middle of the competition period reduced these changes.[103] Analogous changes were confirmed in other studies on endurance athletes.[95-97,104] In weight-lifters the cortisol level as well as the free testosterone level failed to increase during a training period.[95]

H. Adlercreutz et al.[105] considered the free testostrone/cortisol ratio of the plasma to be a tool by which training could be effectively monitored. They proposed using a decrease of this ratio by more than 30% or a decrease below $0.35 \cdot 10^{-3}$ as a criterion for overstrain, connected with extreme prevalence of catabolism. A study of elite speed skaters confirmed the reliability of the criterion proposed by H. Adlercreutz and collaborators. By the results obtained, a decrease by 30% or more in the free testosterone/cortisol ratio indicates temporary incomplete recovery from intensive training and residual weakness and, consequently, reduced effectiveness for competitive purposes.[102]

The link between the testosterone level and anabolic changes in the organism is indicated by a correlation between changes in the testosterone level and training effectiveness in elite weight-lifters. This correlation was used for a prognostic model by which the blood testosterone level may be used for prognostics of the progress in strength improvement.[106]

However, the elevated cortisol level may have various functions. In the training process, it appears not only as a result of heavy training loads. It may also appear after reduction of training loads. In young rowers (mean age 17.6 years) during training with high volume, the serum urea content and creatine kinase activity increased, free testosterone decreased, and cortisol remained constant. After reduction in training volume, urea and creatine kinase normalized and free testosterone increased to a level above the initial value. An increase was also found in the cortisol level.[107]

When a drop in the organism's adaptivity is ignored, continued training with high loads results in a chronic overexertion syndrome called overtraining. The manifestation of this syndrome precludes any doubt that this is causally related to general changes on the level of the whole organism.[108-112] Overtraining may show as an Addisonoid or a Basedowoid syndrome.[108,111] The hypothalamic dysfunction has been described as well.[113]

In track and field athletes a low level of somatotropin was found when they were close to the state of overtraining.[114]

Some evidence of the essential role of a general reason for exhausted adaptivity is provided by changes in immune activity and resistance to various other stressors. A suppression of immune activities and an increased susceptibility to infections appear in sportsmen not only in case of the overtraining syndrome,[115-117] but also as a common phenomenon during the use of high training loads.[118-124]

CONCLUSION

The planning of training macrocycles depends on competition demands as well as the levels of performance capacities of a sportsman. The main standpoints and facts that have to be taken into consideration are:[125]

1. The design of a macrocycle should closely follow the long-term training plan. Emphasis, according to this, should be placed on the planned changes to the body and the development of the planned physical capacities in a given year. If there is a conflict between the long-term plan and the competition demands, the first must take priority.
2. There are limits to the intensity of the adaptation of the body to training and the adaptation capacity has to be restored by relative recoveries (reduced training load). Continuation of intensive training and competition without restoration leads to a drop in performance and even overtraining. It is, therefore, wrong to expect an athlete to be in top form for 6 months or more during a year.
3. Practical experience and studies by Y.V. Verhoshansky[48] have led to the conclusion that high-level athletes have sufficient adaptation energy for 18 to 22 weeks. After this time period, it is necessary to change the contents of training and plan for a restoration phase.
4. The temporary loss of adaptivity has made it necessary to employ a cyclic structure in training. The structure is based on changes in the training loads and recoveries in the microcycles (4 to 7 days) and mezocycles (4 to 6 microcycles) that make up a macrocycle.
5. It is recommended to divide long competition seasons into separate stages to best exploit the adaptivity.
6. The two major tasks of all macrocycles are the creation of movement potential and its realization. The first refers to the fulfillment of certain quantitative demands, and the second to the improvement of technique to correspond to the newly acquired level of physical capacities.

REFERENCES

1. **Matveyev, L.P.**, *Foundations for Sport Training*, FiS, Moscow, 1977 (in Russian).
2. **Nabatnikova, N.Y.**, Evolution of scientific foundations for the adolescnce sports, *Teor. Prakt. Fiz. Kult.*, 11, 45, 1983 (in Russian).

3. **Filin, V.P., and Fomin, N.A.**, *Foundations for Adolescence Sports*, FiS, Moscow, 1980 (in Russian).
4. **Platonov, V.N., and Vaitsekhovski, S.M.**, *Training of High Class Swimmers*, FiS, Moscow, 1985 (in Russian).
5. **Illingworth, R.S., and Lister, J.**, The critical or sensitive periods, with special reference to certain feeding problems in infants and children, *J. Pediatrics*, 65, 839, 1964.
6. **Svetlov, P.B.**, Ontogenesis as a purposeful (telenomal) process, *Arkh. Anat. Gistol. Embriol.*, 63(8), 5, 1972 (in Russian).
7. **Korobkov, A.V., Shurdoda, V.A., Yakovlev, N.N., and Yakovleva, E.S.**, *Physical Culture of Humans of Various Ages*, FiS, Moscow, 1962 (in Russian).
8. **Kuznetsova, Z.I.**, *Critical Periods of Development of Speed, Strength and Endurance in School Children*, Acad. Ped. Sci. USSR, Moscow, 1972 (in Russian).
9. **Filin, V.P.**, *Development of Physical Abilities in Young Sportsmen*, FiS, Moscow, 1974 (in Russian).
10. **Guzalovski, A.A.**, Rate of improvement of physical abilities as a criterion for selection of young sportsmen, *Teor. Prakt. Fiz. Kult.*, 9, 28, 1979 (in Russian).
11. **Malina, R.M., and Bouchard, C.**, *Growth, Maturation, and Physical Activity*, Human Kinetics Books, Champaign, 1991.
12. **Voitenko, Y.L.**, Dynamics of Training Loads and Working Capacities in Young Swimmers, Thesis acad. diss., Cent. Inst. Phys. Cult., Moscow, 1985.
13. **Adams, G.**, Coaching the growing child, *Track Tech. Annu.* 81, 21, 1981.
14. **Farfel, V.S.**, *Development of Movements in School Children*, Acad. Ped. Sci. USSR, Moscow, 1959 (in Russian).
15. **Handelsman, A.B., and Smirnov, K.M.**, *Physical Education of School Children*, FiS, Moscow, 1966 (in Russian).
16. **Vrijens, J.**, Muscle strength development in the pre- and post-pubescent age, in *Medicine and Sport*. Vol. 11, Pediatric Work Physiology, Bornes, J. and Hebbelinck, M., Eds., Karger, New York, 1978, 152.
17. **Pfeiffer, R.D., and Francis, R.S.**, Effects of strength training on muscle development in prepubescent, pubescent and postpubescent males, *Phys. Sportmed.*, 14, 134, 1986.
18. **Sailors, M., and Berg, K.**, Comparison of response to weight training in pubescent boys and men, *J. Sports Med.*, 27, 30, 1987.
19. **Siegel, J.A., Camaione, D.N., and Manfredi, T.G.**, The effects of upper body resistance training on prepubescent children, *Pediatr. Exerc. Sci.*, 1, 145, 1989.
20. **Ramsay, J.A., Blimkie, C.J.R., Smith, K., Garner, S., MacDougall, J.D., and Sale, D.G.**, Strength training effects in prepubescent boys, *Med. Sci. Sports Exerc.*, 22, 605, 1990.
21. **Biryukovich, A.A., and Korol, V.M.**, *Functional Tests of Cardiovasculr System in School Children*, Acad. Ped. Sci. USSR, Moscow, 1963 (in Russian).
22. **Motôlyanskaya, R.B., Stogova, L.I., and Jordanskaya, F.A.**, *Physical Culture and Age*, FiS, Moscow, 1967 (in Russian).
23. **Viru, E.**, Informativity of functional test with auscultatory assessment of arterial pressure, *Acta Comment. Univ. Tartuensis*, 814, 93, 1988.
24. **Hollmann, W., Mader, A., Liesen, H., Dufaux, B., Rost, R., Heck, H., Weber, K., and Völner, K.**, Hemodynamic and metabolic aspects in top-athletes, *Int. J. Sports Med.*, Suppl. 22nd World Congr. Sports Med., 1982, 1.
25. **Rost, R., Gerharden, H., and Schmidt, K.**, Auswirkungen eines Hochleistungstrainings im Schwimmsport mit beginn im kinderalter auf den Herz-Kreislaufsystem, *Med. Welt*, 36(4), 65, 1985.
26. **Volkov, V.M., Lugovtsev, V.P., and Romashov, A.V.**, *Ontogenetic Physiology of Physical Exercises*, Smolensk Institute of Physical Culture, Smolensk, 1978 (in Russian).
27. **Davies, C.T.M.**, Metabolic cost of exercise and physiological performance in children with some observations on external loading, *Eur. J. Appl. Physiol.*, 45, 95, 1980.
28. **Utkin, V.L., Zaitseva, V.V., and Fedotkina, O.I.**, Optimal regimes of cyclic locomotations in humans of various age, *Novel Res. Ontogen. Physiol.* (Moscow), 1(24), 62, 1985.
29. **Bar-Or, O.**, *Pediatric Sports Medicine for the Practitioner: From Physiologic Principles to Clinical Application*, Springer-Verlag, New York, 1983.
30. **Kemaley, J.A., and Boileau, R.A.**, The onset of the anaerobic threshold at three stages of physical maturity, *J. Sports Med. Phys. Fitness*, 28, 367, 1988.
31. **Åstrand, P.-O.**, *Experimental Study of Physical Capacity in Relation to Sex and Age*, Munksgaard, Copenhagen, 1952.
32. **Krahenbuhl, J.S., Skinner, J.S., and Kahrt, W.M.**, Developmental aspects of maximal aerobic power in children, *Exerc. Sport Sci. Rev.*, 13, 503, 1985.
33. **Pärnat, J., and Viru, E.**, Aerobic and anaerobic work capacity and indices of cardiorespiratory system during graduated loads in boys from 10 to 18 years of age, *Acta Comment. Univ. Tartuensis*, 921, 86, 1991.
34. **Sallo, M.**, Aerobic working capacity in 4 to 6 years old children, *Pediatr. Exerc. Sci.*, 5, 465, 1993.

35. **Rowland, T.W.**, Developmental aspects of physiological functions relating to aerobic exercise in children, *Sports Med.*, 10, 255, 1990.
36. **Labitzke, H.**, Trainingsbedingte Anpassungfähigkeit der Herz-Kreislauf-System bei 11 jahrigen Kindern, *Med. Sport*, 9, 244, 1962.
37. **Daniels, J., and Olbridge, N.**, Changes in oxygen comsumption of young boys during growth and running training, *Med. Sci. Sports*, 3, 161, 1971.
38. **Lussier, L., and Buskirk, E.R.**, Effects of an endurance training regimen on assessment of work capacity in prepubertal children, *Ann. N.Y. Acad. Sci.*, 301, 734, 1977.
39. **Sallo, M.**, Trainability of the cardiovascular system in preschool children, *Acta Comment. Univ. Tartuensis*, 967, 110, 1994.
40. **Haffor, A.-S.A., Harrison, A.C., and Kirk, P.A.**, Anaerobic threshold alterations caused by interval training in 11-year-old, *J. Sports Med. Phys. Fitness*, 30, 53, 1990.
41. **Bar-Or, O.**, Trainability of the prepubescent child, *Physician Sportmed.*, 17, 65, 1989.
42. **Volkov, V.M., and Filin, V.P.**, Selection of Sportsmen, FiS, Moscow, 1983 (in Russian).
43. **Erikson, B.O., Karlsson, J., and Saltin, B.**, Muscle metabolites during exercise in pubertal boys, *Acta Paediatr. Scand. Suppl.*, 217, 154, 1971.
44. **Motylyanskaya, P.B.**, Opportunities for investigation of the problems of development of endurance in young sportsmen, in *Endurance in Young Sportsmen*, FiS, Moscow, 1969, 5 (in Russian).
45. **Platonov, V.N.**, *Training in Qualified Sportsmen*, FiS, Moscow, 1986 (in Russian).
45a. **Thayer, R.**, Planning a training program, *Track Tech. Annu.* 83, 4, 1983.
46. **Harre, D.**, *Trainingslehre*, Sportverlag, Berlin, 1973.
47. **Kantola, H.**, Kilpailuun valmistautuminen ja kunnon ajoitus, in *Suomalainen Valmennusoppi. Harjoittelu*, Kantola, H., Ed., Gummerus Kirjapaino OY, Jyväskylä, 1989, 380.
48. **Verhoshansky, Y.V.**, *Programming and Organization of Training Process*, FiS, Moscow, 1985 (in Russian).
49. **Verhoshansky, Y.I., and Viru, A.**, Einige Geretzmäßigkeiten der langfristigen Adaptation des Organismus von Sportlern an körperliche Belastungen, *Leistungssport*, 3, 10, 1990.
50. **Neufer, P.D.**, The effect of detraining and reduced training on the physiological adaptation to aerobic exercise training, *Sports Med.*, 8, 302, 1989.
51. **Houston, M.E., Bentzen, H., and Larsson, H.**, Interrelationships between skeletal muscle adaptations and performance as studied by detraining and retraining, *Acta Physiol. Scand*, 105, 163, 1979.
52. **Klausen, K., Andersen, L.B., and Pelle, I.**, Adaptive changes in work capacity, skeletal muscle capillarization and enzyme levels during training and detraining, *Acta Physiol. Scand.*, 113, 9, 1981.
53. **Coyle, E.F., Martin, W.H., Sincore, D.R., Joyner, M.J., Hagberg, J.M., and Holloszy, J.O.**, Time course of loss of adaptations after stopping prolonged intense endurance training, *J. Appl. Physiol.*, 57, 1857, 1984.
54. **Coyle, E.F., Hammert, N.K., and Coggan, A.R.**, Effects of detraining on cardiovascular response to exercise: role of blood volume, *J. Appl. Physiol.*, 60, 95, 1986.
55. **Henriksson, J., and Reitman, J.S.**, Time course of changes in human skeletal muscle succinate dehydrogenase and cytochrome oxidase activities and maximal oxygen uptake with physical activity and inactivity, *Acta Physiol. Scand.*, 99, 91, 1977.
56. **Ehsani, A.A., Hagberg, J.M., and Hickson, R.C.**, Rapid changes in left ventricular dimensions and mass in response to physical conditioning and deconditioning, *Am. J. Physiol.*, 42, 52, 1978.
57. **Reddy, A.E., and Quinney, H.A.**, Alterations in anaerobic threshold as the result of endurance training and detraining, *Med. Sci. Sports Exerc.*, 14, 292, 1982.
58. **Murase, Y., Kabayashi, K., Kamei, S.. and Matsui, H.**, Longitudinal study of aerobic power in superior junior athletes, *Med. Sci. Sports Exerc.*, 13, 180, 1981.
59. **Coyle, E.F., Martin, W.H., Bloomfield, S.A., Lowry, O.H., and Holloszy, J.O.**, Effect of detraining on responses to submaximal exercise, *J. Appl. Physiol.*, 59, 853, 1985.
60. **Pederson, P.K. and Jørgensen, K.**, Maximal oxygen uptake in young women with training, inactivity and retraining, *Med. Sci. Sports*, 10, 233, 1978.
61. **Hickson, R.C., Kanakis, C., Davis, J.R., Moore, A.M., and Rich, S.**, Reduced training duration effects on aerobic power, endurance, and cardiac growth, *J. Appl. Physiol.*, 53, 225, 1982.
62. **Dickhuth, H.H., Reindell, H., Lehmann, M. and Keul, J.**, Rückbildungsfähigkeit des Sportherzens, *Z. Kardiol.*, 74 (Suppl.), 135, 1985.
63. **Cullinams, E.M., Sady, S.P., Vadeboncoeur, L., Burke, M., and Tompson, P.D.**, Cardiac size and VO_2max do not decrease after short-term exercise cessation, Med. *Sci. Sports Exerc.*, 18, 420, 1986.
64. **Chi, M.M.Y., Hintz, C.S., Coyle, E.F., Martin, W.H., Ivy, J.I., and Holloszy, J.O.**, Effects of detraining on enzymes of energy metabolism in individual human muscle fibers, *Am. J. Physiol.*, 244, C276, 1983.
65. **Costill, D.L., Fink, W.J., Hargreaves, M., King, D.S., Thomas, R., and Fielding, R.**, Metabolic characteristics of skeletal muscle during detraining from competitive swimming, *Med. Sci. Sports Exerc.*, 17, 339, 1985.

66. **Simoneau, J.-A., Lortie, G., Boulay, M.R., Marcotte, M., Thibault, M.-C., and Bouchard, C.**, Effects of two high-intensity intermittent training programs interspaced by detraining on human skeletal muscle and performance, *Eur. J. Appl. Physiol.*, 56, 516, 1987.

67. **Booth, F.**, Effects of endurance exercise on cytochrome c turnover in skeletal muscle, *Ann. N.Y. Acad. Sci.*, 301, 431, 1977.

68. **Brynteson, P., and Sinning, W.E.**, The effect of training frequencies on the retention of cardiovascular fitness, *Med. Sci. Sports*, 5, 29, 1973.

69. **Kemakis, C., Coehlo, A., and Hickson, R.C.**, Left ventricular responses to strenuous endurance training and reduced training frequencies, *J. Cardiac Rehabil.*, 2, 141, 1982.

70. **Snoeckx, L.H.E.H., Abeling, H.F.M., Lambregts, J.A.C., Schmitz, J.J.F., Verstappen, F.T.J., and Reneman, R.S.**, Cardiac dimensions in athletes in relation to variations in their training program, *Eur. J. Physiol.*, 52, 20, 2983.

71. **Hickson, R.C., and Rosenkoetter, M.A.**, Reduced training frequencies and maintenance of increased aerobic power, *Med. Sci. Sports Exerc.*, 13, 13, 1981.

72. **Hickson, R.C., Foster, C., Pollock, M.L., Gallassi, T.M., and Rich, S.**, Reduced training intensities and loss of aerobic power, endurance, and cardiac growth, *J. Appl. Physiol.*, 58, 492, 1985.

73. **Houmard, J.A., Kirwan, J.P., Flynn, M.G., and Mitchell, J.B.**, Effects of reduced training on submaximal and maximal running responses, *Int. J. Sports Med.*, 10, 30, 1989.

74. **Houmard, J.A., Costill, D.L., Mitchell, J.B., Park, S.H., Fink, W.J., and Burns, J.M.**, Testosterone, cortisol, and creatine kinase levels in male distance runners during reduced training, *Int. J. Sports Med.*, 11, 41, 1990.

75. **Zimkin, N.V.**, Qualitative features of motor activity, in *Physiology of Muscular Activity, Work and Sports*, Smirnov, K.M., Ed., Nauka, Leningrad, 1969, 377 (in Russian).

76. **Houston, M.E., Froese, E.A., Valerote, St. P., Green, H.J., and Ranney, D.A.**, Muscle performance, morphology and metabolic capacity during strength training and detraining: a one leg model, *Eur. J. Appl. Physiol.*, 51, 25, 1983.

77. **Groves, J.E., Pollock, M.L., Leggett, S.H., Braith, E.W., Carpenter, D.M., and Bishop, L.E.**, Effect of reduced training frequency on muscular strength, *Int. J. Sports Med.*, 9, 316, 1988.

78. **Neufer, P.D., Costill, D.L., Fielding, R.A., Flynn, M.G., and Kirwan, J.P.**, Effect of reduced training on muscular strength and endurance in competitive swimmers, *Med. Sci. Sports Exerc.*, 19, 486, 1987.

79. **Saltin, B., and Gollnick, P.D.**, Skeletal muscle adaptability: significance for metabolism and performance, in *Handbook of Physiology*, Sect. 10: Skeletal Muscle, Peach, L.D., Adrian, R.H. and Geiger, S.R., Eds., Williams & Wilkins, Baltimore, 1983, 555.

80. **Jackson, C., Ratzin, G., Dickson, A.L., and Ringe, S.P.**, Skeletal musle fiber area in two opposing modes of resistance-exercise training in the same individual, *Eur. J. Appl. Physiol.*, 61, 37, 1990.

81. **Nurmekivi, A.**, *Use of Continuous and Up-Hill Running in Training of Middle- and Long-Distance Runners during the Preparatory Period*, Thesis acad. diss., Tartu University, Tartu, 1974.

82. **Myers, B.**, Principles of strength training in athletics, *Track Tech. Annu.* 83, 20, 1983.

83. **Marks, R.**, Specialized strength & technique training for shot and discus, *Track Tech. Winter*, 2898, 1985.

84. **Kantola, H.**, Valmenkuksen suunittelu ja ohjelmointi, in *Suomalainen Valmennusoppi. Harjoittelu*, Kantola, H., Ed., Gummerus Kirjapaino OY, Jyväskylä, 1989, 133.

85. **Hirvonen, J.**, Nopeuskestävyyden harjoittaminen, in *Suomalainen Valmennusoppi. Harjoittelu*, Kantola, H., Ed., Gummerus Kirjapaino OY, Jyväskylä, 1989, 182.

86. **Prokop, L.**, *Erfolg im Sport*, Vol. 1, Fürlinger, Wien-München, 1959.

87. **Klimov, V.M., and Koloskov, V.I.**, *Guidance of the Training in Ice Hockey Players*, FiS, Moscow, 1982 (in Russian).

88. **Vermulst, L.J.M., Vervoorn, C., Boelens-Quist, A.M., Koppeschaar, H.P.F., Erich, W.B.M., Thijssen, J.H.H., and deVries, W.R.**, Analysis of seasonal training volume and working capacity in elite female rowers, *Int. J. Sports Med.*, 12, 567, 1991.

89. **Bannister, E.W., Morton, R.H., and Fitzclarke, J.**, Dose/response effects of exercise modeled from training: physical and biochemical measures, *Ann. Physiol. Antrop.*, 11, 345, 1992.

90. **Neary, J.P., Martin, T.P., Reid, D.C., Burnham, R., and Quinney, H.A.**, The effects of a reduced exercise duration taper programme of performance and muscle enzymes of endurance cyclists, *Eur. J. Appl. Physiol.*, 65, 30, 1992.

91. **Costill, D.L., Flynn, M.G., Kirwan, J.P., Houmard, J.A., Thomas, R., Mitchell, J., and Park, S.H.**, Effects of repeated days of intensified training on muscle glycogen and swimming performance, *Med. Sci. Sports Exerc.*, 20, 249, 1988.

92. **Kirwan, J.P., Costill, D.L., Flynn, M.G., Mitchell, J.B., Fink, W.J., Neufer, P.D., and Houmard, J.A.**, Physiological responses to successive days of intense training in competitive swimmers, *Med. Sci. Sports Exerc.*, 20, 255, 1988.

93. **Costill, D.L., King, D.S., Thomas, R., and Hargreaves, M.**, Effects of reduced training on muscular power in swimmers, *Physician Sportmed.*, 13, 95, 1985.

94. **Lehmann, M., Dickhuth, H.H., Gendrisch, G., Lazar, W., Thum, M., Kaminski, R., Aramendi, J.F., Peterke, E., Wieland, W., and Keul, J.**, Training-overtraining. A prospective experimental study with experienced middle and long distance runners, *Int. J. Sports Med.*, 12, 444, 1991.

95. **Häkkinen, K., Keskinen, K.L., Alén, M., Komi, P.V., and Kauhanen, H.**, Serum hormone concentrations during prolonged training in elite endurance trained and strength trained athletes, *Eur. J. Appl. Physiol.*, 59, 233, 1989.

96. **Vervoorn, C., Quist, L., Vermulst, L., deVries, W., and Thijssen, J.**, The behaviour of the plasma free testosterone/cortisol ratio during a season of elite rowing training, *Int. J. Sports Med.*, 12, 257, 1991.

97. **Vervoorn, C., Vermulst, L., Koppenschaar, H.P.E., and Erich, W.B.M.**, Seasonal changes in performance and free testosterone:cortisol ratio of elite female rowers, *Eur. J. Appl. Physiol.*, 64, 14, 1992.

98. **Stupnicki, R., Obuchowicz-Fidelus, B., Jedlikowski, P., and Kuslewicz, A.**, Serum cortisol, growth hormone, and physiological responses to laboratory exercise in male and female rowers, *Biol. Sport*, 9, 17, 1992.

99. **Snegovkaya, V., and Viru, A.**, Elevation of cortisol and growth hormone levels in the course of further improvement of performance capacity in trained rowers, *Int. J. Sports Med.*, 14, 202, 1993.

100. **Snegovskaya, V., and Viru, A.**, Growth hormone, cortisol, and progesterone levels in rowers during a period of high intensity rowing, *Biol. Sport*, 9, 93, 1992.

101. **Tabata, I., Atomi, Y., and Misyashita, M.**, Bi-phasic change of serum cortisol concentration in the morning during high-intensity physical training in man, *Horm. Metab. Res.*, 21, 218, 1989.

102. **Banfi, G., Marinelli, M., Roi, G.S., and Agape, B.**, Usefulness of free testosterone/cortisol ratio during a season of elite speed skating athletes, *Int. J. Sports Med.*, 14, 357, 1993.

103. **Urhausen, A., Kullmer, T., and Kindermann, W.**, A 7-week follow-up study of the behaviour of testosterone and cortisol during the competition period in rowers, *Eur. J. Appl. Physiol.*, 56, 528, 1987.

104. **Urhausen, A.. and Kindermann, W.**, Biochemical monitoring of training, *Clin. J. Sports Med.*, 2, 52, 1992.

105. **Adlercreutz, H., Härkönen, M., Kuoppasalmi, K., Näveri, H., Huhtaniemi, T.M., Tikkanen, H., Remes, K., Dessypris, A., and Karvonen, J.**, Effect of training on plasma anabolic and catabolic steroid hormones and their response during physical exercise, *Int. J. Sports Med.*, 7 (Suppl. 1), 27, 1986.

106. **Busso, T., Häkkinen, K., Pakarinen, A., Carasso, C., Lacour, J.R., Komi, P.V., and Kauhanen, H.**, A systems model of training responses and its relationship to hormonal responses in elite weight-lifters, *Eur. J. Appl. Physiol.*, 61, 48, 1990.

107. **Steinacker, J.M., Laske, R., Hetzel, W.D., Lormes, W., Liu, Y., and Stauch, M.**, Metabolic and hormonal reactions during training in junior oarsmen, *Int. J. Sports Med.*, 14 (Suppl. 1), S24, 1993.

108. **Israel, S.**, Zur Problematik der Übertrainings auf internistischer and leistungsphysiologischer Sicht, *Med. Sport*, 16, 1, 1976.

109. **Dressendorfer, R.H., and Wade, C.E.**, The muscular overuse syndrome in long-distance runners, *Physician Sportmed.*, 11, 116, 1983.

110. **Kindermann, W.**, Das Übertraining-Ausdruck einer vegetativen Fehlsteuerung, *Dtsch. Z. Sportmed.*, 37, 138, 1986.

111. **Kuipers, H., and Keizer, H.A.**, Overtraining in elite athletes, *Sports Med.*, 6, 79, 1988.

112. **Fry, R.W., Morton, A.R., and Keart, D.**, Overtraining in athletes, *Sports Med.*, 12, 32, 1991.

113. **Barron, G.L., Noakes, T.D., Levy, W., Smith, C., and Millar, R.P.**, Hypothalamic dysfunction in overtrained athletes, *J. Clin. Endocrin.*, 60, 803, 1985.

114. **Beyer, P., Knuppen, S., Zehender, R., Witt, D., Rieckert, H., Brack, C., Kruse, K., and Ball, P.**, Changes in spontaneous growth hormone (GH) secretion in athletes during different training periods over one year, *Acta Endocrin.*, 122 (Suppl. 1), 35, 1990.

115. **Jokl, E.**, The immunological status of athletes, *J. Sports Med. Phys. Fitness*, 14, 165, 1974.

116. **Levado, V.A., and Suzdal'nitskii, R.S.**, Current problems of diagnostics, treatment and prophylactics of disease in sportsmen, *Teor. Prakt. Fiz. Cult.*, 3, 21, 1983 (in Russian).

117. **Costill, D.L.**, *Inside Running*, Benchmark Press, Indianapolis, 1986.

118. **Surkina, I.D.**, Stress and immunity in sportsmen, *Teor. Prakt. Fiz. Kult.*, 3, 18, 1981 (in Russian).

119. **Levando, V.A., Suzdal'nitskii, R.S., Pershin, B.B., and Zykov, M.P.**, Study of secretory and antiviral immunity in sportsmen, *Sports Training Med. Rehabil.*, 1, 49, 1988.

120. **Pershin, B.B., Kuzmin, S.M., Suzdal'nitskii, R.S., and Levado, V.A.**, Reserve potential of immunity, *Sports Training Med. Rehabil.*, 1, 53, 1988.

121. **Surkina, I.D., and Gotovtseva, E.P.**, Role of immune systems in adaptation processes in sportsmen, *Teor. Prakt. Fiz. Kult.*, 8, 27, 1991.

122. **Lötzerich, H., and Uhlenbruck, G.**, Sport and Immunologie, in *Sportmedizinische Forschung*, Weiß, M. and Rieder, H., Eds., Springer, Berlin, 1991, 117.

123. **Mackinnon, L.T.**, *Exercise and Immunology*, Human Kinetics Books, Champaign, 1992.

124. **Liesen, H., and Uhlenbruck, G.**, Sports immunology, *Sports Sci. Rev.*, 1, 94, 1992.

125. **Viru, A.**, Strategy of Macrocycles, *Track Tech. Spring*, 3299, 1988.

CONCLUDING REMARKS

The presented results of numerous studies are convincing to conclude the existence of a specific link between training exercises and the results of training. Evaluation of these facts against the background of contemporary theories of adaptation leads to the conclusion that this link is founded on the adaptive protein synthesis, induced by metabolic consequences of performed exercises. There cannot be serious doubts on the participation of hormonal mechanisms in actualization of the adaptive protein synthesis in training. It has been suggested that training exercises determine the choice of proteins for their adaptive synthesis, the load of training session causes activation of endocrine systems and thereby the hormonal amplification of the syntheses. Training microcycles ensure the summing up of influences on the adaptive protein synthesis and the mutual coordination of different influences. Training mezo- and macrocycles determine the distribution of various tasks and goals during a year (Figure CR-1).

Consideration of training as a creation of continuous adaptation raises a question as to whether training alters the organism's adaptivity. Further systematic researches are needed for profound evaluation of this problem. Nevertheless, a rather solid amount of results indicate that during training the organism's adaptivity may change, including its exhaustion in connection with achieving the top performance and its restoration during relief micro- and mezocycles or relief period. It is possible to suggest also the existence of a dependence between individual adaptivity and potential for improvement of the performance capacity. In Figure CR-2 the significance of this problem is emphasized according to the understanding of A. Mader. Future research has to place goals on the evaluation of training's influence on the organism's adaptivity in relation to creation/exhaustion of the potential for improved capacities of the organism.

ACKNOWLEDGMENTS

The author gratefully acknowledges the valuable technical aid by Ms. Amanda Kriit, Ms. Kadri Kivistik and Ms. Aino Luik. The author would like to thank also Professor Bengt Saltin for valuable suggestions.

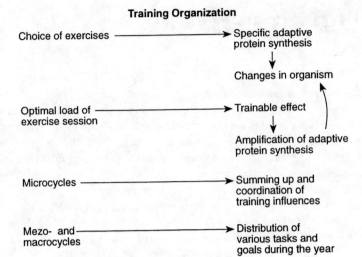

FIGURE CR-1.   An understanding of the training organization.

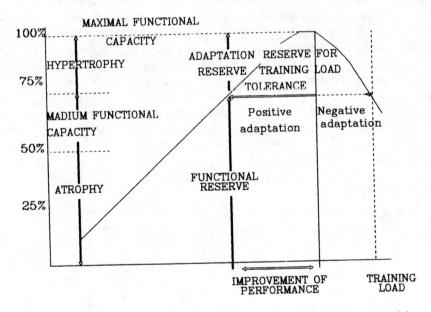

FIGURE CR-2.   Training effect on performance capacity in relation to functional capacity and adaptivity according to A. Mader (Aktive Belastungsadaptation and Regulation des Proteinsynthese auf Zellulär Ebene. Ein Beitrage zum Mechanismus der Trainingswirkung und der Kompensation von funktionellen Mehrbelastungen von Organism, in *Sport: Rettung oder Risiko für die Gesundheit*, Deutsches Arzte Verlag, 1989, 177).

INDEX

A

Acid-base balance, see pH
Actin fibrils, 126
Actomyosins, 107–110, 174–175
Actomyosin ATPase, 129–131
Acute adaptation vs. long-term, 5–6, 27–28
Adaptation, see also Exercise training; Working
    capacity
  acute and long-term, 5–6
  exercise training and, 6–10
  homeostatic regulation, 1
  mechanism of general, 2
  metabolic resource mobilization, 2–5
  nonspecific, 2
  parameters of working capacity, 13–19
  specific, 2
  top-athlete model, 10–13
Adaptive protein synthesis
  alternative theories of, 217–219
  general evidence for, 200–204
  hormonal regulation, 212–217
  metabolic control
    amino acids and, 206–207
    calcium and, 208
    creatine and, 205–206
    of energy balance, 207–208
    muscle satellite cell proliferation and, 210
    muscle stretch and, 208
    prostaglandins and, 209
    protein degradation products and, 205
    specific tRNA, 207
    tissue growth factors and, 209–210
    of transcription, 204–210
  of mitochondrial proteins, 210–212
  myocardial adaptive, 217
  and trainable effect, 249–256
  transcriptional control, 200–212
  translational control, 212
Adaptivity, 292–295
Adenosine triphosphate, see ATP
Adipose tissue, training effects, 54–55
Adrenalectomy studies, 56–59, 63–64, 103, 214
Adrenal hypertrophy, 34
Adrenaline, 256
  blood-glucose utilization and, 61
  glucose tolerance and, 50
  hepatic effects, 57–58
  lipolysis and, 63–64
  in muscle glycogenolysis, 56
Adrenergic receptors, 211, see also Catecholamines
  exercise effects, 50–51
  training effects, 51–52
Adrenocorticocyte activity, 187
Aerobic fitness, see Aerobic working capacity;
    Cardiovascular fitness
Aerobic metabolism, determinants and working
    capacity, 14–15

Aerobic working capacity, 159–177, 245–247, see also
    Cardiovascular system; Working capacity,
    aerobic
  and age, 283–284
  gender differences, 233–234
Age-related aspects of training strategy, 283–286
Alanine activity, 65–68
Aldolase, 139
Aldosterone, see also Renin-angiotensin-aldosterone
    system
  duration and intensity and, 31
  response, 21
Alveolar capillarization, 177
Amenorrhea, 231
Amino acid metabolism, 64–69, 206–207
δ-Aminoevulinic acid synthase, 211–212
Ammonia, blood levels of, 253
Anabolism, in recovery period, 104–107
Anaerobic ATP resynthesis pathways, 137–143
Anaerobic glycogenolysis, 88–90, 245, 252–253
Anaerobic glycolysis, 142
Anaerobic threshold, 159–160
Anaerobic working capacity, 143–147
  lactate analysis and, 252–253
Androgens, see also Testosterone
  deficiency, 215
  in post-exercise strength recovery, 92–93, 106–107
  and protein breakdown, 110–111
  in women, 229
Angiotensin II, 22
Antianabolic activity, 64–69
Applied microcycles, 266
Arginase, 207
Arm vs. leg training, 171
ATP
  and adaptive protein synthesis, 208
  anaerobic resynthesis pathways
    buffer capacity, 141–142
    creatine kinase, 137–138
    glycolytic enzymes, 138–141
  anaerobic working capacity and, 143–144, 159–160,
    245
  in glycogen resynthesis, 98–99
  resynthesis, 10–13
    and anaerobic threshold, 159–160
    interval method and, 245
ATP/ADP ratio, 208
ATPases
  actomyosin, 129–131
  Ca^{2+}, 130
  myofibrillar, 129–131
Atrial natriuretic peptide, 22

B

Beta blockers, 211
Beta-endorphins, see Endorphins
Bioenergetic criteria of working capacity, 13

Blood ammonia, 253
Blood analysis, 252–256
Blood pressure, in recovery period, 86–87
Boys, see Males
Brain, see Central nervous system
Buffer capacity, 141–142, 246

C

Ca^{2+}, see Calcium
Ca-activated proteinases, 111
Calcitonin, 72
Calcium
  and adaptive protein synthesis, 68–71, 208
  hormonal regulation, 72
  proteolysis and, 65
  training effects in skeletal muscle, 129
Calpains, 111
cAMP
  and adaptive protein syntehsis, 211
  synthesis, 52
Cannon, W.B., 200
Capillarization
  alveolar, 177
  hypoxia and, 145
Cardiac cycle, in recovery, 84–86
Cardiac glycogen resynthesis, 102–103
Cardiac hypertrophy, 246, see Hypertrophy, cardiac
Cardiac training effects, 50–51
Cardiovascular fitness
  duration and, 35
  gender differences, 233–234
  heart rate studies, 257–261
  specificity of exercise and, 246
  training effects
    alveolar capillarization, 177
    cardiac performance, 172–174
    myocardial contractility, 174–175
    myocardial energetics, 175–176
CarG-boxes, 209–210
Castration, 214
Catabolic activity, 64–69
  3-methylhistidine studies, 253–256
  in recovery period, 107–111
Catecholamines, 22, 141, 211, 256, see also Adrenaline;
  noradrenaline
    hepatic effects, 57–58
    and insulin binding, 50
    lipolytic activity, 62–63
    in recovery period, 90–91
Central nervous system
  in recovery period, 97–98
  training effects, 191
Children, age-related training aspects, 283–285
Circadian rhythms, hormonal response and, 38
Circuit training, 242–243
Citrate synthase, 135
Collagen synthesis, 204
Competition microcycles, 267
Concentrated unidirectional training, 291–292

Connective tissue, specificity of training effects, 192–194
Continuous (steady) training, 242, 261–262
Contraceptive drugs, 230
Contractility
  myocardial, 174–175
  skeletal muscle, training effects, 127–132
Control functions, specificity of effects, 187–194
Corticotropin
  in recovery period, 91
  response, 21
Cortisol, 96, 256–257
  aerobic fitness and, 35
  and insulin binding, 50
  in recovery period, 91
  variability/stability of response, 22
C-peptides, response, 21
Creatine, 205–206
Creatine kinases, 137–138
Cross-training effects, 191–192
Cushing's disease, 63
Cytochrome c assays, 133–134

D

Detraining effect, 288–291
Development microcycles, 266
Diabetes mellitus, 214
  exercise and insulin binding, 49–50
Diet, hormonal response and, 38
DNA, in skeletal muscle hypertrophy, 127
DNA-dependent protein synthesis, 200–219, see also
        Adaptive protein synthesis
Dudley, G.A., 133
Duration
  hormonal response and, 31–32
  threshold intensity and, 34
Dynamics stereotypes, 219

E

Eftimie, R., 210
Electrolyte homeostasis, 69–72, 129
Electrostimulation training, 190
Emotional strain, hormonal response to, 36–38
Endocrine system, see also Hormonal regulation
  in recovery period, 90–94
Endorphins
  in recovery period, 92
  variability/stability of response, 22–24
Endurance exercises, 250, 263–264
Energy balance, 207–208
Energy reserve regulation
  blood glucose homeostasis, 61–62
  blood glucose utilization, 59–61
  gluconeogenesis, 59
  glycogenolysis, 55–59
  lipids, 62–64
  and working capacity, 16
Engelhardt, W.A., 199